STUDY GUIDE FOR

Medical-Surgical
NURSING

LeMone, Burke, Bauldoff

STUDY GUIDE FOR

Medical-Surgical

NURSING

Critical Thinking in Patient Care

FIFTH EDITION

Emily J. Cannon, RN, MSN
Associate Professor
Ivy Tech Community College
Terre Haute, Indiana

Kim Cooper, RN, MSN
Chair, Nursing Department
Ivy Tech Community College
Terre Haute, Indiana

Pearson

Boston   Columbus   Indianapolis   New York   San Francisco   Upper Saddle River
Amsterdam   Cape Town   Dubai   London   Madrid   Milan   Munich   Paris   Montreal   Toronto
Delhi   Mexico City   Sao Paulo   Sydney   Hong Kong   Seoul   Singapore   Taipei   Tokyo

Publisher: Julie Levin Alexander
Publisher's Assistant: Regina Bruno
Executive Acquisitions Editor: Pamela Fuller
Editorial Assistant: Lisa Pierce/Cynthia Gates
Managing Production Editor: Patrick Walsh
Production Liaison: Cathy O'Connell
Production Editor: GEX Publishing Services
Manufacturing Manager: Ilene Sanford
Director of Marketing: David Gesell
Marketing Manager: Phoenix Harvery
Marketing Specialist: Michael Sirinides
Composition: GEX Publishing Services
Printer/Binder: Bind-Rite Graphics/Robbinsville
Cover Printer: Bind-Rite Graphics/Robbinsville
Cover Image: Rick Brady

Notice: Care has been taken to confirm the accuracy of information presented in this book. The authors, editors, and the publisher, however, cannot accept any responsibility for errors or omissions or for consequences from application of the information in this book and make no warranty, express or implied, with respect to its contents. The authors and publisher have exerted every effort to ensure that drug selections and dosages set forth in this text are in accord with current recommendations and practice at time of publication. However, in view of ongoing research, changes in government regulations, and the constant flow of information relating to drug therapy and drug reactions, the reader is urged to check the package inserts of all drugs for any change in indications of dosage and for added warnings and precautions. This is particularly important when the recommended agent is a new and/or infrequently employed drug.

10 9 8 7 6 5 4 3 2 1

ISBN 10: 0-13-512527-8
ISBN 13: 978-0-13-512527-4

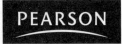

www.pearsonhighered.com

PREFACE

Students entering the field of nursing have a tremendous amount to learn in a very short time. This Study Guide that accompanies *Medical-Surgical Nursing*, **5th Edition** is designed to reinforce the knowledge that you—the student—have gained in each chapter and to help you master the critical concepts.

Each chapter includes a variety of questions and activities to help you comprehend difficult concepts and reinforce basic knowledge gained from textbook reading assignments. Following is a list of features included in this edition that will enhance your learning experience:

- **Matching** exercises that contain key terms and definitions from each chapter.
- Thorough assessment of essential information in the text is provided through the **Fill in the Blank** activities.
- **Multiple Choice** questions that provide you with additional review on key topics.
- More exercises in the **Focused Study** section.
- **Case Studies** and **Care Plans** that apply concepts from the textbook to real nursing scenarios.
- **Interactive activities** test your knowledge of concepts and terminology.
- **NCLEX–RN®** review questions.
- **Answers** are included in the Appendix to provide immediate reinforcement and to permit you to check the accuracy of your work.

In addition to the learning resources you will find in each chapter of the Study Guide, the Pearson Nursing Student Resources offers you access to animations, case studies, and care plans to help you visualize and comprehend difficult concepts. Chapter by chapter, these online resources hone your critical-thinking skills and enable you to apply concepts from the book into practice. http://nursing.pearsonhighered.com.

It is our hope that this Study Guide will serve as a valuable learning tool and will contribute to your success in the nursing profession.

CONTENTS

Medical-Surgical Nursing in the Twenty-first Century

LEARNING OUTCOMES

1. Describe the core competencies for healthcare professionals: patient-centered care, interdisciplinary teams, evidence-based practice, quality improvement, safety, and informatics.

2. Apply the attitudes, mental habits, and skills necessary for critical thinking when using the nursing process in patient care.

3. Explain the importance of nursing codes and standards as guidelines for clinical nursing practice.

4. Explain the activities and characteristics of the nurse as caregiver, educator, advocate, leader and manager, and researcher.

CLINICAL COMPETENCIES

1. Demonstrate critical thinking when using the nursing process to provide knowledgeable, safe, patient-centered care.

2. Provide clinical care within a framework that integrates, as appropriate, the medical-surgical nursing roles of caregiver, educator, advocate, leader/manager, and researcher.

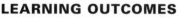

MediaLink

Pearson Nursing Student Resources
Audio Glossary
NCLEX-RN® Review

- Care Plan Activity
  - Nursing Process
- Case Study
  - The Patient with an Advance Directive
- MediaLink Applications
- Links to Resources

TERMS MATCHING

Place the letter of the correct definition in the space next to each term.

1. _____ Patient
2. _____ Code of ethics
3. _____ Core competencies
4. _____ Critical pathway
5. _____ Critical thinking
6. _____ Delegation
7. _____ Dilemma
8. _____ Medical-surgical nursing
9. _____ Nursing process
10. _____ Standard

A. All healthcare professionals should possess these five attributes. They are based on communication, knowledge, clinical reasoning, technical skills, and values related to clinical practice.

B. A choice between two unpleasant, ethically troubling alternatives.

C. A statement or criterion that can be used by a profession and by the general public to measure quality of practice. These established statements make each nurse accountable for his or her nursing practice.

D. Health promotion, health care, and illness care of adults based on knowledge derived from the arts and sciences and shaped by knowledge of nursing.

E. Nursing care is designed and implemented for this person.

F. A healthcare plan that has been designed with a multidisciplinary, managed care focus.

G. The nurse assigns appropriate and effective work activities to other members of the healthcare team.

H. Provides a frame of reference for nurses who want to care for their patients in congruence with the Code for Nurses principles.

I. A series of critical-thinking and clinical-reasoning activities that nurses use as they provide care to patients.

J. The nurse analyzes and synthesizes knowledge from the arts, the sciences, and nursing research and theory to guide decision making.

FOCUSED STUDY

1. Contact your local state board of nursing and request a copy of the Nurse Practice Act. Review the information regarding student nurses.

2. List the five stages of the nursing process. Briefly explain each stage and provide an example of how you may be able to apply each stage of the nursing process in the clinical setting.

_____

_____

_____

_____

_____

3. Use your web browser to go to http://www.nursingworld.org/ethics. You may view the code in sections. Describe how the code of ethics compares to your thoughts about the practice of nursing.

_____

_____

_____

_____

4. Review a list of NANDA nursing diagnoses. Write one nursing diagnosis statement based on your current needs.

_____

_____

CASE STUDY

A 68-year-old female patient has been diagnosed with lung cancer that has metastasized throughout her body. The patient has been admitted to an oncology unit. She has been experiencing an increased amount of pain, and her family has been requesting intravenous morphine for pain control. The patient's respiratory rate has decreased to 9 per minute, but she is still acting as if she's experiencing pain. The physician wrote a p.r.n. order for intravenous morphine that allows the nurses to administer more of the medication per each dose.

1. How may this constitute an ethical dilemma for the nursing staff?

2. What is one NANDA nursing diagnosis that best applies to this patient?

3. What role or roles might the nurse play in helping the patient and the family at this time?

4. How does the code of ethics apply to this patient?

5. Identify two activities the nurse could appropriately delegate to unlicensed personnel in caring for this patient.

6. The patient has become confused and lethargic. What are two NANDA nursing diagnoses that may apply to this patient?

SHORT ANSWERS

Models of Care Delivery

1. Name one type of unit that uses Primary Nursing as its model of care delivery.

_____

2. Name one type of unit or facility that uses Team Nursing as its model of care delivery.

_____

3. Name one type of unit or agency that uses Case Management as its model of care delivery.

_____

NCLEX-RN® REVIEW QUESTIONS

1. Which of the following nursing activities occurs as part of the patient assessment in the nursing process?
   1. developing nursing diagnoses
   2. clarifying subjective data
   3. developing a patient care plan
   4. evaluating patient goals
2. The nurse has determined that the patient has not met the outcome criteria that were established one month ago. Which of the following actions could the nurse reasonably perform at this time? **Select all that apply.**
   1. modify the nursing diagnosis
   2. modify the outcomes
   3. terminate the nursing care plan
   4. continue with the nursing care plan
   5. modify the nursing care plan
3. The nurse is dealing with a patient who is very sick. The nurse requires help from an unlicensed staff member to help meet the needs of the nurse's other patients. Which of the following statements by the nurse is most accurate regarding delegation?
   1. "I realize that I am ultimately accountable for the patient's bath."
   2. "As long as I ensure that the unlicensed staff member understands my directions, I can safely allow this person to perform any nursing duty."
   3. "If the unlicensed staff member has been trained to perform this task, I shouldn't be expected to answer any questions that he or she has about the task."
   4. "When I delegate a task, I should be present to watch the task being completed."

4. The nurse is utilizing critical-thinking skills to solve a problem. Which of the following statements best describes *reasoning*?
   1. "I've been weighing the data about the patient's hypertension with the information provided to me about the medications the patient is currently taking."
   2. "I think the patient is really anxious right now, and that's why the patient's apical heart rate is elevated."
   3. "The last time I cared for a patient with a blood pressure this high, the patient had a myocardial infarction."
   4. "I've been thinking about this situation, and I believe there are two possible solutions to the patient's problem."

5. The nurse is performing an assessment on the patient. Which of the following pieces of information is subjective?
   1. The patient's blood pressure is 142/78.
   2. The patient states that his pain level is a 4 on a scale of 0–10.
   3. The patient's pupils are dilated.
   4. The patient's right knee is erythematous and edematous.

6. The nurse is documenting information about the patient's assessment. Which of the following pieces of documentation indicates that the nurse requires further education?
   1. "Patient is resting quietly in bed."
   2. "Patient was really mean to her husband after the evening meal."
   3. "Patient refused the ordered antiemetic and stated, 'I cannot stay awake when you give me that medication.'"
   4. "Patient turned to the right side and repositioned with pillows."

7. The 87-year-old patient had a cerebrovascular accident that left him paralyzed on the right side of his body. He has been unable to eat without assistance and needs a gastric tube placed. Which of the following are "potential" nursing diagnoses that can most accurately be applied to this patient? **Select all that apply.**
   1. *Impaired Swallowing*
   2. *Potential for Impaired Social Interaction*
   3. *Potential for Altered Nutrition: More than Body Requirements*
   4. *Potential for Impaired Skin Integrity*
   5. *Unilateral Neglect*

8. The nurse is assessing a patient in the emergency department of a large urban hospital to determine whether a critical pathway can be used for this patient. Which of the following patients would most likely be placed on a critical pathway?
   1. The patient has been diagnosed with a sprained left ankle.
   2. The patient has been diagnosed with bilateral cataracts.
   3. The patient has been diagnosed with cholecystitis.
   4. The patient has been diagnosed with an evolving brain attack.

9. The nurse is providing care for a patient based on the facility's established nursing care plan. Which of the following statements indicates that the nurse requires further education about implementing interventions?
   1. "We need to get your bath done right now, but I'll be back later to look at the incision on your abdomen."
   2. "I'm going to show you how to give yourself the insulin injection right now, but the next time you need one, we'll see how much of this you can do."
   3. "I'll be back in a little while because I need to make notes in your chart about the dressing change to your foot."
   4. "It's really good to see your blood pressure coming down with the medication, and I hope it will be within a normal range by tomorrow."

10. The nurse is educating another less experienced nurse about the rules associated with health information privacy. Which of the following statements by the nurse is inaccurate?
    1. "At times, we have posted a patient's name outside his or her room."
    2. "We must have consent from the patient before we treat him or her."
    3. "When the patient has been abused, we must report it."
    4. "At certain times, we have to talk to family members about a patient's care."

Health and Illness in Adults

LEARNING OUTCOMES

1. Define health, incorporating the health–illness continuum and the concept of high-level wellness.
2. Explain factors affecting functional health status.
3. Discuss the nurse's role in health promotion.
4. Describe characteristics of health, disease, and illness.
5. Describe illness behaviors and needs of the patient with acute illness and chronic illness.
6. Describe the primary, secondary, and tertiary levels of illness prevention.
7. Compare and contrast the physical status, risks for alterations in health, assessment guidelines, and healthy behaviors of the young adult, middle adult, and older adult.
8. Explain the definitions, functions, and developmental stages and tasks of the family.

CLINICAL COMPETENCIES

1. Use knowledge of developmental levels and of activities to promote, restore, and maintain health when planning and implementing patient-centered care for adults.
2. Engage patients and family members in active partnerships to promote and maintain health of the adult.

MediaLink

Pearson Nursing Student Resources
Audio Glossary
NCLEX-RN® Review
- Care Plan Activity
  - Family-Centered Care in Chronic Illness
- Case Studies
  - Care Across the Lifespan
  - Health and Illness in the Adult Patient
- Animations/Videos
  - Health Promotion for Young Adults
  - Health Promotion for Older Adults
- MediaLink Applications
- Links to Resources

TERMS MATCHING

Place the letter of the correct definition in the space next to each term.

1. _____ Acute illness
2. _____ Chronic illness
3. _____ Disease
4. _____ Exacerbation
5. _____ Family
6. _____ Health
7. _____ Health–illness continuum
8. _____ Holistic health care
9. _____ Illness
10. _____ Manifestations
11. _____ Remission
12. _____ Wellness

A. A period of time during a chronic condition in which symptoms reappear.

B. A period of time during a chronic condition in which symptoms are not notable.

C. A condition that occurs rapidly, lasts for a relatively short time, and is self-limiting.

D. Alterations in function or structure that cause signs and symptoms.

E. A unit of people related by marriage, birth, or adoption.

F. A state of complete physical, mental, and social well-being and not merely the absence of disease or infirmity.

G. The representation of health as a dynamic process, with high-level wellness at one extreme and death at the opposite extreme.

H. An individual's integrated response to pathophysiologic alterations; psychologic effects of those alterations; effects on roles, relationships, and values; and cultural and spiritual beliefs.

I. An impairment or deviation from normal functioning that is permanent, leaves permanent disability, is caused by nonreversible pathologic alterations, and/or requires special training of the patient for rehabilitation.

J. A philosophy of health care in which all aspects of a person (physical, psychosocial, cultural, spiritual, and intellectual) are considered as essential components of individualized care.

K. A medical term describing alterations in structure and function of the body or mind that may have mechanical, biologic, or normative causes.

L. An integrated method of functioning oriented toward maximizing an individual's potential within the environment

FOCUSED STUDY

1. List and describe factors that affect health.
   a.
   _____
   b.
   _____
   c.
   _____
   d.
   _____
   e.
   _____
   f.
   _____
   g.
   _____

2. Identify the generally accepted common causes of disease.
   a.
   _____
   b.
   _____
   c.
   _____
   d.
   _____
   e.
   _____
   f.
   _____

g.
_____

h.
_____

i.
_____

3. Describe the difference between acute and chronic illness.

_____

_____

_____

_____

4. Define and give examples of primary, secondary, and tertiary illness prevention activities.
   a. Primary Activities:

   _____

   _____

   b. Secondary Activities:

   _____

   _____

   c. Tertiary Activities:

   _____

   _____

CASE STUDY

Jacob is a 50-year-old Black unemployed male with a history of past substance abuse who is being counseled about health promotion activities. Answer the following questions based on your knowledge of the middle-aged adult and Jacob's history.

   1. What alterations in health is Jacob at risk for developing as a middle-aged adult?

   2. What guidelines are useful in assessing the achievement of significant developmental tasks in the middle adult?

   3. How can the nurse promote healthy behaviors in Jacob?

SHORT ANSWERS

Fill in the information table for recommended adult immunizations.

Vaccine	Indications	Do not give to
Measles-mumps-rubella		Pregnant women, immunocompromised people, or anyone with a history of anaphylactic reaction to egg protein or neomycin
Tetanus and diphtheria toxoids		
Hepatitis B		People with a history of anaphylactic reaction to common baker's yeast
Influenza A	Anyone at high risk for complications, healthcare providers, and those wanting immunity.	
Pneumoccal pneumonia	Anyone at high risk for pneumococcal disease and those _____ of age.	
Varicella		Pregnant women, immunocompromised people, those who _____ within five months, or those with a history of anaphylactic reactions to neomycin or gelatin

NCLEX-RN® REVIEW QUESTIONS

1. Identify the acute illness from the following illnesses.
   1. influenza
   2. cancer
   3. hemophilia
   4. sickle cell disease

2. Which of the following relationships is an example of an altered response of health to lifestyle and environmental influences?
   1. cigarette smoking to a sedentary lifestyle
   2. alcoholism to obesity
   3. obesity to hypertension
   4. a sedentary lifestyle to chronic obstructive pulmonary disease

3. Which of the following practices is not known to promote health and wellness?
   1. sleeping five to six hours each day
   2. smoking cessation
   3. keeping sun exposure to a minimum
   4. maintaining recommended immunizations

4. The patient demonstrates behaviors of self-preoccupation during the initial assessment. This behavior is characteristic of what stage of illness?
   1. experiencing symptoms
   2. assuming a dependent role
   3. achieving recovery and rehabilitation
   4. assuming the sick role

5. Given that the patient is 35 years old, the nurse knows that the patient would fall into which stage of adulthood?
   1. young adult
   2. middle adult
   3. older adult
   4. young middle adult

6. Identify the cancer not commonly found in the middle adult.
   1. lung
   2. liver
   3. reproductive
   4. colon

7. Which of the following is not a frequently occurring condition in the older adult?
   1. hypertension
   2. arthritis
   3. sinusitis
   4. obesity

8. Identify the family developmental stage that focuses on transition.
   1. family with infants and preschoolers
   2. family with school-age children
   3. family with adolescents and young adults
   4. family with middle adults

9. The nurse is caring for a 45-year-old Chinese American patient. The nurse is aware that the patient is at risk for all of the following illnesses except one. Identify that illness.
   1. an eye disorder
   2. a cardiovascular disorder
   3. obesity
   4. sexually transmitted diseases

10. Identify the ineffective coping skill of a patient with a chronic illness.
    1. learning to adapt activities of daily living and self-care activities
    2. denying the inevitability of death
    3. complying with a medical treatment plan
    4. maintaining a feeling of being in control

Community and Home Care of Adults

LEARNING OUTCOMES

1. Differentiate community-based care from community health care.
2. Discuss selected factors affecting health in the community.
3. Describe services and settings for healthcare consumers receiving community-based and home care.
4. Describe the components of the home health care system, including agencies, patients, referrals, nursing care, physicians, reimbursement, and legal considerations.
5. Compare and contrast the roles of the nurse providing home care with the roles of the nurse in medical-surgical nursing discussed in Chapter 1.
6. Discuss nursing interventions to deliver safe and competent care to patients in their homes.
7. Explain the purpose of rehabilitation in health care.

MediaLink

Pearson Nursing Student Resources
Audio Glossary
NCLEX-RN® Review
- Care Plan Activity
  - Home Health Assessment
- Case Study
  - Safety First for Home Health
- MediaLink Application
- Links to Resources

CLINICAL COMPETENCIES

1. Assess factors affecting the health of individuals in the community.
2. Provide patient care in community-based settings and the home.
3. Apply the nursing process to care of the patient in the home.

TERMS MATCHING

Place the letter of the correct definition in the space next to each term.

1. _____ Community-based care

2. _____ Contracting

3. _____ Disability

4. _____ Faith community nursing

5. _____ Handicap

6. _____ Home care

7. _____ Hospice care

8. _____ Impairment

9. _____ Referral source

10. _____ Respite care

A. A disturbance in structure or function resulting from physiological or psychologic abnormalities.

B. The degree of observable and measurable impairment.

C. The total adjustment to disability that limits functioning at a normal level.

D. Culturally competent, community-based care that focuses on the patient and the family.

E. Care is provided in the patient's place of residence for the purpose of promoting, maintaining, or restoring health or of maximizing the level of independence while minimizing the effects of disability and illness, including terminal illness.

F. Short-term or intermittent home care that is provided to give the primary caregiver time away from the individual who is ill.

G. Designed to provide medical, nursing, social, psychologic, and spiritual care for terminally ill patients and their families.

H. The negotiation of a cooperative working agreement between the nurse and patient that is continuously renegotiated.

I. A nontraditional community-based way of providing health promotion and health restoration nursing interventions to specific groups of people.

J. A person recommending home care services and supplying the agency with details about the patient's needs.

FOCUSED STUDY

1. What are the primary predictors of the need for home care services?

_____

_____

_____

_____

_____

2. List two nursing interventions that ensure good rapport between the patient and the nurse in community home care.

_____

_____

_____

_____

_____

3. Identify individuals who may benefit from home care services.

_____

_____

_____

_____

4. List services that are available through home care services.

_____

_____

_____

_____

CASE STUDY

Mr. Maxwell Cohen is an 85-year-old male who has been discharged from the acute care hospital after a fall outside his home that was caused by a weak railing. He has multiple bruises and skin tears, as well as a left radial ulnar fracture. The cast limits his mobility, but he is right-handed and does not believe this will be a problem. Mr. Cohen has been a widower for the last year and a half and seems well-adjusted.

During the nurse's first visit, it is evident that Mr. Cohen has many friends in the neighborhood who check on him often. Several stop by during the nurse's visit. The railing has been repaired, and no additional areas appear to be loose. A nonslip mat is at the front and side doors for people to use in wiping their shoes before entering the home. Things appear to be neat and tidy in the home, with little clutter. Two extension cords are visible in the home, one of which runs under the edge of a carpet in an unused corner of the living room.

The kitchen is well-organized and clean. The cookware is heavy, but Mr. Cohen is able to lift it without difficulty using his right hand. The nurse is able to observe Mr. Cohen in the kitchen because he is making lunch at the time the nurse arrives. The patient uses plastic dinnerware and drinking glasses.

Mr. Cohen states that he is healing, but the progress seems to be slower than he expected. He also states that he has had difficulty changing clothes, getting in and out of the bathtub, and opening his medication bottles. His medications are lined up on the counter; none is expired, and he is able to discuss his medications without difficulty.

1. What distractions limited the nurse's ability to assess and care for Mr. Cohen?

2. What safety concerns do you see in Mr. Cohen's home setting? Would these be expensive to repair? Explain.

3. What can you do to improve Mr. Cohen's safety with regard to his medication administration?

CARE PLAN CRITICAL-THINKING ACTIVITY

Use the preceding case study to develop a series of nursing diagnoses in which the most important physiological, psychosocial, teaching, and safety issues are identified.

NCLEX-RN® REVIEW QUESTIONS

1. Which factors affect the health of a community? **Select all that apply.**
    1. the providing of care in a patient's home
    2. the number of extended families in a community
    3. environmental factors such as air and water quality
    4. access to health care
    5. the number of ambulatory care clinics
2. Community-based healthcare services allow patients to remain in the community longer. Which of the following best describes these types of services?
    1. services that allow patients with late stages of Alzheimer's disease to remain at home
    2. programs that encourage physical safety and social, nutritional, and recreational needs
    3. Meals on Wheels
    4. programs that decrease the need for hospitalization days and limit costs
3. Which statement by the nurse is most accurate when discussing home health care?
    1. The purpose of home health care is to promote, maintain, or restore the level of dependence of the patient.
    2. Home health care provides care for patients who need long-term daily care.
    3. The largest single source of reimbursement for home health care is Medicaid.
    4. Home health care is designed for patients who require additional assistance and education in their home.
4. A family member believes that a 43-year-old female patient would benefit from home health care after a trauma. The patient has no health insurance and does not think that she needs this type of care. Which of the following is the most appropriate statement the nurse can make about home health care?
    1. Home health care is inexpensive and will help the patient return to his or her maximum level of wellness earlier than patients who don't have home health care support.
    2. Some home health care agencies have sliding scale or donations payment plans.
    3. Family members cannot request home health care.
    4. A registered nurse can help to keep the cost lower by limiting the involvement of a physician in the patient's aftercare.

5. Which of the following best describes the focus of the initial home health visit?

1. Evaluation of patient outcomes established during the acute care in-hospital stay.
2. The time to obtain a referral and establish the nurse–patient relationship.
3. Assessment of the patient, the physical environment, and support systems.
4. The best time to determine whether this patient will be successful with in-home care.

6. Which of the following statements is the most appropriate outcome statement?

1. Deficient knowledge related to a diagnosis of chronic obstructive pulmonary disease.
2. Patient will use oxygen.
3. Patient will demonstrate application of oxygen by the second home health visit.
4. Apply oxygen per physician order.

7. As a coordinator of services, what will the home health nurse do?

1. Discuss the patient's care with the various members of the healthcare team.
2. Change the treatment plan at the direction of the patient.
3. Document the patient's care to meet the needs of the physician.
4. Fax requests to the physician's office to maintain patient confidentiality.

8. Which of the following can be a challenge in providing care in the patient's home?

1. the patient's independence in the home
2. the blurring of lines between nursing and the family support system
3. establishment of a positive rapport with the patient and family
4. caregivers who share responsibility for the patient's support

9. Education is an important part of home health care. Which statement is most appropriate with regard to patient education?

1. The nurse is the most influential source of information for the home health patient.
2. The nurse can empower the patient to learn by encouraging the patient to listen to his or her body and ask questions.
3. The nurse gives the patient written information about concerns the patient might have in the future.
4. The nurse involves as many people as possible in the learning process.

10. During a home health visit, the nurse notices that the patient is taking expired medications and has no heat. Which would be the most appropriate action of the nurse?

1. Discuss the situation with social services.
2. Ignore the situation and hope it gets better.
3. Encourage the patient to wear warmer clothing and to get the furnace fixed before winter comes.
4. Discuss the issues with the patient.

Nursing Care of Patients Having Surgery

LEARNING OUTCOMES

1. Compare the differences and similarities between outpatient and inpatient surgery.
2. Identify the three phases of perioperative care.
3. Interpret the significance of diagnostic tests used in the perioperative period.
4. Explain nursing implications for medications prescribed for the surgical patient.
5. Identify variations in perioperative care for the older adult.
6. Describe principles of pain management specific to acute postoperative pain control.

MediaLink

Pearson Nursing Student Resources
Audio Glossary
NCLEX-RN® Review
■ Care Plan Activity
  ■ Providing Postoperative Care
■ Case Study
  ■ A Patient Having Surgery
■ Tools
  ■ Stages of Wound Healing
■ MediaLink Applications
■ Links to Resources

CLINICAL COMPETENCIES

1. Assess the physiologic and psychosocial health status of patients for surgery to determine their ability to tolerate surgery and identify risks for complications.
2. Participate in patient and family teaching prior to anesthesia, during postoperative care, and prior to discharge from the facility.
3. Use appropriate communication techniques to minimize risks associated with handoffs among healthcare team members during transitions between phases of the perioperative experience.
4. Observe and participate as appropriate with nursing responsibilities and interventions to promote patient safety and integrity and to prevent hazards in the operating room.
5. Use the nursing process to provide safe and effective nursing care for the patient in the preoperative, intraoperative, and postoperative phases of surgery.

TERMS MATCHING

Place the letter of the correct definition in the space next to each term.

1. _____ Anesthesia
2. _____ Circulating nurse
3. _____ Conscious sedation
4. _____ Dehiscence
5. _____ Equianalgesia
6. _____ Evisceration
7. _____ General anesthesia
8. _____ Informed consent
9. _____ Intraoperative phase
10. _____ Perioperative nursing
11. _____ Positioning
12. _____ Postoperative phase
13. _____ Preoperative phase
14. _____ Regional anesthesia
15. _____ Scrub person
16. _____ Surgery

A. The disclosure of risks associated with the intended procedure or operation to the patient and usually obtained by means of a legal document required for certain diagnostic procedures or therapeutic measures, including surgery.

B. A type of anesthesia providing analgesia, amnesia, and moderate sedation, allowing the patient to respond to verbal and physical stimulation.

C. The period of time beginning when the decision for surgery is made and ending when the patient is transferred to the operating room.

D. The process by which two different medications provide the same degree of pain management to the patient.

E. A separation in the layers of the incisional wound.

F. An experienced registered nurse who coordinates and manages a wide range of activities before, during, and after a surgical procedure. The duties include overseeing the physical aspects of the operating room and equipment, assisting with the transfer and positioning of the patient, preparing the patient's skin, ensuring that no break in aseptic technique occurs, and counting all sponges and instruments.

G. The protrusion of body organs from a wound dehiscence that may result immediately after surgery, from delayed wound healing, or after forceful straining.

H. A specialized area of practice incorporating the three phases of the surgical experience: preoperative, intraoperative, and postoperative.

I. The phase of the surgical experience that begins with the patient's entry into the operating room and ends with admittance to the postanesthesia care unit (PACU), or recovery room.

J. The phase of the surgical experience that begins with the patient's admittance to the PACU and ends with the patient's complete recovery from the surgical intervention.

K. A position requiring manual dexterity and in-depth knowledge of the anatomic and mechanical aspects of a particular surgery. The role may be assumed by a registered nurse or an operating room technician (ORT), depending on hospital policy and the complexity of the surgery.

L. Medications used to produce unconsciousness, analgesia, reflex loss, and muscle relaxation during a surgical procedure.

M. An invasive medical procedure performed to diagnose or treat illness, injury, or deformity.

N. Medications administered for a surgical procedure to provide analgesia, reflex loss, and muscle relaxation but not loss of consciousness.

O. Medications administered by inhalation or intravenous route that produce central nervous system depression resulting in a loss of consciousness, a loss of pain perception, and skeletal muscle relaxation.

P. The anatomic placement of the patient in preparation for a surgical procedure.

FOCUSED STUDY

1. List and describe the three phases of the perioperative experience.

a.

_____

b.

_____

c.

_____

2. Describe the role and responsibilities of the following healthcare providers within the perioperative setting.

a. Surgeon

_____

b. Circulating nurse

_____

c. Scrub nurse

_____

d. Anesthesiologist

_____

e. Phlebotomist

_____

f. X-ray technician

_____

g. Transporter

_____

3. Describe the differences between general anesthesia, regional anesthesia, and conscious sedation.

_____

_____

_____

_____

_____

4. Describe the following postoperative complications and their appropriate nursing interventions.

a. Hemorrhage:

_____

_____

b. Deep vein thrombosis:

_____

_____

_____

c. Pneumonia:

_____

_____

_____

CASE STUDY

Mrs. Elvira, a 28-year-old female, is scheduled to undergo a right radical mastectomy. Mrs. Elvira reports smoking two-and-a-half packs of cigarettes a day and obtaining minimal exercise. She takes aspirin for frequent headaches and herbal supplements to help her lose weight. Answer the following questions based on your knowledge of patient needs for undergoing surgery.

1. Mrs. Elvira's informed consent document includes the surgeon's name, the alternatives and risks of treatments, and the date and time she and her surgeon signed the consent. What is missing?

2. What postoperative complication(s) is Mrs. Elvira at most risk of developing based on her history?

3. What preoperative studies and interventions will Mrs. Elvira undergo to reduce the likelihood of intraoperative and postoperative complications?

4. Prior to discharge, Mrs. Elvira will be instructed to assess her incision site for signs of infection. What are they?

SHORT ANSWERS

1. Complete the following chart.

Classification of Medication	Potential Surgical Complication	Nursing Care
Anticoagulants		
Antidepressants (particularly monoamine oxidase inhibitors)		
Antihypertensives		
Antibiotics (particularly the "mycin" group)		
Diuretics		

NCLEX-RN® REVIEW QUESTIONS

1. Informed consent must include which of the following? **Select all that apply.**
   1. description and purpose of the proposed procedure
   2. alternative treatments or procedures available
   3. date, time, and location of the proposed surgical procedure
   4. right to refuse treatment or withdraw consent
   5. potential complications
2. The nurse is working to orient a new nurse in the postanesthesia care unit. Which of the following actions by the new nurse indicates an understanding of methods to prevent hypothermia?
   1. The nurse monitors the patient's temperature every 15 minutes.
   2. The nurse monitors the patient's blood pressure every 30 minutes.
   3. Upon patient's arrival in postanesthesia care unit and after sterile drapes are removed, the nurse applies warm blankets.
   4. The nurse advises the patient to report feelings of coldness.
3. After the patient has undergone surgery with a spinal anesthetic, she develops a postoperative spinal headache. Which intervention is appropriate for the nurse to implement?
   1. Decrease patient hydration.
   2. Raise the head of the bed 45 degrees.
   3. Prepare the patient for a blood patch procedure.
   4. Restrict all caffeine products.

4. Identify the surgical team member who is responsible for documenting intraoperative nursing activities, medications, blood administration, placement of drains and catheters, and length of the procedure.
   1. surgeon
   2. circulating nurse
   3. Certified Registered Nurse Anesthetist
   4. surgical scrub

5. What is an outcome of improper intraoperative surgical positioning?
   1. nerve damage
   2. hyperthermia
   3. hemorrhage
   4. increased joint flexibility

6. The nurse knows that the patient understood perioperative teaching when the patient demonstrates which of these behaviors?
   1. arrives with freshly painted nails
   2. has eaten a full breakfast before arriving at the hospital
   3. has completed all preoperative testing as ordered
   4. arrives with contacts in place

7. The patient has a positive Homan's sign after surgery. Which of the following interventions by a nursing student indicates the need for further education?
   1. Keep affected extremity at or below heart level.
   2. Ensure that the affected area is not rubbed or massaged.
   3. Record bilateral calf or thigh circumferences every shift.
   4. Teach and support the patient and family.

8. Which of the following is not a common assessment finding of a patient who is experiencing symptoms of a pulmonary embolism?
   1. anxiety
   2. decreased oxygen saturation
   3. decrease in respiratory rate
   4. cough

5 Nursing Care of Patients Experiencing Loss, Grief, and Death

LEARNING OUTCOMES

1. Compare and contrast theories of loss and grief.
2. Explain factors affecting responses to loss.
3. Explain the physiological basis for manifestations associated with the end of life.
4. Discuss legal and ethical issues in end-of-life care.
5. Describe the philosophy and activities of hospice and palliative care.

CLINICAL COMPETENCIES

1. Identify physiological changes in the dying patient.
2. Use assessments, patient values, and evidence to provide nursing interventions to promote a comfortable and dignified death.
3. Effectively communicate with and function within the interdisciplinary team to plan and provide individualized care for patients and families experiencing loss, grief, or death.
4. Adapt individual and cultural values and variations, as well as expressed needs and preferences, into the plan of care for patients and families experiencing loss, grief, or death.

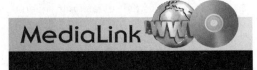

MediaLink

Pearson Nursing Student Resources
Audio Glossary
NCLEX-RN® Review
■ Care Plan Activity
  ■ Anticipatory Grieving
■ Case Study
  ■ Do Not Resuscitate
■ Animation/Video
  ■ End of Life Care or Grieving
■ MediaLink Applications
■ Links to Resources

TERMS MATCHING

Place the letter of the correct definition in the space next to each term.

1. _____ Anticipatory grieving

2. _____ Bereavement

3. _____ Chronic sorrow

4. _____ Death

5. _____ Death anxiety

6. _____ Do-not-resuscitate order

7. _____ Durable power of attorney

8. _____ End-of-life nursing care

9. _____ Euthanasia

10. _____ Grief

11. _____ Grieving

12. _____ Healthcare surrogate

13. _____ Hospice

14. _____ Living will

15. _____ Loss

16. _____ Mourning

17. _____ Palliative care

A. An irreversible cessation of circulatory and respiratory functions.

B. Signifys a killing prompted by some humanitarian motive.

C. Hospice and palliative care.

D. Coordinated care for patients with limited life expectancy.

E. Actions or expressions of the bereaved.

F. Focused on the relief of physical, mental, and spiritual distress for individuals who have an incurable illness.

G. A cluster of predictable responses to an anticipated loss.

H. The emotional response to loss.

I. An individual selected to make medical decisions when another person can no longer make them.

J. An actual or potential situation in which a valued object, person, body part, or emotion that was formerly present is lost.

K. Worry or fear related to death or dying.

L. A document that can delegate the authority to make health, financial, and/or legal decisions on a person's behalf.

M. A document that provides written directions about life-prolonging procedures.

N. The time of mourning experienced after a loss.

O. No cardiopulmonary resuscitation be performed for respiratory or cardiac arrest.

P. The internal process the person uses to work through the response to loss.

Q. A cyclical, recurring, and potentially progressive pattern of pervasive sadness.

FOCUSED STUDY

1. Describe the philosophy and activities of hospice and palliative care.

_____

_____

_____

_____

_____

2. List the manifestations of impending death.

_____

_____

_____

_____

3. Cultural care is as important at the end of life as it is at any other time during the patient's life. Discuss nursing interventions with regard to cultural considerations of a variety of ethnic groups regarding end-of-life care.

_____

_____

_____

_____

_____

_____

CASE STUDY

You are the hospice nurse for 27-year-old Alana Oberan. She recently received a terminal diagnosis of an aggressive form of cancer and has been informed by her physician that a four-month survival rate would be optimistic. Alana's support system consists of both of her parents. Answer the following questions based on your knowledge of grief and end-of-life care.

1. Discuss Spiritual assessment, including questions to consider during this assessment process.

2. Discuss Kübler-Ross's stages of death and dying, including reactions that may occur during the grieving process.

3. What factors will affect the parents' ability to grieve their upcoming loss?

CROSSWORD PUZZLE

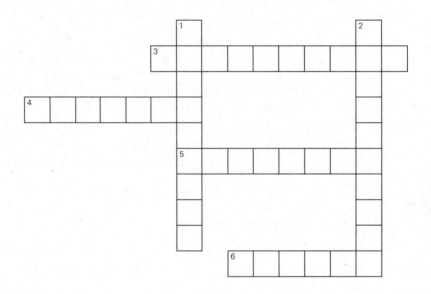

Across

3   Signify a killing prompted by some humanitarian motive

4   Stage of grief in which the person's behavior becomes disorganized

5   A combination of intellectual and emotional responses and behaviors by which people adjust their self-concept in the face of an actual or potential loss

6   Kübler-Ross stage of grief in which individual resists loss

Down

1   A health care _____ is an individual selected to make medical decisions when another person is no longer able to do so

2   Legal documents that allow a person to plan for health care

NCLEX-RN® REVIEW QUESTIONS

1. After the physician leaves the room, the nurse enters and finds the patient crying. Which would be the best statement for the nurse to make to the patient?

1. "The physician said that she told you about your testing tomorrow. Is that true?"
2. "Is there someone I can call for you?"
3. "Tell me what concerns you the most."
4. "Are you upset about tomorrow's testing?"

2. After providing care for a dying patient, the nurse documents the care. Which is the best evaluation statement in regards to the grieving process?

1. Oral care provided, patient repositioned for comfort
2. Mucous membranes moist and intact
3. Oxygen applied via nasal cannula
4. Patient confused, sister at bedside

3. A patient is unresponsive after six months of aggressive treatment for pancreatic cancer. Which document would allow a designated person to make decisions about the patient's health care?

1. advanced directive
2. durable power of attorney
3. living will
4. Patient's Bill of Rights

4. The patient has a do-not-resuscitate order on the chart, and the family has decided to provide palliative care rather than aggressive treatment. Which nursing intervention is an appropriate nursing response to the patient's moans and grimaces?

1. Administer 2 mg IV morphine per the physician's order.
2. Assess for pain, reposition the patient, and then reassess for pain.
3. Ask the family if this is how the patient reacts to pain.
4. Call the physician to seek a long-term pain control medication.

5. A patient asks the nurse about the reputation of the physician who diagnosed his colon cancer. The patient states, "I should get another opinion before I have this surgery tomorrow." In which stage of grief is this patient? **Select all that apply.**

1. Kübler-Ross: anger
2. Engel: acute stage
3. Bowlby: protest
4. Lindemann: morbid grief reaction
5. Caplan: stress and loss

6. The patient chooses palliative care for the end of his life. What would be the most appropriate action for the nurse to take in the last hours of the patient's life?

1. Take vital signs hourly.
2. Reposition the patient every two hours if needed for comfort.
3. Elevate the head of the bed 90 degrees at all times and administer 4 mg of IV morphine.
4. Encourage the patient to eat to keep up his or her strength.

7. The patient is complaining of being short of breath with a respiratory rate of 38 and an oxygen saturation of 92%. Which nursing intervention would be the lowest priority?

1. Administer 2 mg of IV morphine.
2. Administer oxygen 2 L/min via nasal cannula.
3. Elevate the head of bed.
4. Administer oxygen via 100% nonrebreather mask.

8. A patient at the end of life has intractable vomiting and has refused a nasogastric tube. What other nursing interventions may aid the patient's comfort?

1. Encourage the patient to drink ginger ale with ice chips.
2. Administer morphine 1 mg IV.
3. Administer prochlorperazine (Compazine) PO.
4. Administer ondansetron (Zofran) IV.

6 Nursing Care of Patients with **Problems** of **Substance Abuse**

LEARNING OUTCOMES

1. Discuss risk factors associated with substance abuse.
2. Recognize the manifestations of potential substance abuse in coworkers.
3. Describe common characteristics of substance abusers.
4. Explain the effects of addictive substances on physiological, cognitive, psychologic, and social well-being.
5. Support interdisciplinary care for the patient with substance abuse problems, including diagnostic tests, emergency care for overdose, and treatment of withdrawal.

CLINICAL COMPETENCIES

1. Assess functional health status of patients with substance abuse or dependence.
2. Monitor for signs of withdrawal and life-threatening conditions.
3. Provide skilled nursing care during the detoxification period.
4. Collaborate with other disciplines when caring for patients with substance abuse problems.
5. Educate patients about stress management, coping skills, nutrition, relapse prevention, and healthy lifestyle choices.
6. Use the nursing process to provide individualized nursing care for patients experiencing problems with substance abuse.
7. Revise plan of care as needed to promote, maintain, or restore functional health status to patients with substance abuse problems.

MediaLink

Pearson Nursing Student Resources
Audio Glossary
NCLEX-RN® Review

- Care Plan Activities
  - Alcohol Withdrawal
  - Tobacco Cessation
- Case Study
  - Patient with Problems of Substance Abuse
- Animation/Video
  - Substance Abuse
- MediaLink Applications
- Links to Resources

TERMS MATCHING

Place the letter of the correct definition in the space next to each term.

1. _____ Alcohol
2. _____ Cannabis sativa
3. _____ Central nervous system depressants
4. _____ Co-occurring disorders
5. _____ Delirium tremens (DT)
6. _____ Hallucinogens
7. _____ Inhalants
8. _____ Nicotine
9. _____ Opiates
10. _____ Polysubstance abuse
11. _____ Psychostimulants
12. _____ Substance abuse
13. _____ Substance dependence
14. _____ Tolerance
15. _____ Wernicke's encephalopathy
16. _____ Withdrawal

A. A condition in which an individual must use increasing amounts of a substance to produce the desired effect or must use the substance to avoid or relieve uncomfortable symptoms.

B. Substances also referred to as psychedelics, including phencyclidine (PCP), 3,4-methylenedioxy-methamphetamine (MDMA), d-lysergic acid diethylamide (LSD), mescaline, dimethyltryptamine (DMT), and psilocin. Psychedelics bring on the same types of thoughts, perceptions, and feelings that occur in dreams.

C. Severe withdrawal resulting in a medical emergency that usually occurs two to five days following alcohol withdrawal and persists two to three days.

D. Continued use of a chemical substance for at least one month in a fashion inconsistent with medical or social norms, despite related problems.

E. Narcotic analgesics such as meperidine (Demerol®), hydrocodone (Vicodin®), Percocet®, oxycodone (OxyContin®), and Darvon®.

F. Inhaled solvents categorized into three types: anesthetics, volatile nitrites, and organic solvents.

G. A compound found in tobacco that enters the system via the lungs (cigarettes and cigars) and oral mucous membranes (chewing tobacco as well as smoking). In low doses, it stimulates nicotinic receptors in the brain to release norepinephrine and epinephrine, causing vasoconstriction. As a result, the heart rate accelerates and the force of ventricular contractions increases.

H. A central nervous system depressant that is the most commonly abused drug.

I. Highly addictive substances such as cocaine and amphetamines that give the user a sense of euphoria.

J. Concurrent diagnosis of a substance use disorder and a psychiatric disorder.

K. The source of marijuana.

L. The simultaneous use of many substances.

M. An intensive subjective need for a particular psychoactive drug.

N. A condition seen in chronic alcoholism as a result of thiamine (B_1) deficiency that is characterized by nystagmus, ptosis, ataxia, confusion, coma, and possible death.

O. A series of signs and symptoms that occurs in physically dependent individuals when they discontinue the use of a substance.

FOCUSED STUDY

1. Explain the following risk factors as they relate to substance abuse.
   a. Genetic factors

   _____

   _____

   b. Biological factors

   _____

   _____

   c. Psychologic factors

   _____

   _____

   d. Sociocultural factors

   _____

   _____

2. Complete the following table.

Addictive Substance	Effect
Caffeine	
Nicotine	
Cannabis	
Alcohol	
CNS Depressants	
Psychostimulants	
Amphetamines	
Opiates	
Hallucinogens	
Inhalants	

3. Describe the following substance abuse screening tools.
  a. Michigan Alcohol Screening Test (MAST) brief version

_____

_____

  b. CAGE questionnaire

_____

_____

  c. Brief Drug Abuse Screening Test (B-DAST)

_____

_____

4. Identify community-based care options available to patients who suffer from substance abuse.

_____

_____

_____

_____

_____

CASE STUDY

Ryan Dern is a 32-year-old male who suffers from alcoholism. He has taken the initial step of admitting to his problem and seeking medical assistance. Answer the following questions based on your knowledge of alcoholism.

1. How long does Ryan need to have had excessive drinking behaviors to be considered substance-dependent?

2. What factors affect the rate of alcohol absorption?

3. What vitamin deficiency is associated with alcoholism? How will the nurse assist Ryan in meeting his nutritional needs?

4. The nurse will teach Ryan HALT. What is HALT?

CROSSWORD PUZZLE

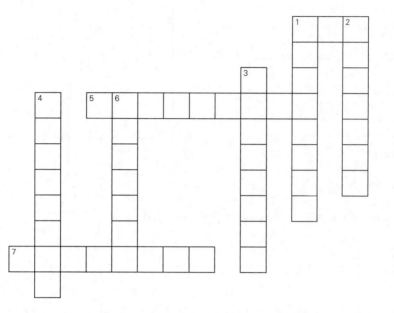

Across

1 The psychoactive component of marijuana

5 Substance referred to as hash

7 Long-term changes in brain neurotransmission that occur after repeated detoxifications

Down

1 Vitamin deficiency commonly seen in alcoholics

2 Street term commonly used to refer to methamphetamine

3 Stimulant found in food and beverages that causes heart rate increases

4 The primary subjective effect associated with cocaine and amphetamines

6 Most commonly abused legal drug in the United States

NCLEX-RN® REVIEW QUESTIONS

1. Identify the neurotransmitter that plays a pivotal role in substance abuse.
   1. dopamine
   2. endorphin
   3. enkephalin
   4. dynorphin
2. Which ethnic group reports the lowest incidence of alcohol abuse?
   1. African Americans
   2. Native Americans
   3. Hispanics
   4. Asians
3. Which addictive substance may be a risk factor in developing future psychotic symptoms?
   1. cocaine
   2. methamphetamine
   3. cannabis
   4. OxyContin®
4. The patient reports to the nurse that he has been using crank. The nurse knows that crank is a form of what substance?
   1. methamphetamine
   2. opiate
   3. hallucinogen
   4. alcohol
5. Which body fluids are often tested for drug content? **Select all that apply**.
   1. saliva
   2. tears
   3. urine
   4. blood
   5. stool
6. Which is the correct form of questioning to use when assessing a patient for substance abuse?
   1. "You don't have any drug abusers in your family, do you?"
   2. "Did you ever abuse a substance in the past?"
   3. "Have you ever been treated in an alcohol or drug abuse clinic?"
   4. "Were you ever arrested for a driving while under the influence (DUI) offense?"
7. Which screening tool is most effective for the nurse to use when the patient does not recognize his or her substance abuse problem?
   1. Brief Drug Abuse Screening Test (B-DAST)
   2. CAGE questionnaire
   3. Michigan Alcohol Screening Test (MAST) brief version
   4. HALT Screening Assessment tool
8. The nurse caring for a patient with a substance abuse addiction should employ which intervention?
   1. Assess the patient's level of disorientation.
   2. Place the patient alone in a private room.
   3. Accept the use of defense mechanisms.
   4. Do not encourage the patient to verbalize anxieties.
9. Nurses have a higher incidence of what type of abuse?
   1. alcohol
   2. hallucinogen
   3. opiate
   4. amphetamine

Nursing Care of Patients Experiencing Disasters

LEARNING OUTCOMES

1. Distinguish the difference between an emergency and a disaster.
2. Describe the types of injuries and manifestations associated with biologic, chemical, or radiologic terrorism.
3. Discuss nursing interventions for the treatment of injuries related to biologic, chemical, or radiologic terrorism.
4. Explain the rationale for reverse triage in disasters versus conventional triage in emergencies.
5. Discuss situations requiring the need for patient isolation or patient decontamination.
6. Discuss the role of the nurse in disaster planning, response, and mitigation.

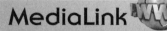

MediaLink

Pearson Nursing Student Resources
Audio Glossary
NCLEX-RN® Review
- Care Plan Activity
  - Biologic Contamination
- Case Studies
  - Triage after a Disaster
  - Bioterrorism
- MediaLink Applications
- Links to Resources

CLINICAL COMPETENCIES

1. Assess health status of patients who have experienced a disaster and monitor, document, and triage to the appropriate level of care.
2. Use evidence-based interventions to plan and implement nursing care for patients with injuries suffered as a result of a disaster.
3. Using assessment skills, determine priority nursing diagnoses, implement, and evaluate individualized nursing interventions for patients who are victims of disasters.
4. Provide safe and knowledgeable nursing care to treat disaster-related injuries.
5. Evaluate and revise plan of care to restore functional health status to patients who have sustained injuries due to a disaster.
6. Provide education to promote prevention of disaster-related injuries.

TERMS MATCHING

Place the letter of the correct definition in the space next to each term.

1. ____ Bioterrorism
2. ____ Cold zone
3. ____ Conventional weapons
4. ____ Disasters
5. ____ Emergency
6. ____ Hot zone
7. ____ Man-made disasters
8. ____ Mass casualty incidents
9. ____ Mitigation
10. ____ Multiple casualty incidents
11. ____ Natural disasters
12. ____ Nonconventional terrorist weapons
13. ____ Personal protective equipment (PPE)
14. ____ Preparedness
15. ____ Radiation sickness
16. ____ Recovery
17. ____ Reverse triage
18. ____ Surge capacity
19. ____ Terrorism
20. ____ Triage
21. ____ Warm zone

A. These include complex emergencies, technologic situations, material shortages, and other situations that are not produced by natural hazards.

B. This refers to when a comprehensive disaster plan that coordinates efforts among many people, agencies, and levels of government is in place.

C. This term refers to an unforeseen combination of circumstances that call for immediate action for a range of victims from one to many.

D. A healthcare system's ability to rapidly expand beyond normal services to meet the increased demand for qualified personnel, medical care, and public health in the event of a large-scale disaster.

E. During a mass casualty event, victims who are least injured would be transferred from the hot zone to the warm zone first. Those victims with minor injuries would be processed next and those with severe injuries would be processed last.

F. The site of the disaster where a weapon was released or where the contamination occurred.

G. This stage is also called *reconstruction*. During this stage, restoration, reconstitution, and mitigation take place.

H. These are events that require extraordinary efforts beyond those needed to respond to everyday emergencies. They may be natural or man-made.

I. These are produced by acts of nature or emerging diseases. They may be predictable through advanced meteorologic technologies or they may be unexpected.

J. The action taken to prevent or reduce the harmful effects of a disaster on human health or property. It involves future-oriented activities to prevent subsequent disasters or to minimize their effects.

K. The kind of equipment used for the protection of personnel. This includes gloves, masks, goggles, gowns, and biologic disposal bags.

L. This can happen when a person is exposed to electrically charged ions. Cells die and diseases can occur as a result of this type of exposure.

M. This can include all types of bombs and guns.

N. The U.S. Department of Defense defines this term as the "calculated use of violence or the threat of violence to inculcate fear; intended to coerce or to intimidate governments or societies in the pursuit of goals that are generally political, religious or ideological."

O. This type of event has occurred when 100 or more people have been injured.

P. This is when etiological agents (disease) are used to cause harm or to kill a population, food, and/or their livestock.

Q. This is a safe area. It is next to the warm zone and where in-depth triage of victims can occur. Survivors may find shelter in this area, and the command and control vehicles would be located here as well.

R. This can include chemicals, biologic agents, and nuclear agents that can be used to harm or kill a population.

S. This area is adjacent to the hot zone. This area is also referred to as the *control zone*. This is where decontamination of victims or triage and emergency treatment can occur.

T. This type of event has occurred when 2 to 100 people have been injured.

U. This is where victims are categorized. Those persons who need the most support and emergency care are classified as "red." Those less critical but still in need of transport to emergency centers for care are classified as "yellow." Victims who have minor injuries and do not warrant transport to an emergency center are categorized as "green."

FOCUSED STUDY

1. Describe the differences between an emergency and a disaster. Provide one example of each.

_____

_____

_____

2. Provide examples of conventional weapons and nonconventional terrorist weapons.

_____

_____

_____

3. What agencies become involved in the following levels of disasters?
   a. Level I

   _____

   b. Level II

   _____

   c. Level III

   _____

4. Describe the difference between triage and reverse triage. Provide an example of when each system should be utilized.

_____

_____

_____

_____

CASE STUDY

Mrs. Deckman, a 72-year-old female, has been trapped in her home as a result of a hurricane and flooding. She is a diabetic who controls her blood sugar with oral hypoglycemics. She has no other significant past medical history. Answer the following questions based on your knowledge of the care of patients experiencing disasters.

1. What is a hurricane?

2. What physical effects of a hurricane is Mrs. Deckman at risk for, regardless of her past medical history?

3. Mrs. Deckman was classified with a triage level of "red" after she was taken to a local shelter. What does this mean?

4. Mrs. Deckman asks the nurse for assistance in developing a disaster box to be used in case of another disaster. What items should the nurse suggest to be kept in the box?

5. What is the role of the nurse who works with the victims of this natural disaster?

6. Of the five stages of disaster preparedness, which stage is being described in this scenario?

7. What should the triage nurse document on the Mass Trauma Data Instrument?

8. A crowd has developed at the site of the shelter where Mrs. Deckman is being treated. What is one consequence of poor crowd management?

SHORT ANSWERS

List types of injuries that may be seen in victims of chemical and radiologic terrorism. Briefly describe three nursing interventions that should be provided for these two types of terrorism.

Type of terrorism	Chemical	Radiologic
Types of injuries	1.	1.
		2.
Nursing interventions	1.	1.
	2.	2.
	3.	3.

NCLEX-RN® REVIEW QUESTIONS

1. Identify the nonconventional terrorist weapon.
   1. incendiary bomb
   2. shoulder-fired missiles
   3. anthrax
   4. hand grenade

2. Which of the following are sources of ionizing radiation? **Select all that apply.**
   1. stars
   2. sun
   3. x-ray machines
   4. cell phones
   5. fire

3. A disaster that requires mutual aid from surrounding communities and regional efforts is what level of disaster?
   1. level I
   2. level II
   3. level III
   4. level IV

4. The pre-disaster stage involves which types of activities?
   1. planning and preparation
   2. warning, preimpact mobilization, and evacuation
   3. the community experiencing the immediate effects
   4. the immediate response to the effects of the disaster

5. The nurse classifies a patient as "yellow" during the triage process. The yellow code identifies the patient as which of the following?
   1. requiring the most support and immediate emergency care
   2. being in less critical condition but still in need of transport to an emergency care center
   3. having only minor injuries, which does not warrant the victim's transport to an emergency center
   4. being least likely to survive or already deceased

6. Which of the following terms refers to the area where a weapon was released or where the contamination has occurred?
   1. cold zone
   2. warm zone
   3. hot zone
   4. danger zone

7. Identify the nursing diagnoses that may apply to victims of a disaster. **Select all that apply.**
   1. *Decisional Conflict*
   2. *Risk for Injury*
   3. *Impaired Verbal Communication*
   4. *Anxiety*
   5. *Ineffective Individual Coping*

8. Overexertion and exhaustion are often associated with which of the following types of disasters?
   1. blast
   2. snow
   3. earthquake
   4. tornado

Genetic Implications of Adult Health Nursing

LEARNING OUTCOMES

1. Discuss the role of genetic concepts in health promotion and health maintenance.
2. Apply knowledge of the principles of genetic transmission and risk factors for genetic disorders.
3. Describe the significance of delivering genetic education and counseling follow-up in a professional manner.
4. Explain the implications of genetic advances on the role of nurses, paying particular attention to spiritual, cultural, ethical, legal, and social issues.
5. Identify the significance of recent advances in human genetics and the effect on healthcare delivery.

MediaLink

Pearson Nursing Student Resources
Audio Glossary
NCLEX-RN® Review
- Care Plan Activity
  - Genetic Implications of Adult Health Nursing Care
- Case Study
  - Genetic Counseling
- Animations/Videos
  - 1988 Human Genome Project
  - Nursing Role in Genetic Testing
- MediaLink Application
- Links to Resources

CLINICAL COMPETENCIES

1. Integrate genetic physical assessment and the use of a pedigree family history into delivery of nursing care.
2. Identify patients or families with actual or potential genetic conditions and initiate referrals to a genetics professional.
3. Prepare patients and their families for a genetic evaluation and facilitate the genetic counseling process.
4. Integrate basic genetic concepts into patient and family education and the reinforcement of information provided to patients by genetics professionals.

TERMS MATCHING

Place the letter of the correct definition in the space next to each item.

1. _____ Alleles
2. _____ Autosomes
3. _____ Biological markers
4. _____ Chromosomes
5. _____ Gene
6. _____ Genotype
7. _____ Heterozygous
8. _____ Homozygous
9. _____ Human genome
10. _____ Meiosis
11. _____ Mitosis
12. _____ Monosomy
13. _____ Penetrance
14. _____ Phenotype
15. _____ Polymorphisms
16. _____ Sex chromosomes
17. _____ Somatic cells
18. _____ Translocation
19. _____ Trisomy 21
20. _____ X-linked dominant
21. _____ X-linked recessive

A. The process of making new cells.
B. The specific sequence of nucleotides (the genes and the variations therein).
C. Describes an individual with two different forms (alleles) of a gene.
D. The reductional division of a cell.
E. The probability that a gene will be expressed phenotypically.
F. Different forms or versions of genes.
G. The loss of a single chromosome from a pair.
H. The observable, outward expression of an individual's entire physical, biochemical, and physiological makeup as determined by his or her genotype (alleles) and by environmental factors.
I. Determine an individual's gender.
J. Seen in hemophilia A.
K. The first 22 pairs of chromosomes.
L. Describes an individual with two identical forms (alleles) of a gene.
M. Tissue cells of the body.
N. Stable segments of DNA.
O. A small portion (segment) of the nucleotide (base) sequence of a chromosome DNA molecule that can be identified as having specific directions for a particular function or characteristic.
P. Seen in vitamin D-resistant rickets.
Q. Down syndrome.
R. Structures in the nucleus containing DNA.
S. The total sum of DNA in a human cell.
T. Chromosomal reshuffling.
U. DNA sequences that are natural variations in a gene in which each possible sequence is present in at least 1% of people.

FOCUSED STUDY

1. Discuss the difference between mitosis and meiosis cell division. What role do they play in chromosomal alteration?

_____

_____

_____

_____

2. Explain the principles of inheritance and discuss how nurses can apply these principles when performing genetic counseling.

_____

_____

_____

_____

3. List specific examples of genetic testing and the condition, disease, or trait for which the test screens.

_____

_____

_____

_____

4. Discuss the importance of performing a thorough patient genetic intake and history. List items that must be included in a comprehensive genetic intake and history.

_____

_____

_____

_____

_____

CASE STUDIES

Case Study 1

Janine Steinman, a 27-year-old married female, is being seen for her first prenatal visit by Dr. Williams. Mrs. Steinman reports that her relatives have a history of Tay-Sachs disease and that she is concerned about her child's potential for developing the disease. Dr. Williams orders a carrier test followed by genetic counseling. Answer the following questions based on your knowledge of Tay-Sachs disease and genetic implications.

1. Why did the physician order carrier testing for Mrs. Steinman?

2. How can the Steinmans be assured of the accuracy of their genetic testing results?

3. Who may obtain the results of the Steinmans' genetic testing?

Case Study 2

Dianne Simmons, a 42-year-old female, is considering having an elective bilateral mastectomy. Ms. Simmons has a strong family history of breast cancer. Ms. Simmons's mother, sister, maternal aunt, and great-grandmother have all been diagnosed and treated for breast cancer. Ms. Simmons is consulting with Dr. Powers and his team to determine whether elective bilateral mastectomies will lessen the likelihood of her developing a form of breast cancer. Answer the following questions based on your knowledge of breast cancer and genetic implications.

1. Describe the predictive genetic testing that Ms. Simmons will have performed.

2. Why is it important to discuss and map Ms. Simmons's family tree in relation to breast cancer?

3. What type of nursing diagnoses will the nurse include in Ms. Simmons's genetic counseling care plan?

4. How can the testing information obtained by Ms. Simmons be used in the care of her extended family members?

CROSSWORD PUZZLE

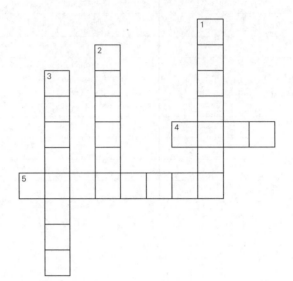

Across

4   The same

5   The loss of a single chromosome from a pair

Down

1   The gain of a single chromosome

2   Different

3   The normal number of 46 chromosomes

NCLEX-RN® REVIEW QUESTIONS

1. A nurse is reviewing the patient's chromosomal report. What is the correct number of chromosomes per nucleus the nurse recognizes?

　　1. 23

　　2. 33

　　3. 46

　　4. 52

2. DNA molecules consist of long sequences of nucleotides or bases represented by what letters?

　　1. A, G, T, and C

　　2. A, H, P, and S

　　3. T, O, D, and P

　　4. A, D, S, and M

3. Down syndrome is better known as what?

　　1. Trisomy 5

　　2. Duosomy 19

　　3. Trisomy 21

　　4. Monosomic 16

4. The nurse is providing inheritance risk assessment and teaching to a patient. Which of the following statements is incorrect?
   1. A family history of multiple male miscarriages may be a sign of an X-linked recessive condition.
   2. The sex chromosome X is unevenly distributed to males and females.
   3. An individual with a recessive condition has inherited one altered gene from his or her mother and one from his or her father.
   4. Homozygous dominant conditions are generally more severe than heterozygous dominant conditions and are often lethal.

5. A newborn undergoes what type of genetic newborn testing for phenylketonuria (PKU)?
   1. predictive genetic testing
   2. pharmacogenetic testing
   3. carrier testing
   4. newborn screening

6. Prior to genetic testing, the nurse discusses all but which of the following with the patient?
   1. risks and benefits of the testing
   2. emotional stress caused by the testing and results
   3. cost of the procedure to be performed and its impact on family resources
   4. verbal consent, the preferred method of consent to avoid disclosing the patient's identity on a written consent

7. A patient has a strong family history for the BRCA1 and BRCA2 tumor suppressor genes. What would be observed in the evaluation of successful genetic counseling in this patient?
   1. undergoes her first mammogram by age 50
   2. keeps the counseling session information private
   3. begins early clinical breast screenings at a young age
   4. does not perform breast self-exams due to unlikelihood of feeling these tumors

8. Mitochondrial genes and any diseases due to DNA alterations on those genes are transmitted by what means?
   1. through the mother in a matrilineal pattern
   2. through the father in a patrilineal pattern
   3. by either parent
   4. Mitochondrial diseases are not transmitted based on a sex link.

9. A genetic counselor has just informed a female patient that carrier testing has confirmed that she, her husband, and her infant daughter are positive for the sickle cell trait. You would expect the patient to express all but which of the following emotions?
   1. survivor guilt
   2. fear
   3. shame
   4. self-image disturbance

9 Nursing Care of Patients in **Pain**

LEARNING OUTCOMES

1. Describe the neurophysiology of pain.

2. Compare and contrast definitions and characteristics of acute, chronic, central, malignant, phantom, and psychogenic pain.

3. Discuss factors affecting individualized responses to pain.

4. Discuss interdisciplinary care for the patient in pain, including medications, surgery, transcutaneous electrical nerve stimulation, and complementary therapies.

5. Use the nursing process as a framework for providing individualized nursing care for patients experiencing pain.

MediaLink

Pearson Nursing Student Resources
Audio Glossary
NCLEX-RN® Review
- Care Plan Activity
  - The Patient in Pain
- Case Study
  - Assessing the Patient in Pain
- MediaLink Applications
- Links to Resources

CLINICAL COMPETENCIES

1. Assess patients' pain intensity, quality, location, pattern, intensifiers, and relievers; side effects of analgesics; and effect on function and mood.

2. Determine patient's expressed desire, values preference, and support for pain management.

3. In collaboration with the healthcare team, intervene with appropriate evidence-based pharmacologic and non-pharmacologic methodologies. Revise plan of care according to patient's response to interventions and need for control.

4. Use equianalgesia tables to select and transition between opioid analgesics.

5. Teach patients about effective self-management of pain.

6. Evaluate effectiveness of interventions to relieve pain and promote comfort; re-treat or adjust doses of medication and interventions as necessary.

TERMS MATCHING

Place the letter of the correct definition in the space next to each term.

1. _____ Addiction

2. _____ Analgesic

3. _____ Breakthrough pain

4. _____ Chronic malignant pain

5. _____ Incident pain

6. _____ Nociceptors

7. _____ Phantom limb pain

8. _____ Titrate

9. _____ Transdermal

A. To increase or decrease medication doses according to a patient's needs.

B. Predictable discomfort that is precipitated by an event or activity such as coughing, changing position, or being touched.

C. Discomfort caused by advance of a life-threatening disease or associated with treatment.

D. A medication used to treat pain.

E. One method used to deliver local anesthetics to treat focal neuropathic pain.

F. One type of pain that can be experienced by a patient who has had a body part amputated.

G. When activated, these generate pain impulses.

H. Discomfort that exceeds baseline levels of discomfort. It is often described as a sudden flare that exceeds the analgesic effect of long-acting pain medications.

I. A primary, chronic neurobiologic disease characterized by compulsive use of a substance despite negative consequences such as health threats or legal problems.

FOCUSED STUDY

1. Describe the differences between acute and chronic pain.

_____

_____

_____

_____

2. List factors that influence a patient's response to pain.

_____

_____

_____

_____

_____

_____

3. Describe the different methods of administering medication.

_____

_____

_____

_____

_____

4. What are the nurse's responsibilities when educating a patient who uses NSAIDs to help control pain?

_____

_____

_____

_____

CASE STUDIES

Case Study 1

John Browning was brought to the emergency room after suffering a traumatic amputation of his right lower leg during a motor vehicle accident. An emergency above-knee amputation was performed soon after his arrival at the hospital.

1. Which nerve fibers will transmit pain sensations from John Browning's injury to his spinal cord?

2. What form of acute pain will he experience immediately after the injury?

3. Which type of pain is Mr. Browning most at risk for developing as a result of his injuries?

4. What strategies will the nurse employ to best assess Mr. Browning's pain?

Case Study 2

Bailey Bowen is a 32-year-old male who suffers from recurrent lower back pain as a result of an injury that occurred at work. Mr. Bowen is a construction worker. Mr. Bowen has come to the physician's office for pain relief.

1. What factors will influence Mr. Bowen's perceived level of pain?

2. What strategies other than medication administration can be used to lessen Mr. Bowen's perceived level of pain?

3. What types of medications would you expect this patient to be prescribed for pain control at home?

4. Mr. Bowen's doctor has discussed placing a transcutaneous electrical nerve stimulation (TENS) unit on the patient. Explain how this may benefit a patient with chronic pain.

CROSSWORD PUZZLE

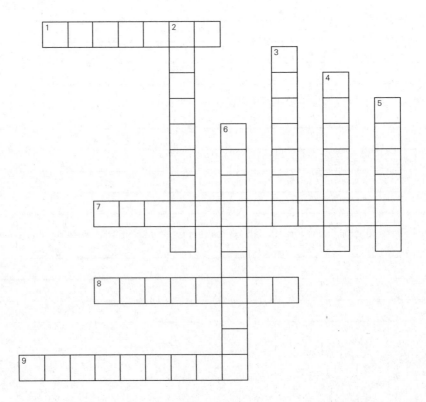

Across

1   The "Q" of the PQRST mnemonic

7   Dull, poorly localized pain arising from body organs

8   Another name for an opioid analgesic

9   The dorsal spinal roots are severed during this type of surgery

Down

2   The amount of pain a person can endure before outwardly responding to the pain

3   A brand name of an analgesic that should be avoided if the patient has a history of alcohol abuse

4   A type of pain with associated changes in sensations that is caused by a lesion or damage to the brain or spinal cord

5   The "T" of the PQRST mnemonic

6   A surgery used to remove or destroy a nerve

NCLEX-RN® REVIEW QUESTIONS

1. The patient is complaining of nausea and a deep cramping pain in the abdomen. The patient is unable to localize the pain. The patient is most likely experiencing what type of pain?
   1. somatic pain
   2. visceral pain
   3. referred pain
   4. hyperesthesia pain

2. When caring for a geriatric patient, the nurse is aware of which of the following?
   1. As a patient ages, the perception of pain decreases.
   2. Opioids cause excessive respiratory depression in older adults.
   3. Older adult patients fear narcotic addiction.
   4. Pain is a part of growing older.

3. Which of the following statements is a common misconception regarding pain?
   1. Pain is a condition and not just a symptom.
   2. Narcotic medication is an appropriate method to help relieve a patient's chronic pain.
   3. Patients rarely lie about their pain.
   4. Pain relief interferes with a healthcare provider's ability to diagnose the source of the patient's pain.

4. The patient has been diagnosed with herpes zoster. The nurse is aware that pain control may be best achieved by administering a medication from which of the following classes?
   1. local anesthetics
   2. anticonvulsants
   3. narcotics
   4. nonsteroidal anti-inflammatory drugs (NSAIDs)

5. Which of the following is an advantage of administering pain medication before the patient experiences pain?
   1. The patient may spend less time in pain.
   2. Frequent administration allows for larger doses.
   3. The patient's fear and anxiety about the return of pain will increase.
   4. The patient will be less physically active.

6. The patient has been ordered a transdermal analgesic patch. Which of the following statements demonstrates that the patient understands the use and application of the patch?
   1. "I will change this patch every 24 hours."
   2. "I should apply it in the same place each time I reapply a new patch."
   3. "A heating pad may increase how fast I absorb the medication."
   4. "I can expect to feel pain relief 10 hours after I apply the patch."

7. The patient is experiencing pain. Which of the following would be an unexpected finding by the nurse?
   1. shallow, rapid breathing
   2. increased blood pressure
   3. increased pulse rate
   4. constricted pupil

10 Nursing Care of Patients with Altered Fluid, Electrolyte, and Acid–Base Balance

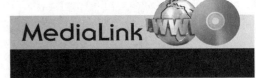

LEARNING OUTCOMES

1. Describe the functions and regulatory mechanisms that maintain water and electrolyte balance in the body.
2. Compare and contrast the causes, effects, and care of the patient with fluid volume or electrolyte imbalance.
3. Explain the pathophysiology and manifestations of imbalances of sodium, potassium, calcium, magnesium, and phosphorus.
4. Describe the causes and effects of acid–base imbalances.

CLINICAL COMPETENCIES

1. Assess and monitor fluid, electrolyte, and acid–base balance.
2. Administer fluids and medications knowledgeably and safely.
3. Determine priority nursing diagnoses, based on assessment data, to select and implement individualized nursing interventions.
4. Use assessed data, patient values, and evidence to provide patient and family teaching about diet and medications used to promote, restore, and maintain fluid, electrolyte, and acid–base balance.
5. Effectively communicate and function within the interdisciplinary team to plan and provide care to patients with altered fluid, electrolyte, and acid–base balance.
6. Adapt individual cultural values and variations and expressed needs and preferences into the plan of care to provide knowledgeable and safe care to patients with fluid and electrolyte imbalances.

MediaLink

Pearson Nursing Student Resources
Audio Glossary
NCLEX-RN® Review
- Care Plan Activity
  - Hypocalcemia
- Case Studies
  - Third Spacing
  - Hypernatremia
- MediaLink Applications
- Links to Resources

TERMS MATCHING

Place the letter of the correct definition in the space next to each term.

1. _____ Acidosis

2. _____ Alkali

3. _____ Alkalosis

4. _____ Anasarca

5. _____ Arterial blood gases (ABGs)

6. _____ Ascites

7. _____ Base excess (BE)

8. _____ Dehydration

9. _____ Dyspnea

10. _____ Edema

11. _____ Fluid volume deficit (FVD)

12. _____ Fluid volume excess

13. _____ Homeostasis

14. _____ Kussmaul's respirations

15. _____ Orthopnea

16. _____ Serum bicarbonate

17. _____ Tetany

18. _____ Third spacing

A. The loss of water from the body.

B. A decrease in interstitial, intravascular, and/or intracellular fluid in the body.

C. A calculated value that reflects the degree of acid–base imbalance by indicating the status of the body's total buffering capacity.

D. When the body's electrolyte composition, fluid volume, and pH of both intracellular and extracellular spaces remain constant within a narrow range to maintain health and life.

E. A shift of fluid from the vascular space into an area such as the abdomen or bowel where it is not available to support normal physiological processes.

F. Another term for a base. This will accept hydrogen ions in solution.

G. Excess fluid collects in the interstitial spaces as a result of conditions that cause retention of sodium and water.

H. Used by the body to buffer excess acid in extracellular fluids.

I. Tonic muscular spasms that can be a result of hypocalcemia.

J. Severe, generalized edema.

K. Deep and rapid respirations.

L. An increase in interstitial, intravascular, and/or intracellular fluid in the body.

M. The hydrogen ion concentration increases to an above-normal level (pH falls below 7.35).

N. The term used to describe excess fluid in the peritoneal cavity.

O. A diagnostic test used to measure acid–base balance.

P. Labored breathing.

Q. The hydrogen ion concentration falls below normal (ph is above 7.45).

R. The patient experiences difficulty breathing when lying down.

FOCUSED STUDY

1. Describe the differences between intracellular fluid (ICF) and extracellular fluid (ECF).

_____

_____

_____

_____

2. Describe the following ways that fluids move within the body:
  a. Osmosis

_____

_____

  b. Diffusion

_____

_____

  c. Filtration

_____

_____

  d. Active transport

_____

_____

3. Describe how each acid or base imbalance is produced.

a. Metabolic acidosis and alkalosis

_____

_____

b. Respiratory acidosis and alkalosis

_____

_____

4. List three expected outcomes for the patient who has been diagnosed with metabolic alkalosis.

1. _____

2. _____

3. _____

CASE STUDY

Mr. Sweeney has been admitted with diabetic ketoacidosis. The patient's arterial blood gas values are abnormal. Answer the following questions based on his diagnosis.

1. Which acid–base imbalance is this patient most at risk for developing?

2. What is a normal pH? What does the nurse expect Mr. Sweeney's pH to be based on his admitting diagnosis and abnormal arterial blood gas values?

3. The nurse would expect Mr. Sweeney's respirations to be of what quality and depth? What is the specific name for this type of breathing?

4. What are the early manifestations of this type of acid–base imbalance?

5. As the nurse reviews the results of this patient's laboratory tests, what are the expected changes that may be seen in potassium and magnesium levels?

6. What are vital teaching areas for Mr. Sweeney?

7. How is the heart's ability to function affected by this type of acid–base imbalance?

SHORT ANSWERS

Fill in the following table.

Condition	Laboratory Values	Short Questions Regarding Clinical Manifestations	
Hyponatremia		Has this patient's blood pressure increased or decreased?	
Hypernatremia		Has this patient gained or lost weight?	
Hypokalemia		Hypokalemia increases the patient's risk of developing toxicity related to which medication?	
Hyperkalemia		Which medication may be ordered to increase renal potassium excretion?	
Hypocalcemia		When should the hypocalcemic patient be instructed to take his or her ordered oral calcium salts?	
Hypercalcemia		Will the hyperkalemic patient develop muscle weakness or tetany?	
Hypomagnesemia		This patient is receiving intravenous magnesium sulfate. The function of which organ should be monitored during this type of therapy?	
Hypermagnesemia		Will deep tendon reflexes be hyperactive or hypoactive in a patient with this condition?	
Hypophosphatemia		Nursing interventions for this patient should be focused on which types of issues?	
Hyperphosphatemia		Is this patient more likely to suffer from complications related to hypotension or hypertension?	

NCLEX-RN® REVIEW QUESTIONS

1. Of the following, which can be immediately replaced intravascularly?
   1. plasma
   2. urine
   3. synovial fluid
   4. perspiration

2. Identify the primary process that controls body fluid movement between the intracellular fluid (ICF) and extracellular fluid (ECF) compartments.
   1. osmosis
   2. diffusion
   3. active transport
   4. filtration

3. Monitoring which of the following in the older adult is a poor indicator of fluid volume deficit?
   1. skin turgor
   2. tongue furrows
   3. blood pressure
   4. weight

4. Your patient is diagnosed with a fluid volume deficit due to a severe burn injury. Which laboratory finding would be unexpected?
   1. decrease in potassium
   2. elevated hemoglobin
   3. increase in urine specific gravity
   4. decreased hematocrit

5. Which of the following is the initial clinical manifestation associated with hypernatremia?
   1. lethargy
   2. weakness
   3. thirst
   4. irritability

6. A buffer prevents major changes in pH by releasing which of the following types of ions?
   1. hydrogen
   2. calcium
   3. sodium
   4. magnesium

11 Nursing Care of Patients Experiencing Trauma and Shock

LEARNING OUTCOMES

1. Define the word *trauma*.
2. Define the components and types of trauma.
3. Describe the result of energy transfer to the human body.
4. Discuss causes, effects, and initial management of trauma.
5. Discuss diagnostic tests used in assessing patients experiencing trauma and shock.
6. Describe collaborative interventions for patients experiencing trauma and shock, including medications, blood transfusion, and intravenous fluids.
7. Discuss organ donation and forensic implications of traumatic injury or death.
8. Discuss cellular homeostasis and basic hemodynamics.
9. Discuss the risk factors, etiologies, and pathophysiologies of hypovolemic shock, cardiogenic shock, obstructive shock, and distributive shock.
10. Use the nursing process as a framework for providing individualized care to patients experiencing trauma and shock.

MediaLink

Pearson Nursing Student Resources
Audio Glossary
NCLEX-RN® Review

- Care Plan Activity
  - Patients Experiencing Trauma and Shock
- Case Studies
  - A Patient Experiencing Trauma
  - Identifying Types of Shock
- Animations/Videos
  - Types of Shock
  - Hypovolemic Shock
  - Hemo/Pneumothorax
- MediaLink Applications
- Links to Resources

CLINICAL COMPETENCIES

1. Describe steps of the primary survey to diagnose and manage life-threatening injuries.
2. Obtain initial subjective and objective data of the trauma patient to include history taking, assessment, review of past medical history, and communication with prehospital and other healthcare providers and family members.
3. Evaluate patient response to medical and surgical interventions for patients sustaining multiple trauma and shock.
4. Provide essential ongoing written communication for patient care and continuity of the trauma patient.
5. Describe the role of the nurse in trauma prevention education and develop a plan of care to restore the functional health status of trauma patients.
6. Communicate significant data and changes in the condition of a patient who has sustained trauma.
7. Identify nursing diagnoses based on signs and symptoms recognized during the nursing assessment.
8. Develop a plan of care for the trauma patient based on scientific knowledge and patient diversity that address the nursing diagnosis.
9. Document quality of care issues associated with the trauma patient.
10. Advocate for the patient's rights as indicated by documents that address end-of-life issues.
11. Comply with guidelines related to the Uniform Anatomical Gift Act.

TERMS MATCHING

Place the letter of the correct definition in the space next to each term.

1. _____ Abrasion
2. _____ Brain death criteria
3. _____ Contusion
4. _____ Laceration
5. _____ Pneumothorax
6. _____ Puncture
7. _____ Shock
8. _____ Tension pneumothorax
9. _____ Transfusion
10. _____ Trauma

A. A systemic imbalance between oxygen supply and demand that results in a state of inadequate blood flow to body organs and tissues, causing life-threatening cellular dysfunction.

B. An open wound that is the result of a sharp cut or tear.

C. Air is present in the potential space between the parietal and visceral pleura.

D. At this point, the human brain is incapable of maintaining the human's life.

E. Can be administered to a patient to increase the amount of hemoglobin that is available to carry oxygen to the cells, improve hemoglobin and hematocrit levels during active bleeding, increase intravascular volume, and replace deficient substances such as platelets and clotting factors.

F. Injury to tissue and organs that is the result of a transfer of energy from the human's environment.

G. A partial-thickness removal of skin, usually occurring as the result of a fall or scrape.

H. An emergent situation that occurs when air has entered the potential space between the parietal and visceral pleura.

I. A superficial tissue injury that is the result of blunt trauma; small blood vessels break, and there is bleeding into the surrounding tissues.

J. An object has penetrated the integument.

FOCUSED STUDY

1. List factors that may influence the host's susceptibility to injury during a traumatic event.

_____

_____

_____

2. When caring for a patient with a possible cervical spine injury, what five criteria indicate that the patient probably did not experience a cervical spine injury?

a.

_____

b.

_____

c.

_____

d.

_____

e.

_____

3. Which blood type is known as the "universal receiver"? Which blood type is known as the "universal donor"?

Universal receiver _____

Universal donor _____

4. According to the Uniform Anatomical Gift Act, who may give consent for organ donation?

_____

_____

_____

CASE STUDY

Mr. Richard Key, a 26-year-old male was involved in a motorcycle accident along a rural road. A passing motorist found him lying next to a tree and his motorcycle. Mr. Key was unconscious. Answer the following questions based on your knowledge about the care of a patient who has suffered trauma.

1. What types of trauma did Mr. Key potentially experience?

2. What method of transportation will most likely be used to transport Mr. Key to the hospital? To what trauma level hospital should he be transported?

3. As healthcare providers assess Mr. Key, what is their highest priority?

4. What diagnostic studies may be performed on Mr. Key once he reaches the trauma center?

5. The physician notes that Mr. Key has developed a tension pneumothorax. What clinical manifestations are associated with this diagnosis?

6. After several days, healthcare providers determine that Mr. Key has experienced brain death. The family wants to donate his organs. Mr. Key is found to be an ineligible donor. What are some possible reasons for this?

7. What criteria are used to determine that Mr. Key has experienced brain death?

NCLEX-RN® REVIEW QUESTIONS

1. What type of energy is most commonly transferred to a host in trauma?
   1. mechanical
   2. gravitational
   3. thermal
   4. electrical

2. The nurse receives a report that the incoming patient has suffered a minor trauma. Of the following, which injury would be classified as a minor trauma?
   1. gunshot wound
   2. compression injury
   3. stab wound
   4. fractured clavicle

3. Identify the organ system that is not involved in multiple organ dysfunction syndrome (MODS).
   1. reproductive
   2. pulmonary
   3. hepatic
   4. cardiovascular

4. The patient has been admitted to the hospital with multiple trauma. Which of the following medication orders would the nurse question?
   1. opioids
   2. vasodilators
   3. inotropic drugs
   4. crystalloids

5. Your patient is experiencing shock. Which of the following clinical manifestations would the nurse not expect to find during the assessment?
   1. apical heart rate of 122 beats per minute
   2. increased carbon dioxide levels
   3. hyperactive bowel sounds and diarrhea
   4. cerebral hypoxia

6. What type of shock is the leading cause of death for patients in intensive care units?
   1. hypovolemic shock
   2. septic shock
   3. distributive shock
   4. neurogenic shock

7. The nurse is administering a blood transfusion. The nurse knows that the goal of blood administration is to keep the hematocrit in what range?
   1. from 20%–25%
   2. from 30%–35%
   3. from 40%–45%
   4. from 50%–55%

Nursing Care of Patients with **Infection**

LEARNING OUTCOMES

1. Explain the components and functions of the immune system and the immune response.

2. Compare antibody-mediated and cell-mediated immune responses.

3. Describe the pathophysiology of wound healing, inflammation, and infection.

4. Identify factors responsible for nosocomial infections.

5. Discuss the purposes, nursing implications, and health education for medications and treatments used to treat inflammations and infections.

6. Explain the nursing care necessary to prevent and/or monitor the status of infections.

MediaLink

Pearson Nursing Student Resources
Audio Glossary
NCLEX-RN® Review
- Care Plan Activity
  - Postoperative Infection
- Case Study
  - The Patient with a Bacterial Infection
- Animations/Videos
  - Prevention: Hand Washing
  - Infection Control
- MediaLink Applications
- Links to Resources

CLINICAL COMPETENCIES

1. Apply standard precautions, particularly hand hygiene, to prevent the spread of infection within the patient, to other patients in the facility, and to members of the interdisciplinary team and visitors.

2. Use the nursing process as a framework to provide safe, effective individualized care to patients with inflammation and infection.

3. Collaborate with the interdisciplinary care team to integrate care of patients with infection.

4. Promote therapeutic levels and complete dosage of anti-inflammatory and anti-infective medication through prompt administration and patient and family teaching.

5. Assess for hypersensitivities to anti-infectives prior to administering and during administration.

6. Participate in quality improvement processes to reduce the rates and risk of infection for a patient group or population.

TERMS MATCHING

Place the letter of the correct definition in the space next to each term.

1. _____ Acquired immunity

2. _____ Active immunity

3. _____ Adaptive immunity

4. _____ Anergy

5. _____ Antibodies

6. _____ Antibody-mediated (humoral) immune response

7. _____ Antigen

8. _____ B lymphocyte (B cell)

9. _____ Cell-mediated (cellular) immune response

10. _____ Cytokines

11. _____ Endotoxins

12. _____ Exotoxins

13. _____ Immunity

14. _____ Immunocompetent

15. _____ Immunoglobulin (Ig)

16. _____ Innate immunity

17. _____ Leukocytosis

18. _____ Leukopenia

19. _____ Macrophages

20. _____ Natural killer cells (NK cells, null cells)

21. _____ Nosocomial infections

22. _____ Passive immunity

23. _____ Pathogens

24. _____ Phagocytosis

25. _____ T lymphocytes (T cells)

26. _____ Vaccines

A. WBC count of greater than 10,000/mm^3.

B. Used to describe the way the body develops immunity to a specific antigen.

C. A substance the immune system recognizes as foreign.

D. A nonspecific defense mechanism; lymphokines are one type of subgroup.

E. An infection acquired while the patient is in a healthcare setting.

F. Found in the cell wall of gram-negative bacteria and released only when the cell is disrupted.

G. One type of lymphocyte; they are part of the innate immune system, provide immune surveillance and infection resistance, and play an important role in the destruction of early malignant cells.

H. Occurs when the body produces antibodies or develops immune lymphocytes against specific antigens.

I. The nonspecific, generic response to threats to the body's immune system.

J. This term can be used interchangeably with *acquired immunity*.

K. The molecule with the ability to bind to and inactivate a specific antigen; comprises the gamma globulin portion of the blood proteins.

L. Temporary protection against disease-producing antigens; the type of immunity that is provided by antibodies produced by other people or animals.

M. Collectively, this is how the body protects itself against major infectious organisms and abnormal or damaged cells.

N. A response employed by the body to prevent or limit the entry of invaders, thereby limiting the extent of tissue damage and reducing the workload of the adaptive immune system.

O. Highly poisonous soluble proteins that are secreted into surrounding tissue by the microorganism.

P. In this immune response, in the form of helper T cells, cytotoxic T cells, and NK cells, the lymphocytes inactivate the antigen either directly or indirectly.

Q. The body exhibits no immune response to an antigen; indicates depressed cell-mediated immunity.

R. One type of lymphocyte that matures in the thymus gland.

S. Molecules that bind with an antigen and inactivate it.

T. A decreased number of circulating leukocytes.

U. One type of lymphocyte that matures in the bone marrow.

V. Virulent organisms.

W. Refers to a fully functioning and adequate immune system.

X. The process of engulfing dead cells, damaged tissue, nonfunctioning neutrophils, and invading bacteria.

Y. Made of killed organisms or of live organisms that have been attenuated or modified to reduce their disease-producing capability.

Z. Mature monocytes that have settled into the tissues of the body.

FOCUSED STUDY

1. Describe the location and function of the following lymphoid tissues.

a. Spleen

_____

_____

b. Thymus gland

_____

_____

c. Bone marrow

_____

_____

2. Provide one example of acquired immunity and one example of passive immunity.
   a. Acquired immunity

_____

_____

   b. Passive immunity

_____

_____

3. Identify the usual indicators of inflammation. How are the clinical manifestations of an infection altered in the older adult?

_____

_____

_____

_____

4. Explain why the administration of antibiotics is ineffective in treating viral pathogens.

_____

_____

CASE STUDY

Sally Chase, a 12-year-old patient, is being seen in the clinic this morning. She is complaining of a sore throat and headache. Upon examination, her throat is found to be reddened with pustules present on each tonsil. After receiving diagnostic test results, the physician has prescribed penicillin. Sally has a streptococcal infection that is sensitive to penicillin. Answer the following questions based on your knowledge regarding the care of patients with infections.

   1. What should the nurse include when educating Sally about taking penicillin?

   2. What test was performed to identify the organism that is causing Sally's infection?

   3. What are the important nursing diagnoses the nurse should use to create Sally's care plan?

   4. While taking penicillin, what types of things should Sally or her parents report to the physician?

   5. Sally is presenting to physician's office in which stage of the infectious process?

   6. If this streptococcal throat infection is prolonged, what specific health problems may Sally be at an increased risk for developing?

SHORT ANSWERS

Fill in the table identifying the Major Chemical Mediators of Inflammation.

Factor	Source	Effect
Histamine		
Kinins (bradykinin and others)		
Prostaglandins		
Leukotrienes		

NCLEX-RN® REVIEW QUESTIONS

1. Identify a function of the vascular response.
   1. Leukocytes marginate and emigrate into the damaged tissue.
   2. It is a process by which a foreign agent or target cell is engulfed, destroyed, and digested.
   3. It involves the introduction of antigens into the body.
   4. It localizes invading bacteria and keeps them from spreading.
2. Identify the correct statement about vaccines.
   1. Vaccines are suspensions of whole or fractionated bacteria or viruses that have been treated to make them pathogenic.
   2. Vaccines are administered to reduce an immune response.
   3. All vaccines are completely effective and entirely safe.
   4. Vaccines stimulate active immunity by inducing the production of antibodies and antitoxins.
3. Which statement demonstrates that the patient understands self-care activities that can be used to promote healing?
   1. "I must restrict my intake of water."
   2. "I have to stay as active as possible."
   3. "I will eat a well-balanced diet."
   4. "I should take an anti-inflammatory medication at the first sign of swelling."
4. The nurse is explaining to the student nurse the nursing interventions that can be used to help promote tissue integrity. Which of the following nursing interventions would be questioned by the student nurse?
   1. Clean inflamed tissue gently.
   2. Keep the inflamed area moist and prevent exposure to air as much as possible.
   3. Balance rest with the tolerable degree of mobility.
   4. Provide protection and support for inflamed tissue.
5. Identify the most common type of nosocomial infection.
   1. urinary tract infection
   2. pneumonia
   3. bacteremia
   4. *Clostridium difficile*-associated diarrhea
6. The hospital is undergoing a biologic weapon drill. Which pathogen is least likely to be used as a biologic weapon?
   1. anthrax
   2. smallpox
   3. botulism
   4. hepatitis
7. The nurse is assessing the patient for an opportunistic infection. Which finding would be unexpected?
   1. complaints of constipation
   2. fuzzy growth on the tongue
   3. increased vaginal discharge
   4. blood in the urine

Nursing Care of Patients with **Altered Immunity**

LEARNING OUTCOMES

1. Review the normal anatomy and physiology of the immune system.
2. Compare and contrast the four types of hypersensitivity reactions.
3. Explain the pathophysiology of autoimmune disorders and tissue transplant rejection.
4. Discuss the characteristics of immunodeficiencies.
5. Identify laboratory and diagnostic tests used to diagnose and monitor immune response.
6. Describe interdisciplinary therapies and medications used to treat patients with altered immunity.
7. Correlate the pathophysiological alterations with the manifestations of HIV/AIDS infection.

MediaLink

Pearson Nursing Student Resources
Audio Glossary
NCLEX-RN® Review
- Care Plan Activity
  - A Patient with AIDS
- Case Study
  - HIV Prevention
- Animations/Videos
  - Hypersensitivity
  - Anaphylaxis
  - HIV/AIDS
- MediaLink Application
- Links to Resources

CLINICAL COMPETENCIES

1. Assess functional health status of patients with altered immunity and monitor, document, and report abnormal manifestations.
2. Assess for hypersensitivities and anticipate interdisciplinary interventions if manifestations develop.
3. Provide patient teaching about hypersensitivities, avoidance of sensitizing agents, and prophylactic treatment.
4. Use appropriate interventions to protect patients who are immune suppressed.
5. Recognize the burden and benefit of highly active antiretroviral drug therapy (HAART) for the patient with HIV infection.
6. Use the nursing process as a framework to provide safe and individualized care to patients with altered immune responses.
7. Revise plan of care as needed to provide safe and knowledgeable interventions to promote or restore functional health status to patients with altered immunity.

TERMS MATCHING

Place the letter of the correct definition in the space next to each item.

1. _____ Acquired immuno-deficiency syndrome (AIDS)

2. _____ Allergy

3. _____ Allograft

4. _____ Anaphylaxis

5. _____ Antigenic substances

6. _____ Autograft

7. _____ Autoimmune disorder

8. _____ Histocompatibility

9. _____ Human immunodefi-ciency virus (HIV)

10. _____ Hypersensitivity

11. _____ Immunosuppression

12. _____ Isograft

13. _____ Kaposi's sarcoma (KS)

14. _____ Seroconversion

15. _____ Xenograft

A. Stimulate the immune system to produce antibodies only against "nonself" agents.

B. A retrovirus first isolated in 1984, it is transmitted by direct contact with infected blood and body fluids.

C. The use of medication to make the immune response less effective.

D. Occurs when the immune system loses the ability to recognize itself as a non-threatening agent.

E. The final, fatal stage of HIV infection.

F. Overreaction of the immune system; allergies are an example of this type of problem.

G. A tumor of the endothelial cells lining small blood vessels; presents as vascular macules, papules, or brown or violet lesions affecting the skin and viscera; associated with HIV infection.

H. A transplant from an animal species to a human.

I. A transplant of the patient's own tissue.

J. The body produces antibodies against viral proteins.

K. A hypersensitive or altered immune response to an environmental or exogenous antigen that results in harm to the patient.

L. The donor of the tissue and the recipient of the tissue are identical twins.

M. The ability of cells and tissues to survive transplantation without immunologic interference by the recipient; determined by tissue typing.

N. Organ and tissue transplants between members of the same species but who have different genotypes and human leukocyte antigens.

O. The acute systemic type I response that occurs in highly sensitive people following injection of a specific antigen.

FOCUSED STUDY

1. Describe the differences among the following types of transplanted tissue rejection.
   a. Hyperacute tissue rejection:

   _____

   _____

   b. Acute tissue rejection:

   _____

   _____

   c. Chronic tissue rejection: _____

   _____

   _____

   d. Graft-versus-host disease: _____

   _____

   _____

2. Provide one example for each type of hypersensitivity response. Note whether each type is due to an antigen–antibody or antigen–lymphocyte interaction.
   a. Type I IgE-mediated hypersensitivity

   Example: _____

   Type of interaction: _____
   b. Type II cytotoxic hypersensitivity

   Example: _____

   Type of interaction: _____

c. Type III immune complex

Example: _____

Type of interaction: _____

d. Type IV delayed hypersensitivity

Example: _____

Type of interaction: _____

3. When caring for a patient who has developed an anaphylactic reaction and has a nursing diagnosis of ineffective airway clearance, describe interventions that should be implemented.

_____

_____

_____

_____

_____

4. List medications that can be used to treat the clinical manifestations associated with hypersensitivity reactions. Briefly list the intended action of each medication.

_____

_____

_____

CASE STUDIES

Case Study 1

Gary Jones is a 25-year-old African American homosexual who was recently diagnosed with AIDS. Answer the following questions based on your knowledge of caring for patients with HIV and AIDS.

1. What are Mr. Jones's specific risk factors for acquiring HIV?

2. How long after exposure would the nurse expect seroconversion to occur in Mr. Jones?

3. A few weeks ago Mr. Jones had nausea, diarrhea, and abdominal cramping. What might this indicate to the nurse?

4. Which opportunistic infections are associated with AIDS?

Case Study 2

Susan Callahan is a registered nurse who has developed contact dermatitis. The hospital where Susan works stocks powdered latex gloves. Susan has been newly diagnosed with a latex allergy. Answer the following questions based on your knowledge of caring for a patient with a latex allergy.

1. Besides latex gloves, what other items commonly made of latex may have contributed to Susan's allergy to latex?

2. How can employers protect their employees from developing latex allergies?

3. Susan wants to know why powdered latex gloves are "worse" than powder-free latex gloves for people with a latex sensitivity. How should the nurse caring for Susan answer this question?

4. If Susan developed a type I systemic allergic reaction as a result of a respiratory exposure, which two diagnostic tests would Susan's nurse expect to see ordered?

SHORT ANSWERS

The nurse is assessing the patient's immune system. Describe the findings that may accompany a patient with an infection or an immune disorder.

General appearance	
Mucous membranes in nose and mouth	
Skin	
Lymph nodes (cervical, axillae, and groin)	
Joints	

NCLEX-RN® REVIEW QUESTIONS

1. The patient is being screened for a hypersensitivity reaction. The nurse would question which of the following orders because it will provide the least amount of information about a hypersensitivity reaction?
   1. red blood cell (RBC) count
   2. blood type and crossmatch
   3. Coombs' Direct
   4. complement assay

2. Which of the following statements indicates that the patient understands the best way to manage her hypersensitivity to bee venom?
   1. "If I take an antihistamine daily, it will prevent a reaction if I am stung."
   2. "If I use penicillin immediately after I am stung, it will stop a reaction."
   3. "I should carry a bee sting kit at all times so that I can have quick access to epinephrine."
   4. "If I take prednisone each day, it will prevent a hypersensitivity reaction."

3. Transplanted cadaver tissue is known as what type of graft?
   1. autograft
   2. isograft
   3. allograft
   4. xenograft

4. Identify the malignancy that is least likely to be associated with HIV/AIDS?
   1. Hodgkin's lymphoma
   2. Kaposi's sarcoma
   3. primary lymphoma of the brain
   4. invasive cervical cancer

5. The patient with HIV has developed a reddened blister due to frequent episodes of diarrhea. Identify the appropriate nursing intervention.
   1. Rub the skin directly over the blister to enhance circulation.
   2. Open and drain the blister.
   3. Apply heat to the area three times daily until healed.
   4. Encourage ambulation to increase circulation and maintain muscle tone.

Nursing Care of Patients with **Cancer**

LEARNING OUTCOMES

1. Define cancer and differentiate benign from malignant neoplasm.
2. Describe the theories of carcinogenesis.
3. Explain known carcinogens and identify risk factors for cancer.
4. Compare the mechanisms and characteristics of normal cells with those of malignant cells.
5. Describe physical and psychological effects of cancer.
6. Describe and compare laboratory and diagnostic tests for cancer.
7. Discuss the role of chemotherapy in cancer treatment and classify chemotherapeutic agents.
8. Compare and contrast the role of surgery, radiation therapy, and biotherapy in the treatment of cancer.
9. Explain causes and discuss the nursing interventions for common oncologic emergencies.
10. Design an appropriate care plan for patients with cancer and their families regarding cancer diagnosis, treatment, and coping strategies.

MediaLink

Pearson Nursing Student Resources
Audio Glossary
NCLEX-RN® Review
- Care Plan Activity
  - Weight Loss and Chemotherapy
- Case Studies
  - Patient with Cancer
  - Chronic Pain
- Animations/Videos
  - Metastasis
  - Genes and Cancer
  - Radiation/Chemotherapy
  - Immunotherapy
- MediaLink Applications
- Links to Resources

CLINICAL COMPETENCIES

1. Assess functional health status of patients with cancer and monitor, document, and report abnormal manifestations.
2. Incorporate evidence-based research into the plan of nursing care for patients with cancer.
3. Prioritize nursing diagnoses based on assessment data and implement appropriate nursing interventions for patients with cancer during cancer diagnosis, treatment, and rehabilitation.
4. Safely administer medications for pain, nausea and vomiting, mucositis, or anemia.
5. Use the nursing process as a framework for planning and providing individualized care and integrating interdisciplinary care for patients with cancer to meet their healthcare needs.
6. Include cultural variation and diverse values in designing and implementing individualized plans of care for patients with cancer.
7. Design and provide individualized patient and family teaching to restore, promote, and maintain patients' functional status.
8. Revise plan of care as needed to provide effective interventions for patients with cancer and their families.

TERMS MATCHING

Place the letter of the correct definition in the space next to each term.

1. _____ Anaplasia
2. _____ Biotherapy
3. _____ Cachexia
4. _____ Cancer
5. _____ Carcinogenesis
6. _____ Carcinogens
7. _____ Cell cycle
8. _____ Chemotherapy
9. _____ Differentiation
10. _____ Dysplasia
11. _____ Hospice
12. _____ Hyperplasia
13. _____ Metaplasia
14. _____ Metastasis
15. _____ Neoplasm
16. _____ Oncogenes
17. _____ Oncologic emergencies
18. _____ Oncology
19. _____ Radiation therapy
20. _____ Tumor marker
21. _____ Xerostomia

A. A group of complex diseases characterized by uncontrolled growth of abnormal cells.

B. The use of cytotoxic medications to cure some types of cancers, to decrease tumor size, and to prevent or treat suspected metastases.

C. The regression of a cell to an immature or undifferentiated cell type.

D. Malignant cells from the primary tumor travel through the blood or lymph to invade other tissues and organs of the body and form a secondary tumor.

E. The patient's immune responses are enhanced to help treat cancer.

F. A protein molecule detectable in serum or other body fluids, it is used as a biochemical indicator of the presence of a malignancy.

G. An increase in the number or density of normal cells.

H. The wasted appearance associated with people who have cancer.

I. A change in the normal pattern of differentiation; dividing cells differentiate into cell types not normally found in that location in the body.

J. Genes that promote cell proliferation and are capable of triggering cancerous characteristics.

K. The type of care that can be provided at home for patients who have been diagnosed with terminal cancer.

L. Certain agents that cause mutations in cellular DNA and transform cells into cancer cells.

M. The study of cancer.

N. Emergency situations that arise when caring for patients diagnosed with cancer.

O. The process by which normal cells are transformed into cancer cells.

P. The loss of DNA control over differentiation occurring in response to adverse conditions; affected cells show abnormal variation in size, shape, and appearance and a disturbance in their usual arrangement.

Q. A collection of cells that grows independently of the surrounding structures and has no physiological purpose.

R. The four phases that are responsible for cellular reproduction.

S. The type of cancer treatment that consists of delivering ionizing radiations of gamma and x-rays.

T. A normal process occurring over many cell cycles that allows cells to specialize in certain tasks.

U. Excessive dryness of the mucous membranes.

FOCUSED STUDY

1. How can a person modify his or her diet to help prevent the occurrence of cancer?

_____

_____

_____

_____

2. How does stress play a role in cancer development?

_____

_____

_____

3. Describe the differences between benign and malignant neoplasms (appearance, growth, and effect on surrounding tissue).

_____

_____

_____

4. Briefly describe the following methods used to treat cancer.
   a. Surgery as a primary treatment for cancer:

   _____

   _____

   b. Chemotherapy:

   _____

   _____

   c. Radiation:

   _____

   _____

   d. Biotherapy:

   _____

   _____

   e. Photodynamic therapy:

   _____

   _____

CASE STUDY

Donna Lee is a 54-year-old female who was diagnosed with carcinoma of her right breast yesterday. She is scheduled for a mastectomy of her right breast. Her current medication includes an estrogen supplement. She has experienced menopause. Answer the following questions based on your knowledge of caring for a patient with cancer.

1. What are the American Cancer Society's guidelines for breast cancer screening?

2. Which ethnic group experiences the highest prevalence of breast cancer?

3. What role does Donna's age play in her cancer?

4. During a mastectomy, the axillary lymph nodes are removed for examination. Why is this done?

5. How will the nurse assist the patient in adjusting to her new body image after the mastectomy?

6. What specific tumor marker is associated with breast cancer? Which laboratory test results may be abnormal?

7. If the physician chose to treat Donna's breast cancer with chemotherapy, which type of chemotherapeutic drugs might the physician prescribe? What side effects are associated with this medication?

SHORT ANSWERS

Cancers Associated with Different Viruses

Indicate which kind of cancer(s) are associated with each type of virus.

Virus	Cancer
Herpes simplex Vvirus types I and II (HSV-1 and HSV-2)	a. b. c.
Human cytomegalovirus (HCMV)	a. b.
Epstein-Barr virus (EBV)	a.
Human herpesvirus 6 (HHV-6)	a.
Hepatitis B virus (HBV)	a.
Papillomavirus	a. b.
Human T-cell lymphotropic viruses (HTLVs)	a. b. c.

NCLEX-RN® REVIEW QUESTIONS

1. Which type of cancer should the nurse screen for more closely in men than in women patients?
   1. skin
   2. bladder
   3. lung
   4. thyroid

2. The patient has a diagnosis of lung cancer. Which imaging technique will provide the greatest accuracy in tumor diagnosis?
   1. ultrasonography
   2. magnetic resonance imaging
   3. computed tomography
   4. nuclear imaging

3. The patient has been newly diagnosed with cancer and is undergoing the first chemotherapy treatment. Which statement indicates that the patient understands an effect of chemotherapy?
   1. "I will not lose my hair."
   2. "My body will respond quicker to an infection."
   3. "I may lose my sense of taste."
   4. "I will become pregnant easily while undergoing chemotherapy."

4. The patient has been diagnosed with an anxiety disorder. Which finding by the nurse would be unexpected?
   1. direct eye contact
   2. hyperactivity
   3. trembling
   4. withdrawal

5. The patient has recently undergone a right radical mastectomy. Which behavior indicates that the patient has maintained a positive body image after surgery?
   1. The patient denies a change in physical body appearance.
   2. The patient is willing to look at the wound.
   3. The patient requests that no visitors be allowed in her room.
   4. The patient prefers that only nursing staff perform care to the affected area.

6. Mr. Packer has recently been diagnosed with cancer. Which oral hygiene practice should be avoided?
   1. using a soft-tipped toothbrush
   2. using an alcohol-based mouthwash
   3. soaking dentures in hydrogen peroxide
   4. using waxed dental floss

7. The patient may have developed tumor lysis syndrome. Which of the following signs would the nurse expect to find?
   1. hypouricemia
   2. hyperphosphatemia
   3. hypokalemia
   4. hyponatremia

Assessing the Integumentary System

LEARNING OUTCOMES

1. Describe the anatomy, physiology, and functions of the skin, hair, and nails.
2. Discuss factors that influence skin color.
3. Identify specific topics for a health history interview of the patient with problems involving the skin, hair, or nails.
4. Explain techniques for assessing the skin, hair, and nails.
5. Give examples of genetic disorders of the integumentary system.
6. Describe normal variations in assessment findings for the older adult.
7. Identify abnormal findings that may indicate impairment of the integumentary system.

CLINICAL COMPETENCIES

1. Conduct and document a health history for patients who have or are at risk for alterations in the skin, hair, or nails.
2. Conduct and document a physical assessment of the integumentary system.
3. Monitor the results of diagnostic tests and report abnormal findings.

MediaLink

Pearson Nursing Student Resources
Audio Glossary
NCLEX-RN® Review
- Care Plan Activity
  - Integumentary Disorders
- Case Studies
  - Patient with Integumentary Disorder
  - Patient with a Bacterial Infection
- MediaLink Applications
- Links to Resources

TERMS MATCHING

Place the letter of the correct definition in the space next to each term.

1. _____ Alopecia
2. _____ Cyanosis
3. _____ Ecchymosis
4. _____ Edema
5. _____ Erythema
6. _____ Hirsutism
7. _____ Jaundice
8. _____ Keratin
9. _____ Melanin
10. _____ Pallor
11. _____ Sebum
12. _____ Urticaria
13. _____ Vitiligo

A. Is often referred to as hives and manifests as patches of pale, itchy wheals in an erythematous area.

B. May be referred to as bruises and are raised bluish or yellowish vascular lesions.

C. A yellow-to-orange color visible in the skin and mucous membranes; it is most often the result of a hepatic disorder.

D. Patches of white spots on the skin that result from a loss of melanocytes.

E. Hair loss.

F. The yellow-to-brown pigment of the skin.

G. A fibrous, water-repellent protein that gives the epidermis its tough protective quality.

H. A bluish discoloration of the skin and mucous membranes.

I. Paleness of the skin.

J. Accumulation of fluid in the body's tissues.

K. An oily substance secreted from glands that provides lubrication to the hair and skin.

L. Excessive hair growth.

M. A reddening of the skin.

FOCUSED STUDY QUESTIONS

1. What factors are responsible for the pigmented color of an individual's skin?

_____

_____

_____

2. Identify the two primary skin layers and their functions.

_____

_____

_____

_____

3. Illnesses may result in color changes in the skin. List two conditions associated with color changes.

_____

_____

_____

CASE STUDY

Forty-two-year-old Cassandra Messersmith was admitted to a medical surgical unit with a diagnosis of bradycardia and hypotension. Her vital signs are as follows: heart rate 28, blood pressure 89/56, and respiratory rate 24. She denies pain at this time. Her past medical history is significant for a small basal cell carcinoma on the side of her nose. The lesion was surgically excised without complication one year ago.

During the morning assessment, the nurse observes a red scaly area with papules on the back of the patient's scalp at the base of the hairline. When the nurse questions the patient about the area, the patient states that it appeared about a week ago and that it bleeds occasionally when she brushes her hair. The nurse measures the area (which is 3 mm), completes the assessment, and makes certain the patient is comfortable. The nurse then documents the findings and calls the physician with the morning lab results.

1. Is the area on the back of the patient's scalp a recurrence of her basal cell carcinoma? Why or why not?

2. What risk factors increase the patient's risk of developing this type of skin disorder?

3. The lesion is located on the back of the patient's head, and she noticed it a week ago. The lesion is 3 mm in size now. Based on knowledge of this type of lesion, has the patient waited too long to seek treatment?

4. Is there a connection between the reason for the patient's admission and the lesion found on the back of her head?

SHORT ANSWERS

Label the following figures.

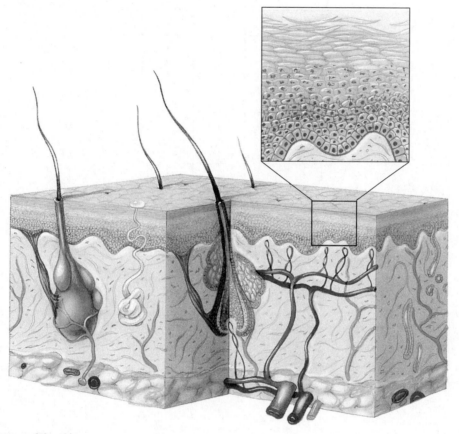

Figure 1 ■ Anatomy of the skin

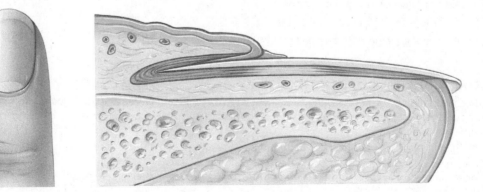

Figure 2 ■ Anatomy of a nail

CROSSWORD PUZZLE

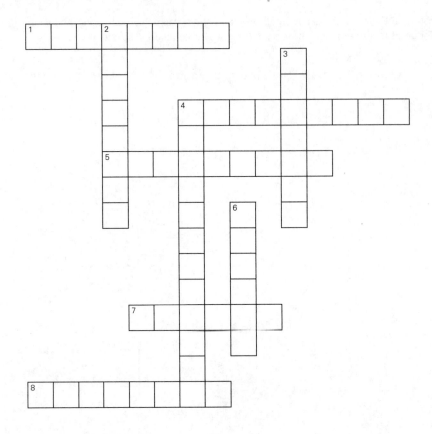

Across

1   Remnant of the sexual scent gland

4   Glands responsible for producing oil

5   The outermost surface of the skin

7   The second layer of skin

8   The total absence of melanin

Down

2   A yellow-to-orange pigment found in the body

3   Glands that regulate heat through perspiration

4   Glands responsible for the production of sweat

6   Retained urochrome pigments in the blood

NCLEX-RN® REVIEW QUESTIONS

1. During a blood pressure screening, the nurse notices that the patient is scratching her abdomen. When the nurse asks about the scratching, the patient states that she has a red itchy rash under her breast. What is the most appropriate response from the nurse?

    1. "That happens in hot weather. It is probably just dry skin from bathing too much."

    2. "Scratching will only make it worse."

    3. "I think it is your new detergent. You should go back to what you were using before."

    4. "How long ago did the itching start?"

2. While assessing a patient, the nurse notices that the patient's ankles and feet are swollen to the point that her shoes are too tight. However, the skin slowly returns to normal when depressed by the nurse's thumb. This finding is most accurately documented as what?
   1. 1+
   2. 2+
   3. 3+
   4. 4+

3. A patient has a significantly receding hairline and a dark suntan. The nurse notices that he has a bandage on top of his head. When asked about it, he states that it is an odd mole that bleeds sometimes. Which of the following factors would increase the patient's risk of skin cancer?
   1. Smoked one pack of cigarettes a day for 15 years
   2. Worked in construction for ten years
   3. Consumed a high-fat diet
   4. Developed hypothyroidism

4. A nurse has been asked to speak to a community group about the risks factors associated with skin cancers. Which statement by the nurse would be most accurate?
   1. "A tendency to sunburn, even with sunscreen, increases your risk."
   2. "Family history is the strongest indicator of your risk."
   3. "Women have twice the risk of skin cancer as do men."
   4. "Your risk of skin cancer is less if you have a mild tan to the skin from a tanning bed."

5. When assessing a patient with dark skin color for jaundice, what is the best place to look?
   1. nail beds
   2. eyes
   3. forearm
   4. mucous membranes

6. The nurse notices that a patient is scratching her head. The nurse assesses the area and finds pustules and some hair loss. The nurse knows that these symptoms are associated with what?
   1. ringworm
   2. head lice
   3. seborrhea
   4. a boil

7. When assessing a patient's nails, the nurse notices that they are thick and yellow in color. The nurse knows that this is associated with what? **Select all that apply.**
   1. fungal infection
   2. trauma to the nail
   3. pseudomonas infection
   4. psoriasis
   5. nutritional deficiency

8. When assessing the skin of a patient, the nurse notices that it is coarse. The nurse knows that coarse, dry skin is associated with what?
   1. hypothyroidism
   2. acne vulgaris
   3. fever
   4. seborrhea

16 Nursing Care of Patients with Integumentary Disorders

LEARNING OUTCOMES

1. Describe the manifestations, self-care, and nursing care of common skin problems and lesions.

2. Compare and contrast the etiology, pathophysiology, interdisciplinary care, and nursing care of patients with infections and infestations, inflammatory disorders, and malignancies of the skin.

3. Explain the risk factors for, pathophysiology of, and nursing interventions to prevent and care for pressure ulcers.

4. Discuss surgical options for excision of neoplasms, reconstruction of facial or body structures, and cosmetic procedures.

5. Explain the pathophysiology of selected disorders of the hair and nails.

6. Discuss the effects and nursing implications of medications and treatments used to treat disorders of the integument.

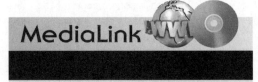

MediaLink

Pearson Nursing Student Resources
Audio Glossary
NCLEX-RN® Review
- Care Plan Activity
  - Pressure Ulcers
- Case Study
  - The Patient with Psoriasis
- Animation/Video
  - Malignant Melanoma
- MediaLink Applications
- Links to Resources

CLINICAL COMPETENCIES

1. Assess functional health status of patients with integumentary disorders and monitor, document, and report abnormal manifestations.

2. Use research to plan and implement evidence-based nursing care for patients with pressure ulcers.

3. Use assessed data, patient values, evidence, and clinical expertise to determine priority nursing diagnoses and select and implement individualized nursing interventions for patients with integumentary disorders.

4. Administer topical, oral, and injectable medications used to treat integumentary disorders knowledgeably and safely.

5. Effectively communicate with and function within the interdisciplinary team to plan and provide care for patients with integumentary disorders.

6. Provide teaching appropriate for prevention and self-care of manifestations and disorders of the integumentary system.

7. Adapt individual and cultural variations, as well as expressed needs and preferences, into the plan of care for patients with integumentary disorders.

8. Revise the plan of care as needed to provide effective interventions to promote, maintain, or restore functional health status to patients with disorders of the integument.

TERMS MATCHING

Place the letter of the correct definition in the space next to each term.

1. _____ Acne
2. _____ Actinic keratosis
3. _____ Angiomas
4. _____ Basal cell cancer
5. _____ Carbuncle
6. _____ Cellulitis
7. _____ Comedones
8. _____ Cysts
9. _____ Dermatitis
10. _____ Dermatophytoses
11. _____ Folliculitis
12. _____ Frostbite
13. _____ Furuncle
14. _____ Herpes simplex
15. _____ Herpes zoster
16. _____ Keloid
17. _____ Keratosis
18. _____ Lichen planus
19. _____ Malignant melanoma
20. _____ Nevus
21. _____ Pemphigus vulgaris
22. _____ Pressure ulcers
23. _____ Pruritis
24. _____ Psoriasis
25. _____ Scabies
26. _____ Skin graft
27. _____ Squamous cell cancer
28. _____ Toxic epidermal necrosis
29. _____ Warts
30. _____ Xerosis

A. A bacterial infection of the hair follicle; most commonly caused by *Staphylococcus aureus*.

B. A group of infected hair follicles.

C. A localized infeciton of dermis and subcutaneous tissue.

D. A subjective itching sensation producing an urge to scratch.

E. Any skin condition in which there is a benign overgrowth and thickening of the cornified epithelium.

F. A disorder of the pilosebaceous (hair and sebaceous gland) structure, which opens to the skin surface through a pore.

G. An injury of the skin as a result of freezing.

H. Dry skin.

I. A chronic disorder of the skin and oral mucous membranes caused by autoantibiodies, resulting in blister formation.

J. Superficial skin infections such as ringworm.

K. A skin lesion known as a mole that arises from a melanocyte.

L. Benign closed sacs in or under the skin surface that are lined with epithelium and contain fluid or a semisolid material.

M. A chronic immune skin disorder characterized by raised, reddened, round circumscribed plaques covered by silvery white scales.

N. A parasitic infestation caused by a mite (*Sarcoptes scabiei*).

O. Also known as shingles, a viral infection of a dermatome section of the skin caused by varicella zoster.

P. An epidermal skin lesion directly related to chronic sun exposure and photodamage.

Q. A rare life-threatening disease in which the epidermis peels off the dermis in sheets, leaving large areas of denuded skin.

R. Lesions of the skin caused by the human papillomavirus (HPV).

S. A malignancy of the skin characterized by erythema, ulcerations, and well-defined borders.

T. An inflammatory disorder of the mucous membranes and skin having no known cause but associated with exposure to drugs or to film processing chemicals.

U. Benign vascular tumors.

V. Noninflammatory acne lesions commonly called pimples, whiteheads, and blackheads.

W. A surgical method of detaching skin from a donor site and placing it in a recipient site, where it develops a new blood supply from the base of the wound.

X. A malignant tumor of the squamous epithelium of the skin or mucous membranes occurring most often on areas of skin exposed to ultraviolet rays and weather.

Y. An acute or chronic inflammation of the skin characterized by erythema and pain or pruritus.

Z. An inflammation of the hair follicle that often begins as folliculitis, but the infection spreads down the hair shaft, through the wall of the follicle, and into the dermis. It may also be referred to as a boil.

AA. A viral infection of the skin and mucous membrane (also called a fever blister or cold sore).

BB. A growth that forms as a result of deposits of excessive amounts of collagen during scar formation.

CC. A serious skin cancer that arises from melanocytes.

DD. Ischemic lesions of the skin and underlying tissues caused by unrelieved pressure that impairs the flow of blood and lymph, resulting in tissue necrosis and eventual ulceration.

FOCUSED STUDY

1. The nurse is instructing a patient about the rationale for prescribed therapeutic baths. What purpose do they serve for patients experiencing integumentary disorders?

_____

_____

_____

2. The nurse is preparing a therapeutic bath for a patient. When preparing the bath, what safety precautions should the nurse institute?

_____

_____

_____

_____

3. The nurse is evaluating a patient and documents the fact that the patient has a stage II pressure ulcer. What assessment findings will confirm this stage of pressure ulcer?

_____

_____

_____

4. The physician has prescribed Retin-A® to manage a patient's acne outbreaks. When providing education to the patient concerning this medication, what information should the nurse include?

_____

_____

_____

_____

CASE STUDY

Chrissy Green is a 30-year-old attorney with blonde hair and green eyes. She is very tan and reports a lot of sun exposure since childhood. She has been seen in the physician's office for a large, dark pigmented area on her right shoulder. The lesion is irregular in shape and has grown in size over the past year. Answer the following questions based on knowledge of malignant melanoma.

1. What factors place Chrissy at risk for developing malignant melanoma?

2. What is Chrissy's prognosis? What factors are used to determine prognosis?

3. What treatments are available to Chrissy?

4. How often must Chrissy be seen for a checkup after removal of the lesion?

SHORT ANSWERS

Review the following types of treatments used to manage integumentary disorders. Complete the table by listing indications and names of products used.

Type	Use	Examples
Creams		
Ointments		
Lotions		
Anesthetics		
Antibiotics		
Corticosteroids		

NCLEX-RN® REVIEW QUESTIONS

1. Upon assessment, the nurse finds a skin lesion that looks like a flat or raised macule or papule with a rounded, well-defined border. The nurse suspects what type of diagnosis?
   1. cyst
   2. nevi
   3. keloid
   4. skin tag

2. The nurse is providing instructions for a patient who has psoriasis. When the nurse is discussing the patient's condition, which of the following should be included? **Select all that apply**.
   1. Avoid exposure to the sun.
   2. Avoid exposure to contagious illnesses.
   3. Avoid trauma to the skin.
   4. Indomethacin and beta-adrenergic blocking agents are known to precipitate exacerbations of psoriasis.
   5. Avoid warm baths and showers.

3. Which of the following is an infection of the skin most often caused by group A streptococci?
   1. cellulitis
   2. carbuncle
   3. furuncle
   4. erysipelas

4. Which behavior demonstrates the patient's understanding of the nurse's teaching about a vaginal *Candida albicans* infection?
   1. The patient wears tight clothing such as jeans and pantyhose.
   2. The patient wears silk or silk-lined underwear.
   3. The patient reports bathing more frequently.
   4. The patient reports not discussing the infection with her sexual partner.

5. Which form of dermatitis is a chronic inflammatory disorder of the skin that involves the scalp, eyebrows, eyelids, ear canals, nasolabial folds, axillae, and trunk?
   1. contact dermatitis
   2. atopic dermatitis
   3. seborrheic dermatitis
   4. exfoliative dermatitis

6. At what temperature does skin freeze?
   1. 0°F–10°F
   2. 14°F–24.8°F
   3. 32°F–50°F
   4. 55°F–72°F

7. The patient has a port wine stain. What treatment will be used to reduce the lesion?
   1. chemical destruction
   2. sclerotherapy
   3. curettage
   4. laser surgery

8. Identify the correct statement about skin grafts.
   1. A split-thickness graft contains both epidermis and dermis.
   2. A common donor site for a skin graft is the posterior thigh.
   3. Skin grafting is an effective way to cover wounds that are infected.
   4. A full-thickness graft is best able to withstand trauma.

17 Nursing Care of Patients with Burns

LEARNING OUTCOMES

1. Discuss the types and causative agents of burns.
2. Explain burn classification by depth and extent of injury.
3. Compare and contrast the pathophysiology and interdisciplinary care of a minor burn and a major burn.
4. Discuss the systemic pathophysiologic effects of a major burn and the stages of burn wound healing.
5. Explain the interdisciplinary care and nursing implications necessary during the emergent/resuscitative stage, the acute stage, and the rehabilitative stage of a major burn.

CLINICAL COMPETENCIES

1. Assess functional health status of patients with burns, and monitor, document, and report abnormal manifestations.
2. Use evidence-based research to plan and implement nursing care for patients with burns.
3. Determine priority nursing diagnoses, based on assessed data, to select and implement individualized nursing interventions for patient with burns.
4. Administer medications knowledgeably and safely to patients with burns.
5. Integrate interdisciplinary care into care of patients with burns.
6. Provide teaching appropriate for prevention of burns.
7. Revise plan of care as needed to provide effective interventions to promote, maintain, or restore functional health status to patients with burns.

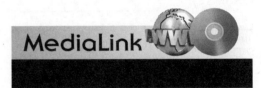

MediaLink

Pearson Nursing Student Resources
Audio Glossary
NCLEX-RN® Review
- Care Plan Activities
  - The Patient with Thermal Burn
  - The Patient Undergoing Autografting
  - The Patient with an Inhalation Burn Injury
- Case Studies
  - The Patient with Electrical Burn
  - The Patient with Burns
  - Contracture Prevention in the Burn Victim
- MediaLink Applications
- Links to Resources

TERMS MATCHING

Place the letter of the correct definition in the space next to each term.

1. ____ Allograft
2. ____ Autografting
3. ____ Burn
4. ____ Burn shock
5. ____ Compartment syndrome
6. ____ Contracture
7. ____ Curling's ulcers
8. ____ Debridement
9. ____ Eschar
10. ____ Escharotomy
11. ____ Fascial excision
12. ____ Fasciectomy
13. ____ Fluid resuscitation
14. ____ Full-thickness burn
15. ____ Heterograft
16. ____ Homograft
17. ____ Hypertrophic scar
18. ____ Keloid
19. ____ Partial-thickness burn
20. ____ Superficial burn
21. ____ Surgical debridement
22. ____ Xenograft

A. A hard crust that forms during the acute stage of an injury. This crust covers the wound and harbors necrotic tissue.

B. Human skin that has been harvested from cadavers.

C. The administration of intravenous fluids to restore the circulating blood volume during the acute period of increasing capillary permeability.

D. Involves all layers of the skin, including the epidermis, dermis, and epidermal appendages. The injury may extend into the subcutaneous fat, connective tissue, muscle, and bone.

E. Acute ulcerations of the stomach or duodenum that form following a burn injury.

F. An overgrowth of dermal tissue that remains within the boundaries of a wound.

G. A scar that extends beyond the boundaries of the original wound.

H. Employing healthy skin from a patient or donor to affect permanent skin coverage.

I. Also known as an allograft.

J. Skin used to cover a wound that has been obtained from an animal such as a pig.

K. An injury resulting from exposure to heat, chemicals, radiation, or electric current. A transfer of energy from a source of heat to the human body initiates a sequence of physiological events that in the most severe cases leads to irreversible tissue destruction.

L. A burn injury involving only the epidermal layer of the skin. This type of burn most often results from damage from sunburn, ultraviolet light, a minor flash injury (from a sudden ignition or explosion), or a mild radiation burn associated with cancer treatment.

M. A massive fluid shift from the intracellular and intravascular compartments into the interstitium (third spacing).

N. The process of excising a wound to the level of fascia or sequentially removing thin slices of a burn wound to the level of viable tissue.

O. A procedure in which a wound is excised to the level of the fascia.

P. Another term used to refer to a fascial excision.

Q. The tissue pressure in a muscle compartment exceeds microvascular pressure, resulting in the interruption of cellular perfusion.

R. A procedure used to prevent circumferential constriction of the torso or an extremity by means of a sterile surgical incision made longitudinally along the trunk or extremity, respectively, to release taut skin and allow for expansion caused by edema formation.

S. The surgical, mechanical, or enzymatic removal of all loose tissue, wound debris, and eschar from a wound.

T. Skin used for grafting that has been obtained from an animal. It is also referred to as a heterograft.

U. A positional deformity that results from prolonged placement in a position of flexion.

V. A burn injury that may be classified as superficial or deep. Both involve the entire dermis and the papillae of the dermis. The deep classified burn injuries extend further into the dermis.

FOCUSED STUDY

1. List and describe the phases and activities that take place in the healing of a burn injury.

_____
_____
_____
_____
_____
_____

2. A patient reports to the ambulatory care clinic with a serious sunburn. When the nurse is planning the patient's care, which of the following will be included?

_____
_____
_____
_____
_____

3. List and describe the four types of burn injuries.

_____
_____
_____
_____

4. What factors are used to determine the classification of a burn injury?

_____
_____
_____
_____

CASE STUDY

Seventy-four-year-old Viola Baker arrives in the emergency department following a fire in her apartment. She has first- and second-degree burns over 50% of her body, including her face, chest, and arms. Viola was cooking when grease caught fire, catching her clothing on fire as well. There are soot marks around her nostrils, and her eyebrows are singed. She is using a 100% nonrebreather mask and has a pulse oximetry reading of 89%. She is being given normal saline solution by IV in addition to the 5 mg morphine sulfate for pain she was given in the ambulance. Her vital signs are as follows: heart rate 116, blood pressure 104/76, and respiratory rate 35. She opens her eyes to verbal stimuli. Her conversation is confused, but she answers some simple questions and withdraws from pain. The patient's past medical history is significant for osteoporosis, bilateral cataract surgery, and type 2 diabetes mellitus that is controlled with diet and exercise. The patient's family was notified by the apartment manager, and they are on their way to the emergency department.

1. What changes need to be made immediately in the patient's care?

2. To what setting will this patient likely be transferred when she is stable?

3. Why would the patient be intubated and placed on a ventilator?

4. Based on the patient's injuries, from what type of immediate surgical intervention might she benefit?

CARE PLAN CRITICAL-THINKING ACTIVITY

The patient arrives in the emergency department with burns suffered while burning leaves. The initial injury reveals that the patient has burns to the arms, hands, and facial area. The nurse is planning care for the patient and providing education to the patient and family.

1. When caring for the patient, what is the greatest concern when he first arrives at the emergency room?

2. What unique burn injuries are the patient at risk for developing as a result of the type of burn injury and related situation? What manifestations are noted with this type of burn injury?

3. Develop a nursing diagnosis consistent with the greatest concern for this patient.

4. In assessing respiratory-related injuries, when does the nurse recognize the greatest time for complications as a result of inflammation to the pulmonary system?

NCLEX-RN® REVIEW QUESTIONS

1. The patient, who weighs 68 kg, has sustained second-degree burns over 40% of his body. Which fluid resuscitation is correct according to the Parkland calculation?
   1. 10.88 liters of lactated Ringer's solution in 24 hours
   2. 5.44 liters of lactated Ringer's (LR) solution in 8 hours and 5.44 liters of LR over the next 16 hours
   3. 5.44 liters of lactated Ringer's solution in 8 hours and 5.44 liters of D5W over the next 16 hours
   4. 10.88 liters of D5W in 24 hours
2. Which nursing intervention holds the highest priority for a patient with burns to her face and upper respiratory tract?
   1. Elevate the head of the bed to at least 30 degrees.
   2. Administer 6 liters of oxygen via nasal cannula.
   3. Medicate the patient prior to repositioning her in bed.
   4. Prevent moving the skin around the burn site.
3. When caring for a patient with chemical burns, which task could the registered nurse assign to unlicensed nursing personnel?
   1. documenting the dressing change and wound bed
   2. overseeing first ambulation of hospital stay
   3. encouraging the patient to use patient-controlled analgesia for pain and the incentive spirometer hourly
   4. checking urinary output for adequacy of fluid resuscitation
4. When teaching a community group about radiation burns, which statement best reflects the goals of treatment?
   1. Radiation burns are usually mild and involve only the surface of the skin.
   2. Severe radiation burns are usually caused by industrial accidents.
   3. Radiation burns are much less common than thermal burns.
   4. Promoting wound and body healing are the most important goals of treatment.
5. Which is an appropriate order when caring for a patient with a burn?
   1. Provide 4000 kcal per 24 hours.
   2. Administer 4 liters of lactated Ringer's solution for a 105 lb patient with a 10% total body surface area.
   3. Administer 6 liters of oxygen via nasal cannula without humidification with a pulse oximetry reading of 99%.
   4. Apply support garments beginning on the fourth day postburn.
6. Which is the highest priority for the nurse when caring for a patient with an electrical burn?
   1. Disconnect the patient from the electrical source.
   2. Ensure that the patient has a cervical collar and is placed on a back board prior to care.
   3. Monitor for cardiac dysrhythmia.
   4. Provide changes in fluid resuscitation as compared to patients with other types of burns.
7. Which patient will require skin grafting for wound closure?
   1. the patient with a 31.5% heavy superficial chemical burn
   2. the patient with a 12 mm full-thickness thermal burn
   3. the patient with a moderate partial-thickness burn
   4. the patient with an 18% partial-thickness burn to the lower limbs

8. How is a major burn defined?
   1. 20% total body surface area in adults less than 40 years of age
   2. 5% total body surface area full-thickness burn in adults greater than 40 years of age
   3. a household electrical burn with a cervical spine injury
   4. a burn that caused the oxygen saturation rate to drop below 95%

9. Document on the diagram below a burn that involves 22.5% of the patient's body surface area.

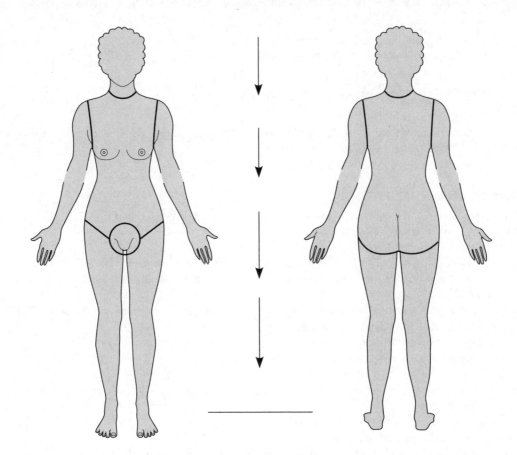

10. Patients with major burns are at risk for many system issues. Which is the highest priority for the nurse caring for a patient with a major burn?
   1. compartment syndrome
   2. hypovolemia
   3. thermal burn and dysrrhythmia
   4. acute renal failure

Assessing the Endocrine System

LEARNING OUTCOMES

1. Describe the anatomy and physiology of the endocrine glands.
2. Summarize the functions of the hormones secreted by the endocrine glands.
3. Describe specific topics to consider during a health history interview of the patient with health problems involving endocrine function.
4. Explain techniques for assessing the thyroid gland and the effects of altered function of thyroid hormones.
5. Describe normal variations in endocrine assessment findings for the older adult.
6. Give examples of genetic disorders of the endocrine glands.
7. Identify abnormal findings that may indicate malfunction of the glands of the endocrine system.

MediaLink

Pearson Nursing Student Resources
Audio Glossary
NCLEX-RN® Review
- Care Plan Activity
  - The Older Adult with Type 2 Diabetes
- Case Study
  - Patients with Endocrine Disorders
- Animation/Video
  - Thyroid Assessment
- MediaLink Application
- Links to Resources

CLINICAL COMPETENCIES

1. Conduct and document a health history for patients who have or are at risk for alterations in the structure or function of the endocrine glands.
2. Monitor the results of diagnostic tests and report abnormal findings.
3. Conduct and document a physical assessment of the structure of the thyroid gland and the effects of altered endocrine function on other body structures and functions.

TERMS MATCHING

Place the letter of the correct definition in the space next to each term.

1. ____ Acromegaly
2. ____ Carpal spasm
3. ____ Chvostek's sign
4. ____ Dwarfism
5. ____ Exophthalmos
6. ____ Goiter
7. ____ Tetany
8. ____ Trousseau's sign

A. A condition characterized by short stature that is associated with growth hormone deficiency.

B. Is elicited by tapping a finger in front of the patient's ear at the angle of the jaw; is indicative of hypocalcemia.

C. Protruding eyes associated with hyperthyroidism.

D. An enlarged thyroid gland.

E. The patient's hand and fingers contract due to hypocalcemia.

F. A response that can be elicited by inflating a blood pressure cuff above the antecubital space to a point greater than systolic blood pressure for 2–5 minutes; in indicative of hypocalcemia.

G. The continued growth of bone from growth hormone hypersecretion.

H. Tonic muscle spasms associated with hypocalcemia.

FOCUSED STUDY

1. Identify which hormones may be altered in the patient without an adequately functioning anterior pituitary.

_____

_____

_____

2. List several questions the nurse, during the health assessment interview, should ask the patient with a suspected endocrine disorder.

_____

_____

_____

3. The patient's adrenal medulla is hypersecreting catecholamines. Identify the findings the nurse would expect to find as he or she assesses the patient.

_____

_____

_____

4. Describe how the nurse should prepare the patient for the water deprivation test.

_____

_____

_____

CASE STUDIES

Case Study 1

Karen Aummert is a 42-year-old female who has come to the physician's office complaining of a decrease in her energy level and feeling sluggish. Her apical heart rate is 56 beats per minute, blood pressure is 98/62, and respiratory rate is 12 per minute. She is recently divorced and is a single parent of a little girl. Answer the following questions based on your knowledge of caring for a patient with an endocrine disorder.

1. Which diagnostic tests might be used to correctly diagnose Ms. Aummert's health problem?

2. Ms. Aummert is diagnosed with hypothyroidism. What can the nurse expect to find during the physical assessment?

3. What are some questions the nurse can ask Ms. Aummert to determine whether she's receiving adequate amounts of sleep and rest?

4. Ms. Aummert states that her 76-year-old mother was recently diagnosed with hypothyroidism. What are some age-related changes that occur in the endocrine system?

Case Study 2

Josh Knight is a 42-year-old male who has been admitted to the hospital with an elevated serum glucose level. The patient collapsed at work and was brought to the hospital via ambulance. Answer the following questions based on your knowledge of caring for a patient with an endocrine disorder.

1. What diagnostic tests may be performed to help the healthcare providers better understand the nature of Mr. Knight's health problem?

2. The nurse questions Mr. Knight regarding his family history of endocrine disorders. Mr. Knight states that his father was diagnosed with diabetes mellitus at the age of 11. Mr. Knight wants to know if other endocrine disorders can be inherited. What is the nurse's best response?

3. Mr. Knight is diagnosed with diabetes mellitus. What are some physical findings associated with this endocrine condition?

SHORT ANSWERS
Glands of the Endocrine System

Label the following figure.

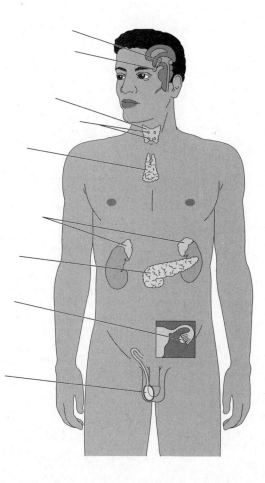

NCLEX-RN® REVIEW QUESTIONS

1. When assessing a patient who is concerned about weight gain, hair loss, and generalized weakness, which of the following is most important?
   1. a focused abdominal assessment
   2. the patient's neck and ability to swallow
   3. the patient's balance and gait
   4. the patient's height and weight
2. The nurse understands that carbohydrate metabolism is most associated with which of the following glands?
   1. pancreas
   2. pituitary
   3. thyroid
   4. parathyroid
3. Epinephrine is produced by which of the following glands?
   1. pancreas
   2. thyroid
   3. adrenal medulla
   4. adrenal cortex
4. A problem with which of the following glands may alter the patient's corticosteroid levels?
   1. thyroid
   2. parathyroid
   3. adrenal cortex
   4. adrenal medulla
5. Which hormone is most responsible for the development of secondary female sexual characteristics?
   1. oxytocin
   2. vasopressin
   3. follicle-stimulating hormone (FSH)
   4. luteinizing hormone (LH)

Nursing Care of Patients with **Endocrine Disorders**

LEARNING OUTCOMES

1. Apply knowledge of normal anatomy, physiology, and assessments of the thyroid, parathyroid, adrenal, and pituitary glands when providing nursing care for patients with endocrine disorders.

2. Compare and contrast the manifestations of disorders that result from hyperfunction and hypofunction of the thyroid, parathyroid, adrenal, and pituitary glands.

3. Explain the nursing implications for medications prescribed to treat disorders of the thyroid and adrenal glands.

4. Provide appropriate nursing care for the patient before and after a subtotal thyroidectomy and an adrenalectomy.

5. Use the nursing process as a framework for providing individualized care to patients with disorders of the thyroid, parathyroid, adrenal, and pituitary glands.

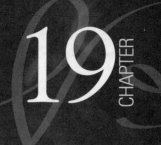

MediaLink

Pearson Nursing Student Resources
Audio Glossary
NCLEX-RN® Review

- Care Plan Activity
  - The Patient with Cushing's Syndrome
- Case Study
  - The Patient with Thyroid Disorder
- Tool
  - Manifestations of Hyperparathyroidism
- MediaLink Application
- Links to Resources

CLINICAL COMPETENCIES

1. Assess functional health status of patients with endocrine disorders and monitor, document, and report abnormal manifestations.

2. Use assessed data, patient values, clinical expertise, and evidence to determine priority nursing diagnoses and select and implement nursing interventions.

3. Effectively communicate with and function within the interdisciplinary team to plan and provide patient care.

4. Administer medications knowledgeably and safely.

5. Plan and provide patient and family teaching to promote, restore, and maintain functional health status.

6. Monitor for respiratory problems and tetany in patients having a thyroidectomy.

7. Adapt individual and cultural values and variations as well as expressed needs and preferences into the plan of care.

8. Evaluate responses to care and use data to revise plan as needed.

TERMS MATCHING

Place the letter of the correct definition in the space next to each term.

1. _____ Acromegaly
2. _____ Addisonian crisis
3. _____ Addison's disease
4. _____ Cushing's syndrome
5. _____ Diabetes insipidus
6. _____ Euthyroid
7. _____ Exophthalmos
8. _____ Gigantism
9. _____ Goiter
10. _____ Graves' disease
11. _____ Hashimoto's disease
12. _____ Hyperparathyroidism
13. _____ Hyperthyroidism
14. _____ Hypoparathyroidism
15. _____ Hypothyroidism
16. _____ Myxedema
17. _____ Myxedema coma
18. _____ Pheochromocytoma
19. _____ Pretibial myxedema
20. _____ Proptosis
21. _____ Syndrome of inappropriate ADH secretion (SIADH)
22. _____ Tetany
23. _____ Thyroid storm or crisis
24. _____ Thyroidectomy
25. _____ Thyroiditis
26. _____ Thyrotoxicosis
27. _____ Toxic multinodular goiter

A. Forward protrusion of the eyeballs that results from an accumulation of inflammation by-products in the retroorbital tissues.

B. A condition that results from abnormally low PTH levels.

C. An enlarged thyroid gland.

D. Inflammation of the thyroid gland.

E. Hyperthyroidism that results from autoimmune stimulation.

F. A condition also known as hyperthyroidism.

G. A condition that results from an increase in the secretion of parathyroid hormone (PTH), which regulates normal serum levels of calcium.

H. A severe state of hypothyroidism characterized by edema around the eyes, hands, and feet.

I. A disorder resulting from destruction or dysfunction of the adrenal cortex that results in chronic deficiency of cortisol, aldosterone, and adrenal androgens.

J. Normal thyroid function.

K. Forward displacement of the eye associated with Graves' disease.

L. The most common cause of goiter and primary hypothyroidism in adults and children; an autoimmune disorder where antibodies develop that destroy thyroid tissue.

M. Tumors of chromaffin tissues in the adrenal medulla, usually benign, that produce catecholamines.

N. A chronic disorder in which hyperfunction of the adrenal cortex produces excessive amounts of circulating cortisol or ACTH.

O. An extreme state of hyperthyroidism.

P. Also called thyrotoxicosis; a disorder caused by excessive delivery of TH to the tissues.

Q. A term that reflects the characteristic accumulation of nonpitting edema in the connective tissues throughout the body in a patient with hypothyroidism.

R. Literally means "enlarged extremities"; occurs in adulthood; most commonly associated with increased levels of growth hormone due to pituitary tumors.

S. A thyroid tumor characterized by small, discrete, independently functioning nodules in the thyroid gland tissue that secrete excessive amounts of TH.

T. A disorder that results when the thyroid gland produces an insufficient amount of TH.

U. A condition that is the result of ADH insufficiency.

V. A continuous spasm of muscles; a sign of hypocalcemia.

W. Surgical removal of all or part of the thyroid gland.

X. A condition characterized by abnormally high levels of ADH.

Y. A condition that occurs when GH hypersecretion begins before puberty and the closure of the epiphyseal plates.

Z. A rare, characteristic skin pathophysiology of Graves' disease; plaques and nodules develop bilaterally over the shins and dorsal surface of the feet.

AA. A life-threatening response to acute adrenal insufficiency.

FOCUSED STUDY

1. Discuss manifestations and treatment of hyperthyroidism.

a. Manifestations

_____

_____

b. Treatment

_____

_____

2. Discuss the manifestations of hypothyroidism.

_____

_____

_____

_____

3. Discuss the treatment for Cushing's syndrome.

_____

_____

_____

_____

4. Compare and contrast gigantism and acromegaly.

_____

_____

_____

_____

5. Discuss the differences between the clinical manifestations associated with diabetes insipidus and syndrome of inappropriate antidiuretic hormone secretion (SIADH).

_____

_____

_____

_____

CASE STUDY

Judy Moss is a 43-year-old white female who was recently diagnosed with Addison's disease. Answer the following questions based on your knowledge of caring for patients with endocrine disorders.

1. How should the nurse explain Addison's disease to Ms. Moss?

2. What manifestations should the nurse look for during the assessment of Ms. Moss?

3. What skin changes should the nurse expect Ms. Moss to experience?

4. What diagnostic testing procedures may have been used to diagnose Ms. Moss's condition?

5. What medications can be used to treat Ms. Moss?

6. What should the nurse include when educating Ms. Moss about self-care techniques?

SHORT ANSWERS

Fill in the missing pieces regarding the pathophysiology of Cushing's syndrome.

Manifestations	Pathophysiology
Fat deposits in the abdominal region, fat pads under the clavicles, a "buffalo hump" over the upper back, and a round "moon" face	
Muscle weakness and wasting, especially in the extremities	
Thinning of skin, abdominal striae, easy bruising, poor wound healing, and frequent skin infections	
Osteoporosis, compression fractures of the vertebrae, and rib fractures	
Hypokalemia	
Hypertension and hypernatremia	
Hyperglycemia, polyuria, and polydipsia	
Increased risk of gastric ulcers	
Hirsutism, acne, and menstrual irregularities	
Emotional instability	

NCLEX-RN® REVIEW QUESTIONS

1. The patient has been diagnosed with hyperthyroidism. As the nurse is reviewing the patient's chart, which of the following would be an unexpected finding?
   1. increased appetite
   2. insomnia
   3. increased sweating
   4. constipation

2. The patient has been diagnosed with thyroid storm. Identify the inappropriate nursing intervention to use with this patient.
   1. Replace fluids.
   2. Reduce body temperature by administering aspirin.
   3. Apply oxygen.
   4. Replace electrolytes.

3. The patient has hyperthyroidism. Which behavior demonstrates that education has been adequate?
   1. The patient participates in almost continuous activity.
   2. The patient practices stress-reduction techniques.
   3. The patient weighs herself weekly.
   4. The patient restricts carbohydrates and protein in her diet.

4. The nurse will administer which medication to the patient with hypothyroidism to increase thyroid function?
   1. anabolic steroids
   2. estrogen
   3. lithium
   4. propranolol

5. The nurse has provided education for the patient regarding Hashimoto's thyroiditis. Which of the following statements by the patient indicates the need for further education?
   1. "It is more common in men."
   2. "It is an autoimmune disorder."
   3. "It causes a goiter to form."
   4. "It has a familial link."
6. The nurse understands that which of the following patient populations is less likely to develop hypercortisolism?
   1. women between the ages of 30 and 50
   2. males who are teenagers
   3. patients prescribed long-term steroids
   4. patients undergoing chemotherapy
7. Identify the behavior that demonstrates the patient's understanding of the education regarding Cushing's syndrome.
   1. The patient refuses to discuss his or her body changes with professionals.
   2. The patient decreases intake of vitamins A and C in his or her diet.
   3. The patient restricts fluids.
   4. The patient uses dim lighting.
8. Patients experience clinical manifestations associated with Addison's disease after what percent of adrenal gland function is lost?
   1. 40%
   2. 50%
   3. 70%
   4. 90%

20 Nursing Care of Patients with Diabetes Mellitus

LEARNING OUTCOMES

1. Describe the prevalence and incidence of diabetes mellitus (DM).
2. Explain the pathophysiology, risk factors, manifestations, and complications of type 1 and type 2 DM.
3. Provide rationale for diagnostic tests used for screening, diagnosis, and monitoring of DM.
4. Discuss the nursing implications for insulin and oral hypoglycemic agents used to treat patients with DM.
5. Discuss best practices of self-care management of DM related to diet planning, sick day management, and exercise.
6. Compare and contrast the manifestations of hypoglycemia, diabetic ketoacidosis (DKA), and hyperosmolar hyperglycemic state (HHS).

CLINICAL COMPETENCIES

1. Assess blood glucose levels and patterns of hyper- and hypoglycemia in patients with DM.
2. Use assessed data, patient values, clinical expertise, and evidence to determine priority nursing diagnoses and select and implement individualized nursing interventions.
3. Administer oral and injectable medications used to treat DM knowledgeably and safely.
4. Assess patients' ability to read markings on syringes and to identify correct insulin doses.
5. Provide individualized care to patients with hypoglycemia, diabetic ketoacidosis, and hyperosmolar hyperglycemic state.
6. Effectively communicate with and function within the interdisciplinary team to plan and provide patient care.
7. Provide appropriate teaching to facilitate self blood glucose monitoring, administration of oral and injectable hypoglycemic medications, diabetic diet, appropriate exercise, and effective foot care.
8. Adapt individual and cultural values and variations as well as expressed needs and preferences into the plan of care for patients with DM.
9. Revise plan of care as needed to provide effective interventions to promote, maintain, or restore normal glucose levels.

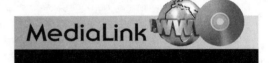

MediaLink

Pearson Nursing Student Resources
Audio Glossary
NCLEX-RN® Review

- Care Plan Activity
    - The Patient with Complications of Diabetes
- Case Study
    - The Patient with Type II Diabetes Mellitus with Hyperglycemic Hyperosmolar Nonketotic Syndrome (HHNS)
- Animations/Videos
    - Type 1 DM
    - Type 2 DM
    - Insulin
- Tools
    - Risk Factors for Development of Type 2 DM in Asymptomatic Adults
- MediaLink Applications
- Links to Resources

TERMS MATCHING

Place the letter of the correct definition in the space next to each term.

1. ____ Diabetes mellitus (DM)
2. ____ Diabetic ketoacidosis (DKA)
3. ____ Endogenous insulin
4. ____ Exogenous insulin
5. ____ Gastroparesis
6. ____ Gluconeogenesis
7. ____ Glycogenolysis
8. ____ Hyperglycemia
9. ____ Hyperosmolar hyperglycemic status (HHS)
10. ____ Hypoglycemia
11. ____ Insulin
12. ____ Ketoacidosis
13. ____ Ketosis
14. ____ Neuropathy
15. ____ Type 1 DM
16. ____ Type 2 DM

A. A delay in gastric emptying.

B. Insulin produced by the body.

C. The breakdown of liver glycogen.

D. An insulin deficit that causes fat stores of the body to break down, resulting in continued hyperglycemia and mobilization of fatty acids.

E. Neurological damage resulting in an alteration or loss in sensation.

F. An accumulation of ketone bodies produced during the oxidation of fatty acids.

G. The formation of glucose from fats and proteins.

H. A metabolic hormone that aids body cells in taking in glucose from the blood.

I. An elevated blood glucose level.

J. Insulin produced outside the body.

K. A metabolic condition in which the body had inadequate insulin to utilize blood glucose levels.

L. A metabolic disorder characterized by plasma osmolarity of 340 mOsm/L or greater (the normal range is 280–300 mOsm/L), greatly elevated blood glucose levels (over 600 mg/dL and often 1000–2000 mg/dL), and altered levels of consciousness.

M. Low blood glucose levels.

N. A metabolic disorder in which the body does not produce insulin, resulting is elevations of blood glucose levels.

O. A metabolic disorder resulting in hyperglycemia as a result of inadequate quantities of insulin or the body's ineffective use of available insulin.

P. A condition that develops when there is an absolute deficiency of insulin and an increase in the insulin counterregulatory hormones (for example, cortisol).

FOCUSED STUDY

1. Describe the differences between type 1 and type 2 diabetes.

_____

_____

_____

_____

_____

2. What diagnostic tests are used to manage diabetes?

_____

_____

_____

_____

_____

3. Describe the different types of insulin preparations.

_____

_____

_____

_____

_____

4. Explain the cause of diabetic ketoacidosis (DKA) and its treatment.

_____

_____

_____

_____

_____

5. Discuss the primary treatment modalities that are used to manage the patient with hyperosmolar hyperglycemic state.

_____

_____

_____

_____

_____

CASE STUDY

Jack Brown is a 56-year-old male who was recently diagnosed with diabetes. He has spent the past three days on the unit with a diagnosis of hypoglycemia secondary to diabetes. He is being discharged with prescriptions for an oral hypoglycemic. Answer the following questions based on your knowledge of caring for patients with diabetes.

   1. With what type of diabetes would Mr. Brown be diagnosed? Why?

   2. How do oral hypoglycemics regulate blood sugar?

   3. What modifications will Mr. Brown need to make to his diet?

   4. How should Mr. Brown be taught to manage an episode of hypoglycemia?

   5. Mr. Brown asks about the types of complications that may accompany his condition. What disorders are linked to diabetes mellitus?

SHORT ANSWERS

Fill in the table.

Drug Name	Classification	Onset (hrs)	Peak (hrs)	Duration (hrs)
Lispro				
Regular				
Humulin R®				
NPH				
Lantus®				

NCLEX-RN® REVIEW QUESTIONS

1. The nurse understands which statement to be true about type 2 diabetes mellitus?
   1. Its onset begins most often in childhood.
   2. It is the nonketonic form of diabetes.
   3. It can be triggered by a viral infection.
   4. An exogenous source of insulin is required.

2. When performing the assessment of a patient with a diagnosis of type 2 diabetes mellitus (DM), the nurse expects which of the following findings to be present?
   1. polydipsia
   2. polyuria
   3. paresthesias
   4. polyphagia

3. What is the normal fasting glucose level?
   1. 40 mg/dL
   2. 60 mg/dL
   3. 100 mg/dL
   4. 200 mg/dL

4. Which syringe is not available for administering insulin?
   1. 0.3 mL (30 U) syringe
   2. 0.5 mL (50 U) syringe
   3. 1.0 mL (100 U) syringe
   4. 1.5 mL (150 U) syringe

5. Identify the incorrect method of insulin injection.
   1. Inject the needle at a 90-degree angle.
   2. Massage the site after administering the injection.
   3. Rotate sites of injection.
   4. Do not inject insulin into an area that will be exercised.

6. The dawn phenomenon is a rise in blood glucose between what hours?
   1. 12 AM–2 AM
   2. 3 AM–8 AM
   3. 4 AM–8 AM
   4. 6 AM–9 AM

7. Which behavior indicates that the patient is following proper foot care?
   1. The patient inspects the feet monthly for changes.
   2. The patient wears tight-fitting shoes to facilitate circulation.
   3. The patient keeps the feet in a dependent position the majority of the day.
   4. After bathing the feet, the patient pats the foot dry and dries the areas between the toes well.

21 Assessing the Gastrointestinal System

LEARNING OUTCOMES

1. Describe the anatomy, physiology, and functions of the gastrointestinal (GI) system and the accessory digestive organs.
2. Identify specific topics to consider during a health history interview of the patient with GI disorders.
3. Explain techniques used for assessing nutritional status and GI function.
4. Give examples of genetic disorders of the GI system.
5. Describe normal variations in GI assessment findings for the older adult.
6. Identify abnormal findings that may indicate alterations in GI function.

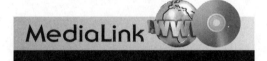

Pearson Nursing Student Resources
Audio Glossary
NCLEX-RN® Review
- Care Plan
  - The Health Assessment Interview
- Case Study
  - Dietary Intake
- Media Link Applications
- Links to Resources

CLINICAL COMPETENCIES

1. Conduct and document a health history for patients who have or are at risk for alterations in GI function.
2. Conduct and document a physical assessment of nutritional status and the GI system.
3. Monitor the results of diagnostic tests and report abnormal findings.

TERMS MATCHING

Place the letter of the correct definition in the space next to each term.

1. ____ Bile
2. ____ Borborygmus
3. ____ Bruit
4. ____ Cheilosis
5. ____ Constipation
6. ____ Diarrhea
7. ____ Flatus
8. ____ Gingivitis
9. ____ Glossitis
10. ____ Hernia
11. ____ Leukoplakia
12. ____ Melena
13. ____ Nutrition
14. ____ Occult blood
15. ____ Ostomy
16. ____ Steatorrhea
17. ____ Striae
18. ____ Valsalva's maneuver

A. Painful lesions in the corners of a patient's mouth; seen with riboflavin and/or niacin deficiency.

B. Intestinal gas.

C. Small white patches that can appear on the buccal mucosa.

D. The process by which the body, via the gastrointestinal system and the accessory digestive organs, ingests, absorbs, transports, uses, and eliminates nutrients in food.

E. Hyperactive high-pitched, tinkling, rushing, or growling bowel sounds; auscultated in patients with diarrhea or bowel obstructions.

F. Performed by closing the glottis and contracting the diaphragm and abdominal muscles to increase intra-abdominal pressure.

G. Black, tarry stools.

H. Greasy, frothy, yellow stools.

I. The frequent passage of loose, watery stools.

J. Swollen, red gums that bleed easily.

K. A surgical opening into a patient's bowel.

L. A smooth, bright red tongue

M. A blowing sound that can be auscultated over arteries in patients who have restricted blood flow through these blood vessels.

N. A positive result of this test requires further testing for colon cancer or GI bleeding due to peptic ulcers, ulcerative colitis, or diverticulosis.

O. The infrequent and often uncomfortable passage of hard, dry stool.

P. Whitish-silver stretch marks that are seen in obese patients and during or after pregnancy.

Q. A substance produced by the liver and stored in the gallbladder; aids in fat digestion and absorption.

R. A defect in the abdominal wall that allows abdominal contents to protrude outward.

FOCUSED STUDY

1. Locate and label the major digestive and accessory digestive organs in the diagram.

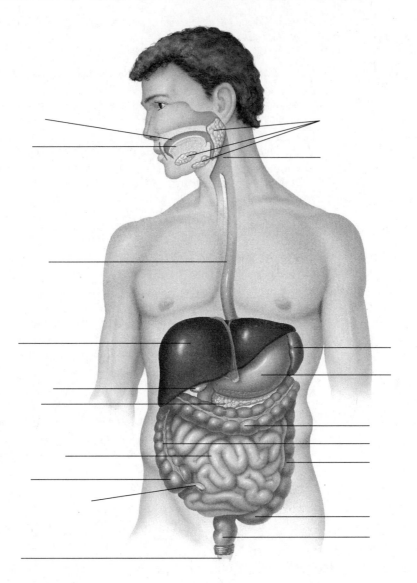

2. Describe the following nutrient categories and provide an example of each.
   a. Carbohydrates

_____

_____

   b. Proteins

_____

_____

   c. Fats

_____

_____

3. Describe how the autonomic nervous system (parasympathetic and sympathetic) influences the production of gastric secretions.

_____

_____

_____

_____

_____

4. Calculate your body mass index.

_____

CASE STUDIES

Case Study 1

During a community health screening, a 36-year-old patient states that he has been experiencing epigastric pain three to five times per week. Answer the following questions based on your knowledge of the digestive system.

1. What questions should the nurse ask this patient?

2. Epigastric pain can be associated with what disorders?

3. The patient has been scheduled for an esophagogastroduodenoscopy. What are the nurse's responsibilities regarding caring for this patient?

Case Study 2

Jerry Parsons is an 86-year-old male who is being seen in the physician's office. He is complaining of constipation. Answer the following based on your knowledge of the digestive system.

1. Mr. Parsons states, "It seems as though my problems with constipation have gotten worse as I have gotten older." How should the nurse respond?

2. What could result from frequent bouts of constipation?

3. What radiographic study may be performed to assess Mr. Parsons' rectum and colon?

SHORT ANSWERS

The nurse is assessing a patient who is experiencing malnutrition. Complete the table by identifying the expected assessment findings.

Body System	Assessment Findings
Nails	
Hair	
Skin	
Eyes	
Nervous system	
Musculoskeletal system	
Cardiovascular system	
GI system	

NCLEX-RN® REVIEW QUESTIONS

1. When obtaining a medical history from a patient, the nurse learns that all of his duodenum and several feet of small intestine were removed. What concerns should the nurse have regarding this patient's nutritional status related to the location of the removal?

   1. malabsorption

   2. loose stools and potential for dehydration

   3. poor production of vitamin D

   4. inadequate bile production

2. During the male patient's assessment, which finding is indicative that he is experiencing malnutrition?

   1. Triceps skin fold thickness is 130 mm.

   2. Midarm muscle circumference is 262 mm.

   3. Body mass index (BMI) is 18.

   4. Midarm circumference (MAC) is 301 mm.

3. When the nurse percusses the lower border of the liver, the dullness ends at the costal margin. What does the nurse know about this finding?

   1. It is indicative of cirrhosis.

   2. It is indicative of venous congestion of the liver.

   3. It is a normal finding.

   4. It is indicative of hepatitis.

4. Which statement regarding the assessment of bowel sounds is accurate?

   1. Bowel sounds are most active in the upper left quadrant.

   2. If bowel sounds are absent in each quadrant, it may take up to 20 minutes to assess.

   3. Bowel sounds should be heard within the first five seconds of auscultation.

   4. Bowel sounds should sound high-pitched, tinkling, or rushing.

5. A patient describes painful vertical fissures on the tongue. With what are these most likely associated?

   1. riboflavin deficiency

   2. dehydration

   3. folic acid deficiency

   4. antibiotic use

6. What is the first step of assessing the abdomen?

   1. auscultate

   2. inspect

   3. percuss

   4. palpate

7. While assessing the anus and rectum, the advanced practice nurse's initial action is to slowly insert a gloved finger into the patient's anus and point it toward:

   1. The descending colon.

   2. The umbilicus.

   3. The right lung.

   4. The liver.

Nursing Care of Patients with **Nutritional Disorders**

LEARNING OUTCOMES

1. Compare and contrast the pathophysiology and manifestations of nutritional disorders.
2. Identify causes and predict effects of nutritional disorders on patient health status.
3. Explain interdisciplinary care for patients with nutritional disorders.
4. Develop strategies to promote nutrition for patient populations.

CLINICAL COMPETENCIES

1. Assess the functional health status of patients with nutritional disorders.
2. Monitor nutritional status and responses to care; document and report abnormal or unexpected responses.
3. Use assessed data to determine priority nursing diagnoses and implement evidence-based nursing interventions.
4. Administer medications and enteral and parenteral nutrition knowledgeably and safely.
5. Integrate interdisciplinary care in the plan of care.
6. Adapt cultural values and variations into the plan of care for patients with nutritional disorders.
7. Plan and provide patient-centered teaching to restore, promote, and maintain functional health status.
8. Evaluate responses to care and use data to revise plan of care as needed.

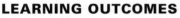

MediaLink

Pearson Nursing Student Resources
Audio Glossary
NCLEX-RN® Review
- Care Plan Activity
  - Malnutrition
- Case Studies
  - Enteral Feeding Complications
  - Nutritional Disorders: Obesity
- Animations/Videos
  - Obesity
  - Eating Disorders
  - Malnutrition
- MediaLink Applications
- Links to Resources

TERMS MATCHING

Place the letter of the correct definition in the space next to each term.

1. _____ Anorexia nervosa
2. _____ Basal metabolic rate (BMR)
3. _____ Binge eating disorder
4. _____ Body mass index (BMI)
5. _____ Bulimia nervosa
6. _____ Catabolism
7. _____ Enteral nutrition
8. _____ Lower body obesity
9. _____ Malnutrition
10. _____ Morbid obesity
11. _____ Nutrients
12. _____ Obesity
13. _____ Protein-calorie malnutrition (PCM)
14. _____ Starvation
15. _____ Total parenteral nutrition (TPN)
16. _____ Triglycerides
17. _____ Upper body obesity
18. _____ Very low caloric diets (VLCDs)

A. Recurring episodes of binge eating followed by purge behaviors.
B. A condition that is the result of an inadequate intake of nutrients.
C. Fat cells stored excess energy.
D. An excess of adipose tissue and a BMI greater than 30 kg/m^2.
E. Both protein and calories are deficient.
F. Diet programs that offer a protein-sparing modified fast (800 kcal/day or less) under close medical supervision.
G. An intense fear of gaining weight or of losing control over food intake.
H. The intravenous administration of amino acids, often with added carbohydrates, fats, electrolytes, vitamins, and minerals.
I. Central obesity.
J. Peripheral obesity.
K. Extreme obesity (BMI of over 40 kg/m^2).
L. The "cost" (in kilocalories) of being alive.
M. Cell and tissue breakdown.
N. Inadequate dietary intake.
O. Provide energy and are the building blocks for growth and tissue repair.
P. A condition that is characterized by eating an excessive amount of food during a defined period of time.
Q. Tube feeding.
R. An indirect measure of the amount of body fat.

FOCUSED STUDY

1. Define obesity and explain its health concerns.

_____

2. Describe the forms of bariatric procedures performed in the United States.

_____
_____
_____
_____

3. Describe the manifestations that patients with malnutrition will experience.

_____
_____
_____
_____

4. Explain the difference between anorexia nervosa and bulimia nervosa.

_____
_____
_____
_____

CASE STUDY

Barbara Spencer is a 50-year-old woman who has been diagnosed with binge-eating disorder. She has been referred to the mental health unit for counseling. Answer the following questions based on your knowledge of caring for patients with a binge-eating disorder.

1. What psychosocial factors may have contributed to Ms. Spencer's eating disorder?

2. What diagnostic studies may be ordered to assess Ms. Spencer's nutritional status?

3. What treatments are instituted for patients with a binge-eating disorder?

4. What role can Ms. Spencer's family play in assisting her to be successful with her treatment regimen?

SHORT ANSWERS

Fill in the table regarding nutritional deficiencies. Identify assessment data related to each nutritional deficiency listed.

Deficiency	Assessment Data
Calorie	
Protein	
Vitamin A	
Thiamine	
Riboflavin	
Vitamin C	
Iron	

NCLEX-RN® REVIEW QUESTIONS

1. The nurse understands that a patient with a BMI of _____ kg/m^2 indicates obesity.
   1. 20
   2. 23
   3. 27
   4. 30

2. What is the most important factor that contributes to obesity?
   1. physical inactivity
   2. genetics
   3. ethnicity
   4. low self-esteem

3. Which is not a manifestation of metabolic syndrome?
   1. increased waist circumference
   2. high HDL cholesterol
   3. hypertension
   4. an increase in fasting blood glucose

4. The patient reports fecal urgency. The nurse recognizes this as a side effect of which medication?
   1. Dexatrim®
   2. AcuTrim®
   3. Meridia® (sibutramine)
   4. Xenical® (orlistat)

5. The patient reports a history of stomach reduction surgery that created a small sac for a stomach. The nurse knows that the patient underwent which of the following procedures?
   1. biliopancreatic diversion
   2. Roux-en-Y gastric bypass
   3. adjustable gastric banding
   4. vertical banded gastroplasty

6. Which nursing intervention is not appropriate for a patient who needs to reduce her weight?
   1. Assist the patient to identify cues to eating.
   2. Establish a weight loss goal of 3–4 pounds per week.
   3. Assist the patient to develop a well-balanced food menu.
   4. Monitor laboratory values.

7. The patient presents with malnutrition. The nurse should assess the patient for which manifestation?
   1. recent acute infection
   2. weight loss of greater than 10% of usual weight
   3. inability to eat for more than two days
   4. affluent lifestyle

8. Which finding requires an immediate intervention when the nurse is monitoring the patient's parenteral nutrition?
   1. The nurse finds that the nutrition is being infused through a central line.
   2. The solution is being administered by gravity.
   3. The patient is afebrile.
   4. The parenteral solution is found to be mixed with intralipids.

9. Dumping syndrome occurs with diets that are high in what nutrient?
   1. fiber
   2. protein
   3. simple carbohydrates
   4. fat

Nursing Care of Patients with Upper Gastrointestinal Disorders

LEARNING OUTCOMES

1. Describe the pathophysiology of common disorders of the mouth, esophagus, and stomach.

2. Relate manifestations and diagnostic test results to the pathophysiologic processes involved in upper gastrointestinal disorders.

3. Explain interdisciplinary care for patients with upper gastrointestinal disorders.

4. Describe the role of the nurse in interdisciplinary care of patients with upper gastrointestinal disorders.

CLINICAL COMPETENCIES

1. Assess the functional health status of patients with upper gastrointestinal disorders.

2. Monitor, document, and, as needed, report manifestations of upper gastrointestinal disorders and their complications.

3. Plan patient-centered nursing care using an evidence base, research, and, as appropriate, decision-support technology.

4. Determine priority nursing diagnoses and interventions based on assessed data.

5. Administer medications and prescribed care knowledgeably and safely.

6. Coordinate and integrate interdisciplinary care into plan of care.

7. Construct and revise individualized plans of care considering the culture and values of the patient.

8. Plan and provide patient and family teaching to promote, maintain, and restore functional health.

MediaLink

Pearson Nursing Student Resources
Audio Glossary
NCLEX-RN® Review

- Care Plan Activity
  - Peptic Ulcer Disease and Pain
- Case Studies
  - GERD
  - Peptic Ulcer Disease
- Animations/Videos
  - Gastroesophageal Reflux Disease
  - Peptic Ulcer Disease
- MediaLink Applications
- Links to Resources

TERMS MATCHING

Place the letter of the correct definition in the space next to each term.

1. ____ Achalasia
2. ____ Acute gastritis
3. ____ Anorexia
4. ____ Cachectic
5. ____ Chronic gastritis
6. ____ Curling's ulcer
7. ____ Cushing's ulcer
8. ____ Diffuse esophageal spasm
9. ____ Dumping syndrome
10. ____ Duodenal ulcer
11. ____ Dysphagia
12. ____ Erosive (stress-induced) gastritis
13. ____ Esophagojejunostomy
14. ____ Gastric lavage
15. ____ Gastric mucosal barrier
16. ____ Gastric outlet obstruction
17. ____ Gastric ulcer
18. ____ Gastritis
19. ____ Gastroduodenostomy (Billroth I)
20. ____ Gastroesophageal reflux
21. ____ Gastroesophageal reflux disease (GERD)
22. ____ Gastrojejunostomy (Billroth II)
23. ____ Hematemesis
24. ____ Hematochezia
25. ____ Hemorrhage
26. ____ Hiatal hernia
27. ____ Melena
28. ____ Nausea
29. ____ Occult bleeding
30. ____ Partial gastrectomy
31. ____ Peptic ulcer disease (PUD)
32. ____ Peptic ulcer
33. ____ Perforation
34. ____ Steatorrhea
35. ____ Stomatitis
36. ____ Total gastrectomy
37. ____ Ulcer
38. ____ Vomiting
39. ____ Zollinger-Ellison syndrome

A. A term that refers to a patient's very poor health and malnourishment.

B. The forceful expulsion of the contents of the upper gastrointestinal tract resulting from contraction of muscles in the gut and abdominal wall.

C. The most lethal complication of peptic ulcer disease; the ulcer extends through the mucosal wall.

D. A disorder characterized by impaired peristalsis of the smooth muscle located in the esophagus and impaired relaxation of the lower esophageal sphincter.

E. This can occur in any area of the gastrointestinal tract exposed to acid-pepsin secretions, including the esophagus, stomach, and duodenum.

F. When the stomach is irrigated or washed out.

G. A condition that occurs when part of the stomach protrudes through the esophageal hiatus of the diaphragm into the thoracic cavity.

H. Inflammation of the stomach lining that results from irritation of the gastric mucosa.

I. A benign, self-limiting disorder associated with the ingestion of gastric irritants such as aspirin, alcohol, caffeine, or foods contaminated with certain types of bacteria.

J. The backward flowing of gastric contents into the esophagus.

K. Visibly bloody stool.

L. A complication that occurs following a gastrectomy procedure; peristalsis is stimulated, and intestinal motility is increased.

M. Black, tarry stool.

N. A severe form of acute gastritis that occurs following a head injury or CNS surgery.

O. The surgical removal of the entire stomach.

P. Protects the stomach from hydrochloric acid and pepsin.

Q. A type of peptic ulcer that is located in the duodenum.

R. A type of peptic ulcer disease that is caused by a gastrinoma, or a gastrin-secreting tumor of the pancreas, stomach, or intestines.

S. Another term used to describe a gastroduodenostomy.

T. A generalized term used to describe severe gastritis that occurs as a complication of other life-threatening conditions such as shock, severe trauma, major surgery, sepsis, burns, or head injury.

U. A severe form of acute gastritis that occurs following a major burn.

V. Difficult or painful swallowing.

W. A vague, unpleasant sensation of sickness or queasiness.

X. A group of disorders characterized by progressive and irreversible changes in the gastric mucosa.

Y. Bleeding that is unnoticed by the patient.

Z. One type of complication that may occur as a result of a peptic ulcer; it may develop from edema surrounding the ulcer, smooth muscle spasm, or scar tissue.

AA. The surgical removal of a portion of the stomach.

BB. During a total gastrectomy, the surgeon forms an anastomosis from the esophagus to the jejunum.

CC. A break in the gastrointestinal mucosa.

DD. Another term used to describe a gastrojejunostomy.

EE. A chronic disease that occurs as a result of a break in the mucous lining of the gastrointestinal tract where it comes in contact with gastric juice.

FF. A chronic condition that results from the backward flowing of gastric contents into the esophagus.

GG. Excess fat in the feces.

HH. A type of peptic ulcer located in the stomach.

II. A significant amount of bleeding; acute.

JJ. Loss of appetite.

KK. A term used to describe inflammation and ulcers of the oral mucosa.

LL. A condition associated with achalasia that results in nonperistaltic contraction of esophageal smooth muscle.

MM. Vomiting blood.

FOCUSED STUDY

1. List several risk factors for developing stomatitis.

_____

_____

_____

_____

2. Discuss the clinical manifestations that can be found in the patient with oral cancer.

_____

_____

_____

_____

3. Discuss the nursing interventions that should be provided for the patient with a disturbed sleep pattern due to peptic ulcer disease.

_____

_____

_____

_____

4. Describe interdisciplinary care that can be provided for the patient with acute or chronic gastritis. Discuss the differences between how acute and chronic gastritis are typically diagnosed.

_____

_____

_____

CASE STUDY

Kevin Hess is a 40-year-old male who has been diagnosed with a duodenal ulcer. He states that he has smoked approximately two packs of cigarettes per day since he was 17 years old. He admits to using ibuprofen in large amounts to ease chronic pain in his right knee. Answer the following questions based on your knowledge of caring for patients with peptic ulcer disease.

1. What role does Mr. Hess's age, smoking history, and ibuprofen use play in his peptic ulcer disease?

2. Why might Mr. Hess be screened for _H. pylori_ infection?

3. As the nurse assesses Mr. Hess, what are some expected findings regarding his description of symptoms?

4. Describe the clinical manifestations Mr. Hess may experience if he develops the most lethal complication of peptic ulcer disease.

5. Mr. Hess's physician has prescribed Prevacid® (lansoprazole). How should the nurse educate Mr. Hess regarding how he should take this medication?

6. During the nurse's assessment of Mr. Hess, he begins to hemorrhage. What are some clinical manifestations the nurse may discover with this?

7. What are several nursing diagnoses the nurse may use when developing Mr. Hess's plan of care?

CARE PLAN CRITICAL-THINKING ACTIVITY

1. Mr. Chavez, a patient diagnosed with oral cancer, states that he quit smoking, but the nurse sees a pack of cigarettes in his shirt pocket and he smells of smoke. What should the nurse do?

2. What techniques can be used to assist Mr. Chavez to communicate during the immediate postoperative period?

3. What behaviors will demonstrate that Mr. Chavez's anxiety has lessened about his speech?

SHORT ANSWERS

Fill in the table. Identify the pathophysiology associated with each clinical manifestation of GERD.

Manifestation	Pathophysiology
Heartburn Chest pain Regurgitation Belching	
Dysphagia	
Pain after eating	
Chronic cough Hoarseness Laryngitis, pharyngitis	

NCLEX-RN® REVIEW QUESTIONS

1. The patient has been diagnosed with oral cancer. Which of the following places in the mouth is an unexpected site for oral cancer to develop?
  1. tongue
  2. upper lip
  3. lower lip
  4. floor of the mouth
2. The nurse expects that the patient will be unable to communicate verbally following oral surgery. Which of the following ways can the nurse communicate most effectively with the patient after surgery?
  1. Have the patient record all questions preoperatively on a tape recorder.
  2. Require that a spokesperson be available at the patient's bedside at all times.
  3. Place a writing tablet and pens next to the bed.
  4. Provide the patient with the cell phone numbers of the nursing staff's unit.
3. The patient has been diagnosed with gastroesophageal reflux disease. Which of the following orders is unexpected by the nurse?
  1. Prepare the patient for a barium enema.
  2. Prepare the patient for 24-hour ambulatory pH monitoring.
  3. Prepare the patient for a barium swallow.
  4. Obtain consent for an upper gastrointestinal endoscopy.
4. Adenocarcinoma is one of two forms of esophageal cancer. Which of the following is the other form of esophageal cancer?
  1. squamous cell
  2. basal cell
  3. epithelial cell
  4. stratus cell

5. The patient has been vomiting for the last six days and has developed the following problems. Which of the following would be an unexpected complication of vomiting?

    1. hyperkalemia

    2. metabolic acidosis

    3. aspiration

    4. tears of the esophagus

6. To help relieve nausea and vomiting, the nurse could suggest using which aromatic root?

    1. anise

    2. catmint

    3. sage

    4. ginger

7. Which patient statement reflects an adequate understanding of how to prevent dumping syndrome?

    1. "I eat three large meals a day."

    2. "I do not drink liquids with my meals."

    3. "I have decreased the amount of protein in my diet."

    4. "I have increased the amount of sugar in my diet."

24 Nursing Care of Patients with Bowel Disorders

LEARNING OUTCOMES

1. Compare and contrast the causes, pathophysiology, manifestations, interdisciplinary and nursing care of patients with disorders of bowel motility.

2. Explain the pathophysiology, manifestations, complications, interdisciplinary care, and nursing care of patients with acute or chronic inflammatory bowel disorders, neoplastic disorders, and structural and obstructive bowel disorders.

3. Discuss the purposes, nursing implications, and health education for the patient and family related to medications used to treat bowel disorders.

4. Explain the rationale for using selected diets, including those for diarrhea and constipation and low-residue, gluten-free, and high-fiber diets.

5. Describe selected surgical procedures of the bowel, including colectomy, colostomy, ileostomy, and perianal surgery.

CLINICAL COMPETENCIES

1. Assess the functional status of patients with bowel disorders, and recognize, document, and report unexpected or abnormal findings.

2. Use assessed data to determine priority nursing diagnoses, identify and implement patient-centered evidence-based nursing interventions, and revise the plan of care for patients with bowel disorders.

3. Integrate interdisciplinary care and administer medications knowledgeably and safely for patients with bowel disorders.

4. Provide skilled care to patients having bowel surgery, an ostomy, or perianal surgery.

5. Provide culturally appropriate teaching to promote nutrition, prevent acute and chronic bowel disorders, encourage screening, and facilitate community-based care related to bowel disorders.

MediaLink

Pearson Nursing Student Resources
Audio Glossary
NCLEX-RN® Review

- Care Plan Activity
  - Irritable Bowel Syndrome
- Case Studies
  - The Patient Complaining of Abdominal Pain
  - Postop Complications
- Animations/Videos
  - Irritable Bowel Syndrome
  - Flexible Sigmoidoscopy
- MediaLink Applications
- Links to Resources

TERMS MATCHING

Place the letter of the correct definition in the space next to each term.

1. ____ Appendicitis
2. ____ Borborygmi
3. ____ Colectomy
4. ____ Colostomy
5. ____ Constipation
6. ____ Crohn's disease
7. ____ Diarrhea
8. ____ Diverticulosis
9. ____ Fecal impaction
10. ____ Gastroenteritis
11. ____ Hematochezia
12. ____ Hemorrhoids
13. ____ Hernia
14. ____ Ileostomy
15. ____ Inflammatory bowel disease (IBD)
16. ____ Irritable bowel syndrome (IBS)
17. ____ Lactose intolerance
18. ____ Malabsorption
19. ____ Paralytic ileus
20. ____ Peritonitis
21. ____ Sprue
22. ____ Steatorrhea
23. ____ Stoma
24. ____ Ulcerative colitis

A. A chronic motility disorder of the lower gastrointestinal tract; also known as spastic bowel and mucous colitis.

B. A defect in the abdominal wall that allows intra-abdominal contents to protrude out of the abdominal cavity.

C. An ostomy made in the ileum of the small intestine.

D. Inflammation of the vermiform appendix; a common cause of acute abdominal pain.

E. A chronic inflammatory bowel disorder that affects the mucosa and submucosa of the colon and rectum.

F. Excessively loud, hyperactive bowel sounds.

G. Inflammation of the stomach and small intestine; also known as enteritis.

H. A group of disorders that includes Crohn's disease and ulcerative colitis; these conditions cause inflammation in the digestive tract.

I. The opening on the surface of the wall of abdominal that is created when an ostomy is created.

J. The surgical resection and removal of the colon.

K. This occurs when the patient is unable to produce the enzyme lactase for the digestion and absorption of lactose.

L. This is when the patient has an increase in the frequency, volume, and fluid content of the stool; the water content of feces is increased.

M. A chronic immune-mediated disorder of the small intestine in which the absorption of nutrients is impaired; characterized by sensitivity to the gliadin fraction of gluten.

N. This is when the patient has two or fewer bowel movements weekly or experiences difficulty passing stools.

O. The hemorrhoidal veins become weak and distended.

P. The impaired propulsion or forward movement of bowel contents.

Q. The patient has diverticula present in the bowel; these form when increased pressure in the bowel lumen causes bowel mucosa to herniate through defects in the colon wall.

R. Stools that are obviously bloody.

S. Inflammation of the peritoneum; a serious complication of many acute abdominal disorders.

T. The surgical creation of an opening from the large bowel on the abdominal wall.

U. A condition in which the intestinal mucosa ineffectively absorbs nutrients, resulting in their excretion in the stool.

V. A chronic, relapsing inflammatory disorder affecting the gastrointestinal tract; also known as regional enteritis.

W. Bulky, foul-smelling stool.

X. A condition that occurs when the patient has a rock-hard or puttylike mass of feces that has formed in the rectum.

FOCUSED STUDY

1. List five risk factors that may contribute to the development of constipation.

_____

_____

_____

2. Describe the clinical manifestations that may be found in a patient who has been diagnosed with peritonitis. Describe the clinical manifestations that may found in a patient who develops a systemic infection due to peritonitis.

_____

_____

_____

_____

3. Describe the different ways diverticular disease can be treated.

_____

_____

_____

4. List the three different types of polyps. Explain how polyps are usually diagnosed.

_____

_____

CASE STUDY

Lynn Bowman is a 16-year-old female who comes into the emergency room with complaints of right lower quadrant pain, nausea, vomiting, and a fever of 101°F. With palpation, she exhibits rebound tenderness at McBurney's point. She is diagnosed with appendicitis. Answer the following questions based on your knowledge of caring for patients with appendicitis.

1. Where is McBurney's point located?

2. What are possible complications of untreated appendicitis?

3. What diagnostic studies may be used to diagnose appendicitis?

4. Prior to an appendectomy, what medications may be ordered for Ms. Bowman?

5. Ms. Bowman undergoes an appendectomy. What should the nurse's postoperative teaching include?

6. What two nursing diagnoses might the nurse use in Ms. Bowman's plan of care following surgery?

SHORT ANSWERS

Fill in the table. Note whether the laboratory value will be "increased," "decreased," or "within normal limits" when the patient has been experiencing severe diarrhea.

Test	Normal Value	Change with Severe Diarrhea
Serum osmolality	280–300 mOsm/kg	
Serum potassium	3.5–5.3 mEq/L	
Serum sodium	135–145 mEq/L	
Serum chloride	95–105 mEq/L	
Blood gases		
pH	Arterial: 7.35–7.45	
PCO$_2$	Arterial: 35–45 mmHg	
Bicarbonate	24–28 mEq/L	
Hematocrit	Males: 40%–54%	
	Females: 36%–46%	
Urine specific gravity	1.005–1.030	

NCLEX-RN® REVIEW QUESTIONS

1. What dietary instruction should the nurse give the patient about managing acute diarrhea?
   1. Eat foods high in fiber.
   2. Eat small, frequent meals.
   3. Avoid drinking electrolyte solutions such as Gatorade®.
   4. Increase the intake of milk products.
2. Which statement demonstrates that the patient understands teaching about managing constipation?
   1. "I should limit my fluid intake."
   2. "I should avoid bran and prunes."
   3. "I should participate in a daily form of exercise."
   4. "I should avoid drinking any warm fluids before breakfast."
3. Which of the following is the best diagnostic test to use when attempting to diagnose acute appendicitis?
   1. ultrasound
   2. x-ray
   3. intravenous pyelogram
   4. urinalysis
4. A urine output of less than _____ mL/hr indicates hypovolemia, decreased cardiac output, and impaired tissue perfusion.
   1. 30
   2. 50
   3. 60
   4. 75

5. Identify the diarrheal illness caused by ingesting raw or improperly cooked meat, eggs, and dairy products in which symptoms develop 8–48 hours after ingestion.

    1. shigellosis

    2. travelers' diarrhea

    3. cholera

    4. salmonellosis

6. Which of the following statements indicates the need for further education about common bowel infections?

    1. Giardiasis is a protozoal infection of the proximal small intestine.

    2. Helminths are parasitic worms capable of causing bowel infections.

    3. Amebiasis is an infection that attacks only the small bowel.

    4. Coccidiosis secretes an enterotoxin that causes watery diarrhea.

7. Which of the following indicates that the patient is not correctly managing his inflammatory bowel disease (IBD)?

    1. The patient has added Ensure® to his diet.

    2. The patient reports drinking less than 1 quart of fluid per day.

    3. The patient takes medication as ordered by his physician.

    4. The patient has started smoking cessation classes.

8. How must patients with celiac disease adjust their diets?

    1. increase in lactose

    2. addition of fats

    3. decrease in calories

    4. elimination of gluten

Nursing Care of Patients with **Gallbladder, Liver,** and **Pancreatic Disorders**

LEARNING OUTCOMES

1. Describe the pathophysiology of commonly occurring disorders of the gallbladder, liver, and exocrine pancreas.
2. Use knowledge of normal anatomy and physiology to understand the manifestations and effects of biliary, hepatic, and pancreatic disorders.
3. Relate changes in normal assessment data to the pathophysiology and manifestations of gallbladder, liver, and exocrine pancreatic disorders.

CLINICAL COMPETENCIES

1. Assess functional health status of patients with gallbladder, liver, or pancreatic disease.
2. Monitor for, recognize, document, and report expected and unexpected manifestations in patients with gallbladder, liver, or pancreatic disease.
3. Provide appropriate, evidence-based teaching about diagnostic tests and test results for patients with gallbladder, liver, and pancreatic disorders.
4. Integrate appropriate dietary, pharmacologic, and other interdisciplinary measures into nursing care and teaching of the patient with a gallbladder, liver, or pancreatic disorder.
5. Provide safe, patient-centered nursing care for the patient who has surgery of the gallbladder, liver, or pancreas.
6. Integrate psychosocial, cultural, and spiritual considerations into the plan of care for a patient with a gallbladder, liver, or pancreatic disorder.
7. Use evidence-based practice, technology, and information management tools to develop, implement, evaluate, and, as needed, revise the plan of care for patients with disorders of the gallbladder, liver, or pancreas.
8. Provide appropriate patient and family teaching to promote, maintain, and restore functional health status for patients with gallbladder, liver, and pancreatic disorders.

MediaLink

Pearson Nursing Student Resources
Audio Glossary
NCLEX-RN® Review
- Care Plan Activity
  - A Patient with Hepatitis A
- Case Studies
  - Hepatitis B
  - Traditional Native American Diet and Gallbladder Disease
- Animations/Videos
  - Cirrhosis
  - Enterohepatic Circulation
- MediaLink Applications
- Links to Resources

TERMS MATCHING

Place the letter of the correct definition in the space next to each term.

1. ____ Alcoholic cirrhosis
2. ____ Ascites
3. ____ Balloon tamponade
4. ____ Biliary colic
5. ____ Cholecystitis
6. ____ Cholelithiasis
7. ____ Chronic hepatitis
8. ____ Cirrhosis
9. ____ Esophageal varices
10. ____ Fulminant hepatitis
11. ____ Gastric lavage
12. ____ Hematochezia
13. ____ Hepatitis
14. ____ Hepatorenal syndrome
15. ____ Jaundice
16. ____ Laparoscopic cholecystectomy
17. ____ Liver transplantation
18. ____ Pancreatitis
19. ____ Paracentesis
20. ____ Portal hypertension
21. ____ Portal systemic encephalopathy
22. ____ Steatorrhea
23. ____ Transjugular intrahepatic porto-systemic shunt (TIPS)

A. Renal failure with azotemia, sodium retention, oliguria, and hypotension that develops in patients with advanced cirrhosis and ascites.

B. Impaired consciousness and mental status due to the accumulation of toxic waste products in the blood as blood bypasses the congested liver.

C. The most common type of cirrhosis in the United States.

D. Irrigation of the stomach with large quantities of normal saline.

E. Visibly bloody stool.

F. Accumulation of plasma-rich fluid in the abdominal cavity.

G. A minimally invasive method to remove the gallbladder.

H. A multiple-lumen nasogastric tube is inserted, and gastric and esophageal balloons are inflated to apply direct pressure on the bleeding varices.

I. An emergency measure used to relieve portal hypertension; a shunt is placed to allow blood to flow directly from the portal vein into the hepatic vein, bypassing the cirrhotic liver.

J. Inflammation of the gallbladder.

K. Fatty, frothy, foul-smelling stools.

L. A severe, steady pain in the epigastric region or right upper quadrant of the abdomen.

M. The surgical procedure indicated for some patients with irreversible, progressive cirrhosis.

N. A condition characterized by fibrosis of liver tissue leading to decreased liver mass, impaired liver function, and altered blood flow.

O. Yellow staining of body tissues.

P. Inflammation of the liver usually caused by a virus, although it may result from exposure to alcohol, drugs and toxins, or other pathogens.

Q. A chronic infection of the liver.

R. Inflammation of the pancreas.

S. Enlarged thin-walled veins that form in the submucosa of the esophagus; formed when blood is shunted from the portal system due to portal hypertension.

T A procedure where fluid is aspirated from the peritoneal cavity.

U. A rapidly progressive disease; liver failure developing within 2–3 weeks after the onset of symptoms.

V. Occurs when there is impaired blood flow through the liver and increased pressure in the portal venous system that drains the gastrointestinal tract, the spleen, and surface veins of the abdomen.

W. The formation of stones in the gallbladder or biliary duct system.

FOCUSED STUDY

1. List 10 risk factors associated with the development of gallstones.

_____

_____

_____

_____

2. Explain the physiological process of jaundice. List the three types of jaundice.

_____

_____

_____

_____

_____

3. Describe the differences between the clinical manifestations associated with chronic versus acute pancreatitis.

_____

_____

_____

_____

_____

4. Describe two nursing interventions that can be performed for a patient who is experiencing acute pain related to cholelithiasis. Include rationale for each intervention.

_____

_____

_____

_____

_____

CASE STUDY

Joseph Wales, a 62-year-old black male has been admitted with a diagnosis of acute pancreatitis. Six months ago he was diagnosed with cholelithiasis and had a laparoscopic cholecystectomy. Mr. Wales has a history of alcoholism. Answer the following questions based on your knowledge of caring for patients with acute pancreatitis.

1. What role does Mr. Wales's past medical history play in his current episode of acute pancreatitis?

2. What clinical manifestations are associated with acute pancreatitis?

3. The nurse is monitoring Mr. Wales for the development of complications related to acute pancreatitis. What are some complications of acute pancreatitis?

4. What is one common nursing diagnosis that is associated with acute pancreatitis?

5. The nurse reviews Mr. Wales's laboratory results. Which laboratory results does the nurse expect to be abnormal?

6. Describe discharge teaching the nurse should provide for Mr. Wales.

CARE PLAN CRITICAL-THINKING ACTIVITY

Please refer to the case study and nursing care plan exercise: A Patient with Cholelithiasis (page 727 in your textbook) to answer the following questions.

1. What role did Mrs. Red Wing's genetic makeup play in the development of cholelithiasis?

2. What nursing interventions may be used to deal with Mrs. Red Wing's recent weight loss?

SHORT ANSWERS

Fill in the blanks regarding the various types of viral hepatitis.

Virus	Hepatitis A (HAV)	Hepatitis B (HBV)	Hepatitis C (HCV)	Hepatitis D (HDV)	Hepatitis E (HEV)
Mode of transmission					
Incubation (in weeks)					
Onset					
Carrier state					
Possible complications					
Laboratory findings					

NCLEX-RN® REVIEW QUESTIONS

1. The nurse knows that most gallstones consist primarily of which of the following?
    1. cholesterol
    2. bile salts
    3. calcium
    4. lecithin

2. The nurse is assessing a patient with a diagnosis of acute cholecystitis. Which of the following is an unexpected sign or symptom?
    1. nausea
    2. fever
    3. right upper quadrant pain
    4. diarrhea

3. The patient presents with abnormal liver function studies and impaired consciousness. The patient is most likely experiencing which of the following problems?
    1. portal systemic encephalopathy
    2. ascites
    3. hepatorenal syndrome
    4. splenomegaly

4. A vaccine is available for which form of viral hepatitis?
    1. hepatitis A
    2. hepatitis C
    3. hepatitis delta
    4. hepatitis E

5. The nurse is creating a care plan for the patient with liver trauma. Which of the following would be an unexpected nursing diagnosis to be used with this patient?
    1. *Deficient Fluid Volume Related to Hemorrhage*
    2. *Risk for Infection Related to Wound or Abdominal Contamination*
    3. *Risk for Bleeding Related to Impaired Coagulation*
    4. *Altered Body Image Related to Bruising*

6. The patient has developed pancreatic cancer. Which of the following is not a known risk factor for the development of pancreatic cancer?
    1. occupational exposure to industrial chemicals
    2. a low-fat diet
    3. diagnosis of diabetes mellitus seven years ago
    4. history of smoking two packs per day for the last 19 years

Assessing the Renal System

26 CHAPTER

LEARNING OUTCOMES

1. Describe the anatomy, physiology, and functions of the renal system.
2. Identify specific topics for consideration during a health history interview of the patient with health problems involving the renal system.
3. Describe techniques used to assess the integrity and function of the renal system.
4. Give examples of genetic disorders of the renal system.
5. Describe normal variations in assessment findings for the older adult.
6. Identify abnormal findings that may indicate alterations in urinary elimination.

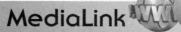

MediaLink

Pearson Nursing Student Resources
Audio Glossary
NCLEX-RN® Review
- Care Plan Activity
  - The Older Adult with UTI
- Case Study
  - The Patient with Renal Disorders
- MediaLink Applications
- Links to Resources

CLINICAL COMPETENCIES

1. Conduct and document a health history for patients who have or are at risk for alterations in renal function.
2. Conduct and document a physical assessment of the renal system.
3. Monitor the results of diagnostic tests and report abnormal findings.

EQUIPMENT NEEDED

- Urine specimen cup
- Disposable gloves
- Stethoscope

TERMS MATCHING

Place the letter of the correct definition in the space next to each item.

1. ____ Calculi   A. Voiding two or more times at night.

2. ____ Dysuria   B. The largest component of urine by weight.

3. ____ Glomerular filtration rate (GFR)   C. Pus in the urine

4. ____ Hematuria   D. The process of urinating or voiding.

5. ____ Micturion   E. Renal stones.

6. ____ Nocturia   F. The presence of blood in the urine.

7. ____ Oliguria   G. Frequent urination.

8. ____ Polyuria   H. Difficulty experienced with urination.

9. ____ Pyuria   I. The amount of fluid filtered from the blood by the kidneys per minute.

10. ____ Urea   J. Urine output of less than 400 mL in 24 hours.

FOCUSED STUDY

1. Discuss the organs of the urinary system.

_____

_____

_____

2. Summarize diagnostic tests for the urinary system.

_____

_____

_____

3. Explain the formation of urine.

_____

_____

_____

CASE STUDY

Anne Sutter is a 64-year-old female patient admitted to the nursing unit. Her skin and mucous membranes are pale. She also has tenderness and pain on percussion of the costovertebral angle.

1. Explain the functions of the kidney.

2. What could tenderness and pain on percussion of the costovertebral angle suggest?

3. What could pallor of the skin and mucous membranes indicate?

CROSSWORD PUZZLE

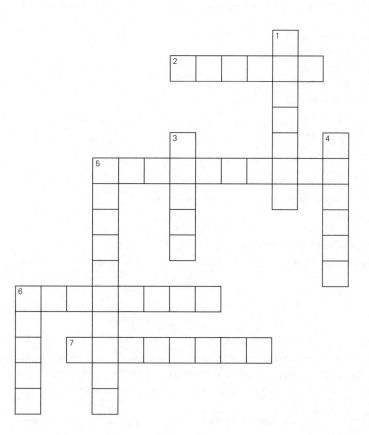

Across

2   Channels urine from the kidney to the bladder

5   The test used to directly visualize the bladder wall

6   Urine remaining in the bladder after voiding

7   The substance necessary for the absorption of calcium

Down

1   The functional unit of the kidney

3   The color of normal urine

4   Milky urine is the result of this

5   The by-product of muscle breakdown that is excreted by the kidney

6   Acts on a plasma globulin, angiotensinogen, to release angiotensin I, which in turn is converted to angiotensin II

NCLEX-RN® REVIEW QUESTIONS

1. The patient contacts the ambulatory care clinic with concerns about her urine appearing discolored. The nursing interview determines that the urine is a bright orange color. Which of the following questions by the nurse is indicated at this time?
   1. "Are you currently sexually active?"
   2. "Is your dietary intake high in saturated fats?"
   3. "Are you taking iron supplements?"
   4. "Are you currently taking any medications?"
2. Which of the following is a function of the kidney?
   1. to form urine
   2. to conserve metabolic waste products
   3. to destroy nutrients
   4. to secrete solutes
3. Which of the following statements about glomerular filtration is true?
   1. Hydrostatic pressure forces fluid and solutes through a membrane.
   2. It is a passive, selective process.
   3. Glomerular filtration rate (GFR) is not influenced by the total surface area available for filtration.
   4. The glomerulus is less efficient than most capillary beds.
4. Urine is composed, by volume, of about _____% water and _____% solutes.
   1. 95, 5
   2. 85, 15
   3. 75, 25
   4. 65, 35
5. Which of the following is correct about renal proteins?
   1. The stimulus for the production of erythropoietin by the kidneys is increased oxygen delivery to kidney cells.
   2. Erythropoietin stimulates the bone marrow to produce red blood cells in response to tissue hypoxia.
   3. Hormones activated or synthesized by the kidneys include the active form of vitamin E, erythropoietin, and natriuretic hormone.
   4. Vitamin D is necessary for the absorption of calcium and phosphate by the large intestine.
6. What are the layers of the bladder wall (from internal to external)?
   1. the epithelial mucosa lining the inside, the connective tissue submucosa, the smooth muscle layer, and the fibrous outer layer
   2. the fibrous outer layer, the connective tissue submucosa, the epithelial mucosa lining the inside, and the smooth muscle layer
   3. the fibrous outer layer, the epithelial mucosa lining the inside, the connective tissue submucosa, and the smooth muscle layer
   4. the connective tissue submucosa, the epithelial mucosa lining the inside, the smooth muscle layer, and the fibrous outer layer
7. Which of the following statements about the bladder is correct?
   1. It holds about 600–800 mL of urine before internal pressure rises and signals the need to empty the bladder through micturition.
   2. It is posterior to the symphysis pubis and serves as a storage site for urine.
   3. In females, the bladder lies immediately in front of the rectum.
   4. Openings for the ureters and the urethra are outside the bladder.
8. The nurse is reviewing the patient's history and physical information and notes the physician's indication that the patient has been experiencing oliguria. What does the nurse recognize about the patient?
   1. There is blood in the patient's urine.
   2. The patient gets up frequently at night to urinate.
   3. The patient is voiding excessive amounts of urine.
   4. The patient is voiding scant amounts of urine.
9. The nurse is reviewing the patient's most recent urinalysis. Which of the findings indicate the need for further action?
   1. a light straw color
   2. a pH of 5.5
   3. WBCs 3
   4. ketones +1

Nursing Care of Patients with **Urinary Tract Disorders**

LEARNING OUTCOMES

1. Identify populations at risk for common urinary tract disorders and behaviors that increase the risk.
2. Explain the pathophysiology of common urinary tract disorders.
3. Describe the manifestations of urinary tract disorders, relating manifestations to the pathophysiology of the disorder.
4. Discuss the nursing implications of medications and treatments prescribed for patients with urinary tract disorders.
5. Describe invasive and surgical procedures used in treating urinary tract disorders.

MediaLink

Pearson Nursing Student Resources
Audio Glossary
NCLEX-RN® Review

- Care Plan Activity
  - Urinary Tract Infection
- Case Studies
  - The Patient with Cystitis
  - The Patient with Urinary Tract Disorders
- Animation/Video
  - Kidney Stones
- MediaLink Applications
- Links to Resources

CLINICAL COMPETENCIES

1. Assess the functional health status of patients with urinary tract disorders, using data to determine priority nursing diagnoses and select individualized nursing interventions.
2. Identify, report, and document abnormal or unexpected assessments, monitoring patient status.
3. Use evidence-based research to plan and implement nursing care for patients with urinary tract disorders.
4. Integrate the interdisciplinary plan of care into care for patients with urinary tract disorders.
5. Knowledgeably and safely administer prescribed medications and treatments for patients with urinary tract disorders.
6. Provide effective nursing care for patients undergoing invasive procedures or surgery of the urinary tract.
7. Plan and provide appropriate teaching for prevention of and self-care of urinary tract disorders.
8. Evaluate patient responses, revising plan of care as needed to promote, maintain, or restore functional health of patients with urinary tract disorders.

TERMS MATCHING

Place the letter of the correct definition in the space next to each item.

1. _____ Cystectomy

2. _____ Cystitis

3. _____ Dysuria

4. _____ Extracorporeal shock wave lithotripsy (ESWL)

5. _____ Hematuria

6. _____ Hydronephrosis

7. _____ Lithiasis

8. _____ Lithotripsy

9. _____ Neurogenic bladder

10. _____ Nocturia

11. _____ Nosocomial

12. _____ Pyelonephritis

13. _____ Reflux

14. _____ Renal colic

15. _____ Ureteral stent

16. _____ Ureteroplasty

17. _____ Urgency

18. _____ Urinary calculi

19. _____ Urinary diversion

20. _____ Urinary drainage system

21. _____ Urinary incontinence (UI)

22. _____ Urinary retention

A. Distention of the renal pelvis and calyces.

B. The preferred treatment for urinary calculi.

C. Stones in the urinary tract.

D. Inflammation of the kidney and renal pelvis.

E. Disruption of the CNS that interferes with normal bladder function.

F. Surgical removal of the bladder.

G. The kidney pelvis, ureters, bladder, and urethra.

H. A sudden, compelling need to urinate.

I. The involuntary loss of urine.

J. A noninvasive technique for fragmenting kidney stones using shock waves.

K. Inflammation of the urinary bladder.

L. A condition in which urine moves from the bladder back toward the kidney.

M. Surgical repair of a ureter.

N. Blood in urine.

O. Hospital-acquired.

P. Painful or difficult urination.

Q. The surgical technique used when urination cannot be managed using conservative measures.

R. Voiding two or more times at night.

S. Stone formation.

T. The inability to empty the bladder completely.

U. Acute, severe flank pain that develops when a stone obstructs the ureter, causing ureteral spasm.

V. A thin catheter inserted into the ureter to provide for urine flow.

FOCUSED STUDY

1. Summarize the surgical procedures used to treat urinary tract disorders.

_____

_____

_____

_____

2. Discuss three diagnostic tests used to diagnose disorders that affect the urinary tract.

_____

_____

3. Summarize the pathophysiology of common urinary tract disorders.

_____

_____

4. List the risk factors of a urinary tract infection (UTI).

_____

_____

_____

CASE STUDY

Christine Scott is a 37-year-old female patient who came to the clinic today. She is complaining of dysuria, hematuria, and urgency. She is diagnosed with cystitis. Answer the following questions based on your knowledge of cystitis.

1. Explain cystitis.

2. What can occur if cystitis is left untreated?

3. Why does cystitis occur more frequently in adult females?

4. List the manifestations of cystitis.

SHORT ANSWERS

Fill in the table regarding manifestations of acute pyelonephritis. Give examples of each.

Urinary	Systemic

NCLEX-RN® REVIEW QUESTIONS

1. Which of the following statements about urinary tract infections (UTIs) is correct?
   1. More than 10 million people are treated annually for UTI.
   2. Community-acquired UTIs are not common in young women and are unusual in men over the age of 50.
   3. Most community-acquired UTIs are caused by *Escherichia coli*, a common gram-positive enteral bacteria.
   4. Catheter-associated UTIs often involve other gram-negative bacteria such as *Proteus, Klebsiella, Serratia,* and *Pseudomonas.*

2. Which of the following statements by a student nurse reflects the need for further clarification concerning the urinary tract?
   1. "The urinary tract is normally sterile below the urethra."
   2. "Adequate urine volume, a free flow from the kidneys through the urinary meatus, and complete bladder emptying are the most important mechanisms for maintaining sterility."
   3. "Pathogens that enter and contaminate the distal urethra are washed out during voiding."
   4. "Other defenses for maintaining sterile urine include its normal acidity and bacteriostatic properties of the bladder and urethral cells."

3. Which of the following types of incontinence is the loss of urine associated with increased intra-abdominal pressure during sneezing, coughing, or lifting in which the quantity of urine lost is usually small?
   1. urge
   2. stress
   3. overflow
   4. functional

4. The nurse is evaluating a student nurse who is providing education to a patient who is receiving a urinary anti-infective. Which of the following statements would be correct?

   1. "These drugs are used along with hygiene practices to prevent recurrent urinary tract infection (UTI). Take as directed, even when no symptoms are present."
   2. "Drink 10–12 glasses of water or fluid per day while taking these drugs."
   3. "Take the drug before meals or food to reduce gastric effects and drink one glass of milk after taking the drug."
   4. "Nitrofurantoin (Furadantin®, Nitrofan) turns the urine blue. This is not harmful and subsides when the drug is discontinued."

5. When discussing the management of urolithiasis, the nurse should recommend which of the following?

   1. Collect and strain all urine, saving any stones.
   2. Do not report stone passage to the physician or bring the stone in for analysis.
   3. Report to physician only the changes in the amount of urine output.
   4. Increase fluid intake to 1550–2450 mL per day.

6. The nurse is evaluating a student nurse's understanding of bladder cancer. Which of the following statements indicates a need for further teaching?

   1. An estimated 70,980 new cases of bladder cancer were diagnosed in the United States in 2009, and 14,330 people died as a result of the disease.
   2. The incidence of bladder cancer is about four times higher in women than it is in men and about twice as high in whites as it is in blacks.
   3. Cigarette smoking is the primary risk factor for bladder cancer.
   4. Most people who develop bladder cancer are over age 60.

7. Diet modifications are often prescribed to change the character of the urine and prevent further lithiasis. The spouse of the patient with lithiasis asks the nurse which of the following foods are high in oxalate?

   1. beans and lentils, dried fruits, canned or smoked fish except tuna, flour, milk and milk products
   2. asparagus, beer and colas, beets, cabbage, celery, fruits, green beans, nuts, tea, and tomatoes
   3. goose, organ meats, sardines and herring, venison; moderate consumption of beef, chicken, crab, pork, salmon, and veal
   4. cheese, cranberries, eggs, grapes, meat and poultry, plums and prunes, tomatoes, and whole grains

8. Which of the following actions is inappropriate for the nurse who is providing urinary stoma care?

   1. Remove old pouch, pulling it away from the skin gently. Use warm water or adhesive solvent to loosen the seal if necessary.
   2. Gather all supplies: a clean, disposable pouch; a liquid skin barrier or barrier ring; 4×4 gauze squares; a stoma guide; an adhesive solvent; clean gloves; and a clean washcloth.
   3. Cleanse skin around the stoma with soap and water, rinse, and pat or air-dry.
   4. Apply the bag with an opening no more than 3–4 mm wider than the outside of the stoma.

9. The nurse is discussing the following points with a patient to help prevent UTI and UI in an older adult. Which statement is correct?

   1. "Maintain a generous fluid intake. Increase fluid intake after the evening meal to reduce nocturia."
   2. "Perform pelvic muscle exercises (Kegel exercises) two times a day to increase perineal muscle tone."
   3. "Increase the consumption of caffeine-containing beverages (coffee, tea, colas), citrus juices, and artificially sweetened beverages that contain NutraSweet®."
   4. "Use behavioral techniques such as scheduled toileting, habit training, and bladder training to reduce the frequency of incontinence."

Nursing Care of Patients with **Kidney Disorders**

LEARNING OUTCOMES

1. Describe the pathophysiology of common kidney disorders, relating pathophysiology to normal functions and manifestations of the disorder.

2. Discuss risk factors for kidney disorders and nursing measures to reduce these risks.

3. Explain diagnostic studies used to identify disorders of the kidneys and their effects.

4. Discuss the effects of and nursing implications for medications and treatments used for patients with kidney disorders.

5. Compare and contrast renal replacement therapies, including dialysis and kidney transplant, to manage acute and chronic renal failure.

MediaLink

Pearson Nursing Student Resources
Audio Glossary
NCLEX-RN® Review

- Care Plan Activity
  - The Patient Undergoing IVP
- Case Studies
  - Patient Having a Kidney Transplant
  - Patient with Kidney Disorder: Acute Glomerulonephritis
- Animations/Videos
  - Acute Renal failure
  - Chronic Renal failure
- MediaLink Applications
- Links to Resources

CLINICAL COMPETENCIES

1. Assess the functional health status of patients with kidney disorders.

2. Recognize, monitor, document, and report unexpected or abnormal manifestations in patients with kidney disorders.

3. Provide safe and effective nursing care for patients undergoing renal replacement therapies, surgery involving the kidneys, or renal transplant.

4. Using assessed data and current standards of practice, determine priority nursing diagnoses and interventions for patients with renal disorders.

5. Plan and implement evidence-based nursing care for patients with renal disorders using research and best practices.

6. Collaborate and coordinate with the patient and other members of the interdisciplinary team to prioritize and implement care.

7. Provide teaching appropriate to the patient and the situation for patients with kidney disorders.

8. Evaluate patient responses to care, revising the plan of care as needed to promote, maintain, or restore functional health status for patients with renal disorders.

TERMS MATCHING

Place the letter of the correct definition in the space next to each item.

1. ____ Acute renal failure (ARF)
2. ____ Acute tubular necrosis (ATN)
3. ____ Azotemia
4. ____ Chronic kidney disease (CKD)
5. ____ Continuous renal replacement therapy (CRRT)
6. ____ Dialysate
7. ____ Dialysis
8. ____ End-stage renal disease (ESRD)
9. ____ Glomerular filtration rate (GFR)
10. ____ Glomerulonephritis
11. ____ Hematuria
12. ____ Hemodialysis
13. ____ Nephrectomy
14. ____ Nephrotic syndrome
15. ____ Oliguria
16. ____ Peritoneal dialysis
17. ____ Plasmapheresis
18. ____ Polycystic kidney disease
19. ____ Proteinuria
20. ____ Renal artery stenosis
21. ____ Renal failure
22. ____ Ultrafiltration
23. ____ Uremia

A. The amount of filtrate made by the kidneys per minute.
B. The diffusion of solute molecules across a semipermeable membrane.
C. Proteins in the urine.
D. Blood in the urine.
E. Removal of the kidney.
F. Urine output of less than 400 mL in 24 hours.
G. A rapid decline in renal function.
H. A condition in which the kidneys are unable to remove accumulated metabolites from the blood.
I. Is defined by the presence of kidney damage for three or more months.
J. Uses the peritoneum surrounding the abdominal cavity as the dialyzing membrane.
K. Gradual occlusion caused by plaque, affecting blood flow to the kidney.
L. A procedure that removes damaging antibodies from the plasma.
M. Destruction of tubular epithelial cells, causing an abrupt and progressive decline of renal function.
N. Blood is continuously circulated through a highly porous hemofilter.
O. Inflammation of the glomerular capillary membrane.
P. A term meaning "urine in the blood" that refers to the syndrome or group of symptoms associated with ESRD.
Q. Increased blood levels of nitrogenous waste.
R. A hereditary disease characterized by formation of fluid-filled cysts and massive kidney enlargement.
S. Excess water is removed by creating a higher hydrostatic pressure of the blood moving through the dialyzer than of the dialysate, which flows in the opposite direction.
T. A procedure in which blood passes through a semipermeable membrane filter outside the body.
U. A solution used for dialysis.
V. A condition marked by massive proteinuria, hypoalbuminemia, hyperlipidemia, and edema.
W. The final phase of chronic renal failure in which little or no kidney function remains.

FOCUSED STUDY

1. Summarize the dialysis procedures used to manage acute and chronic renal failure.

_____

_____

_____

_____

2. Define polycystic kidney disease.

_____

_____

3. List the diagnostic studies used to identify disorders of the kidneys.

_____

_____

_____

_____

_____

4. List the risk factors for acute renal artery thrombosis.

_____

_____

_____

_____

_____

CASE STUDY

Brent Brelle is a 67-year-old male patient admitted to the unit this morning. The physician thinks he might have a renal tumor. His spouse Nancy has several questions about his condition for the nurse. Answer the following questions based on your knowledge of renal tumors.

1. "Why didn't my husband have any signs or symptoms until the last few days?"

2. "What tests might the physician order to determine whether Brent has a renal tumor?"

3. "What is the treatment of choice for a renal tumor?"

SHORT ANSWERS

List possible manifestations associated with each of the following electrolyte imbalances.

Electrolyte Imbalance	Manifestations
Hyperkalemia	
Hyponatremia	
Hyperphosphatemia	

NCLEX-RN® REVIEW QUESTIONS

1. Which of the following statements about glomerular disorders are false? **Select all that apply.**
   1. Glomerular disorders and diseases are the leading cause of chronic kidney disease in the United States.
   2. Hematuria, proteinuria, and hypertension often are late manifestations of glomerular disorders.
   3. Acute poststreptococcal glomerulonephritis (also called acute proliferative glomerulonephritis) is the least common primary glomerular disorder.
   4. Diabetes mellitus, hypertension, and systemic lupus erythematosus (SLE) are common causes of primary glomerulonephritis.

2. You are evaluating a student nurse's understanding of polycystic kidney disease. Which of the following statements by the student nurse indicates a need for further teaching?
   1. Polycystic kidney disease is slowly progressive.
   2. Symptoms usually develop by age 40 to 50.
   3. Common manifestations include flank pain, microscopic or gross hematuria (blood in the urine), proteinuria (proteins in the urine), and polyuria and nocturia because the kidney's concentrating ability is impaired.
   4. The progression to end-stage renal disease tends to occur more rapidly in women than in men.

3. When discussing the nutrition and fluid management with a patient who has chronic kidney disease, the nurse would recommend which of the following?
   1. Water intake of 2–3 L per day is generally recommended to maintain water balance.
   2. Sodium is restricted to 4 g per day initially.
   3. Potassium intake is increased to more than 80 mEq/day.
   4. Daily protein intake is limited to 0.6 g/kg of body weight, or approximately 40 g/day for an average male patient.

4. A nurse is planning a seminar about dialysis. Which of the following is an incorrect statement made by the nurse?
   1. For the patient who is not a candidate for renal transplantation or who has had a transplant failure, dialysis is life-sustaining.
   2. Hemodialysis for end-stage renal disease (ESRD) typically is done three times a week for a total of 9–12 hours.
   3. Patients on long-term dialysis have a higher risk for complications and death than does the general population.
   4. Serum triglyceride levels decrease with peritoneal dialysis.

5. Which of the following is not a risk factor for acute renal failure (ARF)?
   1. major trauma or surgery
   2. infection
   3. hemorrhage
   4. personal hygiene practices

6. A nurse is evaluating a patient's understanding of chronic kidney disease (CKD). Which of the following statements indicates a need for further teaching?
   1. The incidence of CKD and ESRD is significantly higher in people aged 65 and older.
   2. People of Hispanic origin have a higher incidence of CKD and ESRD than do non-Hispanics.
   3. Hypertension is the leading cause of CKD, followed by diabetes mellitus.
   4. Men are more likely to be affected by CKD and ESRD than are women.

7. The nurse who is evaluating a kidney transplant class recognizes that further teaching is necessary when a participant makes which of the following statements?
   1. The donor kidney is placed in the upper abdominal cavity of the recipient, and the renal artery, vein, and ureter are anastomosed.
   2. Kidney transplant improves both survival and quality of life for the patient with end-stage renal disease (ESRD).
   3. Most transplanted kidneys are obtained from deceased donors.
   4. Hypertension is a possible complication of a kidney transplant.

8. Which of the following phases is not typically included in the course of acute renal failure due to acute tubular necrosis (ATN)?
   1. intrarenal
   2. initiation
   3. maintenance
   4. recovery

Assessing the Cardiovascular and Lymphatic Systems

29 CHAPTER

LEARNING OUTCOMES

1. Describe the anatomy, physiology, and functions of the cardiovascular and lymphatic systems.
2. Describe normal variations in cardiovascular assessment findings for the older adult.
3. Give examples of genetic disorders of the cardiovascular system.
4. Identify specific topics for consideration during a health history assessment interview of the patient with cardiovascular or lymphatic disorders.
5. Explain techniques used to assess cardiovascular and lymphatic structure and function.
6. Identify manifestations of impaired cardiovascular structure and functions.

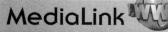

MediaLink

Pearson Nursing Student Resource
Audio Glossary
NCLEX-RN® Review
- Care Plan Activity
  - Cardiac Catheterization
- Case Study
  - Chest Pain
- MediaLink Application
- Links to Resources

CLINICAL COMPETENCIES

1. Assess an ECG strip and identify normal rhythm and cardiac events and abnormal cardiac rhythm.
2. Conduct and document a health history for patients having alterations in the structure and functions of the cardiovascular or lymphatic systems.
3. Conduct and document a physical assessment of cardiovascular and lymphatic status.
4. Monitor the results of diagnostic tests and report abnormal findings.

TERMS MATCHING

Place the letter of the correct definition in the space next to each term.

1. ____ Apical impulse
2. ____ Cardiac index (CI)
3. ____ Cardiac output (CO)
4. ____ Dysrhythmia
5. ____ Heave
6. ____ Ischemic
7. ____ Korotkoff's sounds
8. ____ Lifts
9. ____ Lymphadenopathy
10. ____ Lymphedema
11. ____ Murmur
12. ____ Orthostatic hypotension
13. ____ Retraction
14. ____ Thrill
15. ____ Thrust

A. An abnormal heart rate or rhythm.

B. Deprived of oxygen.

C. A decrease in systolic BP of more than 10–15 mmHg and a drop in diastolic BP upon standing.

D. The cardiac output that is adjusted for the patient's body size; provides meaningful data about the heart's ability to perfuse the tissues; a more accurate indicator of the effectiveness of the circulation.

E. A visible pulsation.

F. The amount of blood pumped by the ventricles into the pulmonary and systemic circulations in one minute.

G. A palpable vibration over the precordium or an artery.

H. Enlargement of lymph nodes.

I. The sounds that can be auscultated when the nurse takes the patient's blood pressure.

J. An abnormal blowing sound that is heard during auscultation of blood vessels.

K. Pulsations that cannot be classified as normal apical pulsations; also known as lifts.

L. Swelling that occurs due to lymphatic obstruction.

M. A pulling in of tissue.

N. A normal, visible pulsation in the area of the midclavicular line in the left fifth intercostal space.

O. Pulsations that cannot be classified as normal apical pulsations; also known as heaves.

FOCUSED STUDY

1. Describe the cardiac cycle.

_____

_____

_____

2. Describe how the following factors can influence arterial blood pressure.

Sympathetic and parasympathetic nervous systems: _____

_____

Baroreceptors and chemoreceptors: _____

_____

Kidneys: _____

_____

Temperature: _____

_____

Chemicals, hormones, and drugs: _____

_____

Diet: _____

3. Explain how red blood cells are destroyed.

_____

_____

_____

4. List four topics the nurse should ask the patient regarding possible genetic influences on the patient's health.

_____

_____

_____

_____

CASE STUDY

Jonathan Drake is a 63-year-old male patient who is scheduled for an electrocardiogram and a treadmill test (stress test). Mr. Drake has had recent episodes of chest pain with activity. Answer the following questions based on your knowledge of caring for patients who require a cardiovascular assessment and diagnostic testing.

1. What is an electrocardiogram (ECG)?

2. How are ECG waveforms recorded?

3. The experienced nurse who works in cardiovascular testing has been asked to interpret Mr. Drake's ECG results. What six steps are used to interpret an ECG?

4. Mr. Drake is preparing for the stress test. About what should the nurse educate Mr. Drake prior to the test?

5. During the stress test, Mr. Drake complains of chest pain. What are some common ways that patients describe chest pain?

6. With further testing, the physician determines that Mr. Drake's heart rate is 92 beats per minute and his stroke volume is 40 mL/ beat. Calculate Mr. Drake's cardiac output.

7. Mr. Drake has blood drawn to determine his lipid levels. His cholesterol is 392 mg/dL, and triglycerides are 210 mg/dL. What are normal values?

SHORT ANSWERS

Fill in the blanks noting the significance of each age-related change in the patient.

Age-Related Change	Significance
Myocardium: ⬇ efficiency and contractibility Sinus node: ⬆ in thickness of shell surrounding the node and ⬇ in the number of pacemaker cells	
Left ventricle: Slight hypertrophy, prolonged isometric contraction phase and relaxation time; ⬆ time for diastolic filling and systolic emptying cycle	
Valves and blood vessels: Elongated and dilated aorta, thicker and more rigid valves, and increase in resistance to peripheral blood flow by 1% per year	
Bone marrow: ⬇ ability of bone marrow to respond to need for increased RBCs, WBCs, and platelets	
Blood vessels: Tunica intima: fibrosis, calcium and lipid accumulation, cellular proliferation Tunica media: thins, elastin fibers calcify; increase in calcium results in stiffening. Baroreceptor function is impaired, and peripheral resistance increases.	
Immune system: Impaired function of B and T lymphocytes; ⬇ production of antibodies	

NCLEX-RN® REVIEW QUESTIONS

1. What covers the entire heart and great vessels and then folds over to form the parietal layer that lines the pericardium and adheres to the heart surface?
   1. endocardium
   2. myocardium
   3. epicardium
   4. parietal pericardium

2. You are evaluating a student nurse's understanding of the heart. Which of the following statements indicates the need for further education?
   1. The right atrium receives deoxygenated blood from the veins of the body.
   2. The left ventricle receives deoxygenated blood from the left atrium and pumps it through the pulmonary artery to the pulmonary capillary bed for oxygenation.
   3. The left atrium receives freshly oxygenated blood from the lungs through the pulmonary veins.
   4. The superior vena cava returns blood from the body area above the diaphragm, the inferior vena cava returns blood from the body below the diaphragm, and the coronary sinus drains blood from the heart.

3. The greater the volume, the greater the stretch of the cardiac muscle fibers and the greater the force with which the fibers contract to accomplish emptying. This principle is called _____ law of the heart.
   1. Stuart's
   2. Starling's
   3. Sarton's
   4. Schell's

4. Which of the following statements by a student nurse reflects an accurate understanding regarding the conduction system of the heart?
   1. The AV node acts as the normal "pacemaker" of the heart, usually generating an impulse 60–100 times per minute.
   2. The AV node is located at the junction of the superior vena cava and right atrium.
   3. The cellular action potential serves as the basis for electrocardiography, a diagnostic test of cardiac function.
   4. The electrical stimulus decreases the permeability of the cell membrane, which creates an action potential (electrical potential).

5. Which of the following conditions may lead to an increase in red blood cell production? **Select all that apply.**
   1. coronary artery disease
   2. renal failure
   3. emphysema
   4. cirrhosis
   5. pneumonia

6. Which of the following statements indicates the need for further education regarding white blood cells?
   1. Neutrophils are active phagocytes.
   2. Immature neutrophils are called bands.
   3. Lymphocytes are phagocytic cells that mature into macrophages.
   4. Basophils and eosinophils increase in number during allergic reactions.

Nursing Care of Patients with **Coronary Heart Disease**

LEARNING OUTCOMES

1. Discuss the coronary circulation and electrical properties of the heart.

2. Compare and contrast the pathophysiology and manifestations of coronary heart disease and common cardiac dysrhythmias.

3. Describe interdisciplinary and nursing care for patients with coronary heart disease and or cardiac dysrhythmias.

4. Relate the outcomes of diagnostic tests and procedures to the pathophysiology of cardiac disorders and implications for patient responses to the disorder.

5. Discuss nursing implications for medications and treatments used to prevent and treat coronary heart disease and dysrhythmias.

6. Describe nursing care for the patient undergoing diagnostic testing, an interventional procedure, or surgery for coronary heart disease or a dysrhythmia.

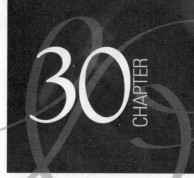

MediaLink

Pearson Nursing Student Resources
Audio Glossary
NCLEX-RN® Review
- Care Plan Activity
  - The Patient with a Temporary Pacemaker
- Case Study
  - The Patient with Coronary Artery Disease: Myocardial Infarction
- Animations/Videos
  - Acute Coronary Syndrome
  - Atherosclerosis
  - Acute MI
- MediaLink Applications
- Links to Resources

CLINICAL COMPETENCIES

1. Assess functional health status of patients with coronary heart disease and/or a dysrhythmia, including the impact of the disorder on the patient's ability to perform activities of daily living and usual tasks.

2. Use knowledge of the normal anatomy and physiology of the heart in caring for patients with coronary heart disease.

3. Monitor patients with coronary heart disease or dysrhythmias for expected and unexpected manifestations, reporting and recording findings as indicated.

4. Use assessed data to select nursing diagnoses, determine priorities of care, and develop and implement individualized nursing interventions for patients with coronary heart disease and dysrhythmias.

5. Administer medications and treatments for patients with coronary heart disease and dysrhythmias safely and knowledgably.

6. Integrate interdisciplinary care into nursing care planning and implementation for patients with coronary heart disease and dysrhythmias.

7. Provide appropriate teaching for prevention, health promotion, and self-care related to coronary heart disease and dysrhythmias.

8. Evaluate the effectiveness of nursing interventions, revising or modifying the plan of care as needed to promote, maintain, or restore functional health for patients with coronary heart disease or dysrhythmias.

TERMS MATCHING

Place the letter of the correct definition in the space next to each term.

1. ____ Acute coronary syndrome (ACS)

2. ____ Acute myocardial infarction (AMI)

3. ____ Angina pectoris

4. ____ Atherosclerosis

5. ____ Atrial kick

6. ____ Cardiac arrest

7. ____ Cardiac rehabilitation

8. ____ Cardiovascular disease (CVD)

9. ____ Collateral channels

10. ____ Coronary heart disease (CHD)

11. ____ Dysrhythmia

12. ____ Ectopic beats

13. ____ Heart block

14. ____ Ischemia

15. ____ Pacemaker

16. ____ Paroxysmal

17. ____ Sudden cardiac death

A. A term used to describe the small coronary arteries that join together to increase blood flow to the myocardium.

B. Chest pain that results from reduced coronary blood flow, which causes a temporary imbalance between myocardial blood supply and demand.

C. Disorders of myocardial blood flow.

D. Myocardial tissue death.

E. A block in the heart's normal conduction pathways.

F. A problem that may develop when the oxygen supply is inadequate to meet metabolic demands.

G. A progressive disease characterized by atheroma formation, which affects the intimal and medial layers of large and midsize arteries.

H. A disturbance or irregularity of the heart's rhythm.

I. An emergency condition where the ventricles are not contracting and there is no cardiac output.

J. A term used to describe when a condition abruptly begins or ends.

K. A long-term program that includes medical evaluation, education, exercise, counseling, and risk factor modification; designed to reduce the psychologic and physical effects associated with cardiac illness.

L. An unexpected death that occurs within one hour of the onset of cardiovascular symptoms.

M. The AV nodal delay that allows the atria to contract and for an extra bolus of blood to be delivered to the ventricles before they contract.

N. Aberrant impulses may originate outside normal conduction pathways and cause this to occur; this interrupts the normal conduction sequence and may not initiate a normal muscle contraction.

O. A device or cells in the heart that have the ability to spontaneously initiate an electrical impulse.

P. A generic term for disorders of the heart and blood vessels.

Q. A condition of unstable and severe cardiac ischemia.

FOCUSED STUDY

1. Describe coronary circulation.

_____

_____

_____

2. Briefly describe the following diagnostic tests that can be performed to diagnose or assess risk factors associated with coronary heart disease.

Total serum cholesterol: _____

_____

C-reactive protein: _____

_____

Ankle-brachial blood pressure index: _____

_____

Exercise electrocardiogram (ECG) testing: _____

_____

Electron beam computed tomography (EBCT): _____

_____

Myocardial perfusion imaging: _____

_____

3. List the medications that can be used to treat acute and chronic types of angina. Briefly describe how each type of medication works.

_____

_____

_____

_____

_____

_____

_____

4. Discuss the nursing interventions that should be included in the care plan of a patient who is experiencing acute chest pain. Include rationale for each intervention.

_____

_____

_____

_____

_____

_____

CASE STUDY

Bradley Baldwin's elderly mother was recently diagnosed with coronary heart disease. He and his mother have created a list of questions to ask during a scheduled office visit. Answer the following questions based on your understanding of coronary heart disease.

1. What are some modifiable and nonmodifiable risk factors for coronary heart disease (CHD)?

2. What are atheromas?

3. What are some characteristics of metabolic syndrome?

4. Mr. Baldwin received training on how to perform cardiopulmonary resuscitation (CPR) 10 months ago. He asks the nurse to refresh his memory about how to perform CPR.

5. Mr. Baldwin's mother states, "I quit smoking three months ago. Will that have any effect on my lipid levels?" How should the nurse respond?

6. Mr. Baldwin requests information about how eating fish can reduce his mother's risk factors.

7. Mr. Baldwin's mother requests information about how exercise can reduce her risk factors.

CARE PLAN CRITICAL-THINKING ACTIVITY

1. Explain synchronized cardioversion.

_____

_____

_____

2. Why is diazepam used during synchronized cardioversion?

_____

_____

_____

3. Why is it important to know that Ms. Vasquez had rheumatic fever as a child?

_____

_____

SHORT ANSWERS

Fill in the blanks regarding dietary recommendations to reduce CHD risk.

Nutrient	Recommendation
Calories	
Total fat	
Saturated fats	
Polyunsaturated fat	
Monounsaturated fat	
Cholesterol	
Carbohydrate (primarily complex carbohydrates such as whole grains, fruits, and vegetables)	
Dietary fiber	
Protein	

NCLEX-RN® REVIEW QUESTIONS

1. The nurse is teaching a course about coronary heart disease (CHD). The nurse recognizes that further teaching is necessary when which of the following statements is made by a participant in the class?
1. CHD is caused by impaired blood flow to the myocardium.
2. CHD is always associated with signs or symptoms.
3. CHD affects 13.2 million people in the United States and causes more than 500,000 deaths annually.
4. Accumulation of atherosclerotic plaque in the coronary arteries is the usual cause of CHD.

2. The patient has been diagnosed with metabolic syndrome. Which of the following would be an unexpected finding during the nurse's assessment of this patient?
1. hypertension
2. elevated fasting blood glucose
3. high HDL
4. abdominal obesity

3. A nurse is providing education to a patient about antianginal medications. Which of the following statements would demonstrate to the nurse that the patient needs further education?
1. "If the first nitrate dose does not relieve angina within five minutes, I'll take a second dose. After five more minutes, I may take a third dose if needed. If the pain is unrelieved or lasts 20 minutes or longer, I'll seek medical assistance immediately."
2. "I'll carry a supply of nitroglycerin tablets with me. I should dissolve sublingual nitroglycerin tablets under my tongue or between the upper lip and gum. I cannot eat, drink, or smoke until the tablet is completely dissolved."
3. "I'll keep the sublingual tablets in any plastic bottle and I'll replace the supply every 12 months."
4. "I'll rotate the ointment or transdermal patch application sites. I'll apply to a hairless area; I'll spread ointment evenly without rubbing or massaging. I'll remove the patch or residual ointment at bedtime daily and apply a fresh dose in the morning."

4. Which of the following is a cause of sudden cardiac death? **Select all that apply.**
   1. dissecting aortic aneurysm
   2. choking
   3. mitral valve prolapse
   4. pulmonary embolism
   5. myocarditis
5. When a nurse is performing CPR on an adult patient, which of the following actions is correct?
   1. Open the airway using the head-thrust, chin-thrust maneuver.
   2. Check the brachial artery for a pulse.
   3. Provide two breaths after every 30 compressions.
   4. Assess for responsiveness by flicking the patient's foot.
6. What is a deficient blood flow to tissue that may be caused by partial obstruction of a coronary artery, a coronary artery spasm, or a thrombus?
   1. atrial kick
   2. angina pectoris
   3. ectopic beats
   4. ischemia
7. A nurse is presenting a seminar about myocardial infarction (MI) to patients who have been diagnosed with coronary heart disease. Which of the following statements by a patient demonstrates the need for further teaching?
   1. MI occurs when blood flow to a portion of cardiac muscle is completely blocked, which results in prolonged tissue ischemia and irreversible cell damage.
   2. MI usually affects the right ventricle because it is the major "workhorse" of the heart; its muscle mass and oxygen demands are greater.
   3. MIs are described by the damaged area of the heart.
   4. Risk factors for MI are the same as those for coronary heart disease: age, gender, heredity, race, smoking, obesity, hyperlipidemia, hypertension, diabetes, sedentary lifestyle, and diet, among others.

31 Nursing Care of Patients with Cardiac Disorders

LEARNING OUTCOMES

1. Compare and contrast the etiology, pathophysiology, and manifestations of common cardiac disorders including heart failure, structural disorders, and inflammatory disorders.

2. Explain risk factors and preventive measures for cardiac disorders such as heart failure, inflammatory disorders, and valve disorders.

3. Discuss indications for and management of patients with hemodynamic monitoring.

4. Discuss the effects and nursing implications for medications commonly prescribed for patients with cardiac disorders.

5. Describe nursing care for the patient undergoing cardiac surgery or cardiac transplant.

CLINICAL COMPETENCIES

1. Apply knowledge of normal cardiac anatomy and physiology and assessment techniques in caring for patients with cardiac disorders.

2. Assess functional health status of patients with cardiac disorders, documenting and reporting deviations for expected findings.

3. Based on patient assessment and knowledge of the disorder, determine priority nursing diagnoses.

4. Plan, prioritize, and provide evidence-based, individualized care for patients with cardiac disorders.

5. Safely and knowledgeably administer prescribed medications and treatments to patients with cardiac disorders.

6. Actively participate in planning and coordinating interdisciplinary care for patients with cardiac disorders.

7. Provide appropriate teaching and community-based care for patients with cardiac disorders and their families.

8. Evaluate the effectiveness of nursing care, revising the plan of care as needed to promote, maintain, or restore functional health status of patients with cardiac disorders.

MediaLink

Pearson Nursing Student Resources
Audio Glossary
NCLEX-RN® Review
- Care Plan Activity
  - Acute Pulmonary Edema
- Case Study
  - The Patient with Cardiac Disorders
- Animations/Videos
  - Heart Failure Symptoms
  - Pericarditis
- MediaLink Applications
- Links to Resources

TERMS MATCHING

Place the letter of the correct definition in the space next to each term.

1. _____ Aortic valve
2. _____ Cardiac tamponade
3. _____ Cardiomyopathy
4. _____ Endocarditis
5. _____ Heart failure
6. _____ Hemodynamics
7. _____ Mean arterial pressure (MAP)
8. _____ Mitral valve
9. _____ Myocarditis
10. _____ Orthopnea
11. _____ Paroxysmal nocturnal dyspnea
12. _____ Pericarditis
13. _____ Pulmonary edema
14. _____ Pulmonic valve
15. _____ Regurgitation
16. _____ Rheumatic fever
17. _____ Rheumatic heart disease
18. _____ Stenosis
19. _____ Tricuspid valve
20. _____ Valvular heart disease

A. A valve of the heart that lies between the left atrium and the left ventricle.

B. This occurs when the valve fails to close properly, allowing blood to flow back through it.

C. A condition where the heart becomes compressed.

D. The average pressure in the arterial circulation throughout the cardiac cycle; an indicator of tissue perfusion.

E. The patient awakens at night acutely short of breath.

F. A valve of the heart that lies between the right ventricle and the pulmonary artery.

G. A condition that interferes with the smooth flow of blood through the heart; blood flow becomes turbulent, causing a murmur.

H. A diverse group of disorders that affect the myocardium.

I. A valve of the heart that is located between the right atrium and the right ventricle.

J. An abnormal accumulation of fluid in the interstitial tissue and alveoli of the lung.

K. The study of forces involved in blood circulation.

L. This occurs when a narrowed fused valve obstructs forward blood flow through it.

M. A slowly progressive valvular deformity that may follow acute or repeated attacks of rheumatic fever.

N. Inflammation of the endocardium.

O. Inflammation of the pericardium.

P. A systemic inflammatory disease caused by an abnormal immune response to pharyngeal infection by group A beta-hemolytic streptococci.

Q. Inflammation of the heart muscle.

R. The patient experiences difficulty breathing while lying down.

S. The valve that lies between the left ventricle and the aorta.

T. The most common cardiac disorder; the heart is unable to pump enough blood to meet the metabolic demands of the body.

FOCUSED STUDY

1. Describe the four stages of heart failure.

_____

_____

_____

_____

_____

2. Discuss the differences between acute and subacute infective endocarditis.

_____

_____

_____

_____

3. Discuss the different causes and clinical manifestations associated with dilated, hypertrophic, and restrictive cardiomyopathies.

_____

_____

_____

_____

_____

4. Explain the nursing responsibilities associated with administering positive inotropic agents.

_____

_____

_____

_____

CASE STUDY

James Hacking is a 76-year-old patient who has been admitted to the hospital with left-sided heart failure. A student nurse is observing the nurse care for Mr. Hacking. The student nurse asks the following questions about Mr. Hacking's condition.

1. What is heart failure?

2. What are the causes of heart failure?

3. What are some clinical manifestations associated with left-sided heart failure?

4. What are the complications of heart failure?

5. How is heart failure diagnosed?

6. Mr. Hacking's physician states that she wants a Swan-Ganz catheter to be placed. The student nurse requests information about this catheter and an explanation as to how it can be used to monitor Mr. Hacking's condition.

7. Mr. Hacking's physician writes an order for the nurse to administer fosinopril (Monopril®). The student nurse requests information about what type of medication this is and how it works.

CARE PLAN CRITICAL-THINKING ACTIVITY

Please refer to the case study and nursing care plan exercise: A Patient with Heart Failure (page 987 in your textbook) to answer the following questions.

1. Why is it important for Ms. Snow to keep a weekly record of symptoms and their frequency for one month?

2. List two drinks or food items that contain caffeine.

3. What is a complication of mitral valve prolapse about which Ms. Snow should be educated?

CROSSWORD PUZZLE

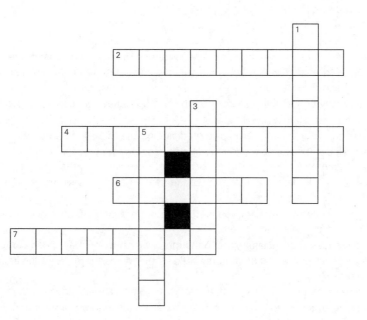

Across

2   The force needed to eject blood into the circulation

4   When the _____ nervous system is stimulated, the heart rate and contractility increase.

6   The amount of blood that returns to the ventricles

7   The ventricular filling time

Down

1   The ability of the heart to increase cardiac output to meet demand is the _____ reserve.

3   The volume of blood ejected with each heartbeat is the _____ volume.

5   The volume of blood in the ventricles prior to contraction

NCLEX-RN® REVIEW QUESTIONS

1. A new nurse is providing education about prosthetic heart valves to a patient. Which of the following is considered an advantage of a prosthetic heart valve?
    1. long-term durability
    2. low incidence of thromboembolism
    3. no need for long-term anticoagulation
    4. quietness

2. During discharge planning, the nurse is teaching the patient with heart failure about home activity guidelines. Which of the following instructions is correct?
    1. "Eat three large meals each day."
    2. "It is okay to lift heavy objects."
    3. "Eat a low-fiber diet and restrict fluid intake."
    4. "Begin a graded exercise program."

3. A nurse is evaluating a patient's understanding about managing valvular disease. Which of the following patient statements indicates the need for further teaching?

   1. "I will notify all of my healthcare providers about my valve disease."
   2. "I should have adequate rest to prevent fatigue."
   3. "I need to call my healthcare provider if I think I'm bleeding anywhere."
   4. "I will follow the diet restrictions to increase my body's ability to retain fluid."

4. The nurse is preparing to educate the patient about how to reduce the risk factors associated with heart failure. Which of the following nursing interventions would be an unexpected addition to the patient's plan of care?

   1. Teach about coronary heart disease, which is a primary cause of heart failure.
   2. Stress the relationship between effective management of cirrhosis and reduced risk of heart failure.
   3. Discuss the importance of monitoring weight daily.
   4. Discuss the importance of taking antihypertensive medications as ordered to reduce the risk for heart failure.

5. A nurse is providing an educational seminar about pulmonary edema for nurses who work in the intensive care unit. Which of the following statements from one of the participants demonstrates the need for further education?

   1. "In cardiogenic pulmonary edema, the contractility of the right ventricle is severely impaired."
   2. "Pulmonary edema is a medical emergency."
   3. "Immediate treatment for acute pulmonary edema focuses on restoring effective gas exchange and reducing fluid and pressure in the pulmonary vascular system."
   4. "The patient often is restless and highly anxious, although severe hypoxia may cause confusion or lethargy."

6. Which of the following statements by a student nurse reflects the needs for further education regarding rheumatic fever and rheumatic heart disease?

   1. "Rheumatic heart disease frequently damages the heart valves and is a major cause of mitral and aortic valve disorders."
   2. "Rheumatic fever is a systemic inflammatory disease caused by an abnormal immune response to pharyngeal infection by group A beta-hemolytic streptococci."
   3. "The peak incidence of rheumatic fever is in patients aged 22 to 35."
   4. "Rheumatic fever and rheumatic heart disease remain significant public health problems in many developing countries."

Nursing Care of Patients with **Vascular** and Lymphatic Disorders

LEARNING OUTCOMES

1. Compare and contrast the manifestations and effects of disorders affecting large and small vessels, arteries, and veins.
2. Explain risk factors for and measures to prevent peripheral vascular disorders and their complications.
3. Explain the nursing implications for medications and other interdisciplinary treatments used for patients with peripheral vascular disorders.
4. Describe preoperative and postoperative nursing care of patients having vascular surgery.
5. Relate the manifestations and diagnostic test results to the etiology, and pathophysiology of common peripheral vascular and lymphatic disorders.

CLINICAL COMPETENCIES

1. Assess patients with peripheral vascular disorders using data to select and prioritize appropriate nursing diagnoses and identify desired outcomes of care.
2. Identify the effects of peripheral vascular disorders on the functional health status of assigned patients.
3. Use research and an evidence base to plan and provide individualized care for patients with peripheral vascular disorders.
4. Collaborate with the interdisciplinary care team in planning and providing care for patients with peripheral vascular disorders.
5. Safely and knowledgably administer medications and prescribed treatments for patients with peripheral vascular disorders.
6. Provide patient and family teaching to promote, maintain, and restore health in patients with common peripheral vascular disorders.

MediaLink

Pearson Nursing Student Resources
Audio Glossary
NCLEX-RN® Review

- Care Plan Activity
  - Peripheral Vascular System
- Case Studies
  - The Patient with Hematologic and Peripheral Vascular Disorders
  - The Patient Experiencing Disseminated Intravascular Coagulation
  - The Patient with Peripheral Vascular Disease
- Animations/Videos
  - Aortic Aneurysm
  - DVT
  - HTN
- MediaLink Application
- Links to Resources

TERMS MATCHING

Place the letter of the correct definition in the space next to each term.

1. ____ Aneurysm
2. ____ Atherosclerosis
3. ____ Blood pressure
4. ____ Chronic venous insufficiency
5. ____ Deep venous thrombosis (DVT)
6. ____ Diastolic blood pressure
7. ____ Dissection
8. ____ Embolism
9. ____ Hypertension
10. ____ Intermittent claudication
11. ____ Lymphedema
12. ____ Mean arterial pressure (MAP)
13. ____ Peripheral vascular disease (PVD)
14. ____ Primary hypertension
15. ____ Pulse pressure
16. ____ Raynaud's disease/phenomenon
17. ____ Secondary hypertension
18. ____ Systolic blood pressure
19. ____ Thromboangiitis obliterans
20. ____ Thromboembolus
21. ____ Thrombus
22. ____ Varicose veins
23. ____ Vasoconstriction
24. ____ Vasodilation
25. ____ Venous thrombosis

A. An occlusive vascular disease in which small and midsize peripheral arteries become inflamed and spastic, which causes clots to form; also called Buerger's disease.

B. Irregular, tortuous veins with incompetent valves.

C. An abnormal dilation of a blood vessel, commonly at a site of a weakness or tear in the vessel wall.

D. Narrowing of the vessel lumen.

E. A form of arteriosclerosis in which deposits of fat and fibrin obstruct and harden the arteries.

F. The tension or pressure exerted by blood against arterial walls.

G. Disorders characterized by episodes of intense vasospasm in the small arteries and arterioles of the fingers and sometimes the toes.

H. A disorder of inadequate venous return over a prolonged period.

I. A condition that occurs when fat and fibrin obstruct and harden the arteries that affect the peripheral circulation.

J. The sudden obstruction of a blood vessel by debris.

K. Expansion of a vessel.

L. An elevated blood pressure that results from an identifiable underlying process.

M. A tear in the intima of an artery with hemorrhage into the media.

N. This can be calculated by subtracting the diastolic blood pressure from the systolic blood pressure.

O. A term used to describe the minimum amount of pressure that is needed during diastole to maintain blood flow through the capillary beds.

P. The average pressure in the arterial circulation throughout the cardiac cycle.

Q. The sudden obstruction of a blood vessel by a thrombus.

R. Cramping or pain in the leg muscles brought on by exercise and relieved by rest.

S. This can be auscultated when the blood pressure rises as the heart contracts during systole, ejecting its blood.

T. A persistently elevated systemic blood pressure; also known as essential hypertension.

U. Excess pressure in the arterial portion of systemic circulation.

V. A disorder characterized by extremity edema due to accumulation of lymph.

W. A condition in which a blood clot forms on the wall of a vein, accompanied by inflammation of the vein wall and some degree of obstructed venous blood flow; also known as thrombophlebitis.

X. When thrombi form in superficial or deep veins; a common complication of hospitalization, surgery, and immobilization.

Y. A blood clot.

FOCUSED STUDY

1. Discuss the complex interactions and factors that result in primary hypertension.

_____

_____

_____

_____

2. Identify the ways that varicose veins can be diagnosed.

_____

_____

_____

_____

_____

3. Explain the nursing interventions that should be included in the plan of care for a patient who has developed fluid volume excess due to lymphedema.

_____

_____

_____

4. Describe the clinical manifestations associated with progressive lymphedema.

_____

_____

_____

_____

CASE STUDIES

Case Study 1

Josh Bradley is a 32-year-old patient who was admitted to the hospital yesterday with a hypertensive emergency. He tells the nurse that his physician was in early this morning and told him something about an arterial blood pressure, PVR, and MAP, but he can't remember what the physician said about each of them. Answer the following questions based on your knowledge of caring for a patient with a vascular disorder.

1. What factors influence arterial blood pressure?

2. Explain peripheral vascular resistance (PVR) and mean arterial pressure (MAP).

3. What are some common clinical manifestations found in patients experiencing hypertensive emergencies?

Case Study 2

Elizabeth Drake is a 44-year-old female patient who is visiting her physician's office to have her blood pressure checked. She is 5'5" and weighs 125 pounds. She states that she currently smokes one pack per day and drinks alcohol socially. The physician diagnoses her with primary hypertension. Answer the following questions based on your knowledge of caring for a patient with primary hypertension.

1. Discuss the manifestations of primary hypertension.

2. Explain the complications of primary hypertension.

3. Briefly summarize the lifestyle changes Ms. Drake should enact to help control her hypertension.

SHORT ANSWERS

Fill in the information regarding arterial ulcers and venous ulcers.

Factor	Arterial Ulcers	Venous Ulcers
Location		
Ulcer appearance		
Skin appearance		
Skin temperature		
Edema		
Pain		
Gangrene		
Pulses		

NCLEX-RN® REVIEW QUESTIONS

1. Which of the following is felt as the peripheral pulse and heard as Korotkoff's sounds during blood pressure measurement?
   1. diastolic blood pressure
   2. systolic blood pressure
   3. pulse pressure
   4. mean arterial pressure

2. The nursing instructor asks the student nurse to provide the formula used to calculate the MAP. Which of the following formulas should the student nurse provide for the instructor?
   1. [diastolic BP + 2 (systolic BP)] / 2
   2. [systolic BP + 2 (diastolic BP)] / 2
   3. [systolic BP + 2 (diastolic BP)] / 3
   4. [diastolic BP + 2 (systolic BP)] / 3

3. The nurse is implementing nursing interventions that can be used to reduce the risk of aneurysm rupture. Which of the following would be an unexpected addition to the patient's care plan?
   1. Maintain bed rest with legs elevated.
   2. Maintain a calm environment and implement measures to reduce psychologic stress.
   3. Instruct patient to prevent straining during defecation and to avoid holding his or her breath while moving.
   4. Administer beta blockers and antihypertensives as prescribed.

4. Which of the following statements by a student nurse reflects an adequate understanding of Raynaud's disease?
   1. "The disease affects primarily older women between the ages of 60 and 80."
   2. "It is characterized by episodes of intense vasospasm in the small veins of the fingers and sometimes the toes."
   3. "It has no identifiable cause."
   4. "It has been called the 'red-yellow-white' disease."

5. A nurse is planning an educational program about varicose veins. Which of the following statements is correct?
   1. Elastic stockings should be removed eight times a day for 15 minutes.
   2. Complications of varicose veins include venous insufficiency and stasis ulcers.
   3. Prolonged sitting, the force of gravity, lack of leg exercise, and incompetent venous valves all weaken the muscle-pumping mechanism, which reduces arteriole blood return to the heart.
   4. Varicose veins may be asymptomatic, but most cause manifestations such as severe aching leg pain, leg spasms, leg lightness, itching, or feelings of coldness in the legs.

6. During discharge planning, the nurse is teaching the patient about factors that contribute to hypertension. Which of the following is considered a modifiable risk factor?
   1. obesity
   2. age
   3. race
   4. family history

7. The patient has been diagnosed with lymphangitis. Which of the following statements by the patient indicates that she has an adequate understanding about this condition?
   1. "I just have some enlarged lymph nodes."
   2. "These red streaks and my fever are related to an infection."
   3. "The lymphangiography for which I'm scheduled can also be curative."
   4. "I really need to drink more fluids."

Nursing Care of Patients with Hematologic Disorders

33 CHAPTER

LEARNING OUTCOMES

1. Relate the physiology and assessment of the hematologic system and related systems to commonly occurring hematologic disorders.

2. Describe the pathophysiology of common hematologic disorders.

3. Explain nursing implications for medications and other treatments prescribed for hematologic disorders.

4. Discuss indications for and complications of bone marrow or stem cell transplantation, as well as related nursing care.

5. Compare and contrast the pathophysiology, manifestations, and management of bleeding disorders.

6. Describe the major types of leukemia and the most common treatment modalities and nursing interventions.

7. Differentiate Hodgkin's disease from non-Hodgkin's lymphomas.

MediaLink

Pearson Nursing Student Resources
Audio Glossary
NCLEX-RN® Review

- Care Plan Activity
  - Acute Myelocytic Leukemia
- Case Study
  - Disseminated Intravascular Coagulation
- Animations/Videos
  - Iron Deficiency Anemia
  - Sickle Cell Anemia
- MediaLink Applications
- Links to Resources

CLINICAL COMPETENCIES

1. Assess effects of hematologic disorders and prescribed treatments on patients' functional health status.

2. Monitor and document continuing assessment data, including laboratory test results, subjective and objective information, and reporting data outside the normal or expected range.

3. Based on knowledge of pathophysiology, prescribed treatment, and assessed data, identify and prioritize nursing diagnoses for patients with hematologic disorders.

4. Use nursing research and evidence-based practice to identify and implement individualized nursing interventions for the patient with a hematologic disorder.

5. Safely administer prescribed medications and treatments for patients with hematologic disorders.

6. Collaborate with the interdisciplinary care team to plan and provide coordinated, effective care for patients with hematologic disorders.

7. Provide appropriate teaching for patients with hematologic disorders, evaluating learning and the need for continued reinforcement of information.

8. Use continuing assessment data to revise the plan of care as needed to restore, maintain, or promote functional health in the patient with a hematologic disorder.

TERMS MATCHING

Place the letter of the correct definition in the space next to each term.

1. ____ Anemia
2. ____ Aplastic anemia
3. ____ Bone marrow transplant
4. ____ Disseminated intravascular coagulation (DIC)
5. ____ Hemolytic anemia
6. ____ Hemophilia
7. ____ Hemostasis
8. ____ Iron-deficiency anemia
9. ____ Leukemia
10. ____ Lymphoma
11. ____ Multiple myeloma
12. ____ Myelodysplastic syndrome
13. ____ Pernicious anemia
14. ____ Polycythemia
15. ____ Sickle cell anemia
16. ____ Sickle cell crisis
17. ____ Stem cell transplant
18. ____ Thalassemia
19. ____ Thrombocytopenia

A. A group of hereditary clotting factor disorders that lead to persistent and sometimes severe bleeding.

B. A malignancy in which plasma cells multiply uncontrollably and infiltrate the bone marrow, lymph nodes, spleen, and other tissues.

C. The stem cells in the bone marrow are dysfunctional, resulting in anemia, thrombocytopenia, and agranulocytosis.

D. An alternative to a bone marrow transplant; results in complete and sustained replacement of the recipient's blood cell lines with cells derived from the donor stem cells.

E. Bone marrow is infused through a central venous line into the patient.

F. An excess of red blood cells characterized by a hematocrit higher than 55%; also known as erythrocytosis.

G. Inherited disorders of hemoglobin synthesis in which the alpha or beta chain of the hemoglobin molecule is missing or defective.

H. The ability of the body to control bleeding.

I. This can occur when the body is unable to absorb adequate amounts of vitamin B_{12}.

J. A condition that is a disruption of hemostasis characterized by widespread intravascular clotting and bleeding.

K. A platelet count of less than 100,000 per milliliter of blood.

L. The most common type of anemia; often caused by poor nutritional intake.

M. This may occur in the patient who has sickle cell anemia; characterized by severe episodes of fever and intense pain.

N. A malignancy of lymphoid tissue.

O. A group of blood disorders characterized by abnormal-appearing bone marrow and cytopenia; it is not a single disease.

P. A proliferation of abnormal white blood cells.

Q. A hereditary, chronic hemolytic anemia; characterized by episodes of sickling.

R. A condition that is characterized by premature destruction of red blood cells.

S. A condition that has an abnormally low RBC count or reduced hemoglobin content; it is the most common RBC disorder.

FOCUSED STUDY

1. List the names of some medications used to replace iron and treat iron-deficiency anemia. Briefly describe information the nurse should provide the patient who is receiving one of these medications.

_____

_____

_____

2. List some clinical manifestations associated with polycythemia.

_____

_____

_____

_____

3. List some clinical manifestations associated with disseminated intravascular coagulation.

_____

_____

_____

_____

_____

4. Describe the differences between Hodgkin's disease and non-Hodgkin's lymphoma.

_____

_____

_____

_____

_____

CASE STUDY

Jonathan Obermark is a 13-year-old male patient who was diagnosed today with acute lymphoblastic leukemia (ALL). His mother was recently diagnosed with iron-deficiency anemia. Jonathan and his mother have some questions for the nurse and physician regarding these two conditions. Answer the following questions based on your knowledge of anemias and ALL.

1. What are the different types of anemias?

2. What are some dietary sources of heme and nonheme iron?

3. What are some common causes of iron-deficiency anemia?

4. Which population is most at risk for developing ALL?

5. What are the associated clinical manifestations of ALL?

6. Jonathan has been scheduled for a chest x-ray to rule out pneumonia. How may pneumonia be related to ALL?

7. The nurse studies Jonathan's laboratory results and determines that his platelet count is low. What problems may arise because of this?

8. The physician spoke with Jonathan and his mother about how ALL is treated. Which medications are typically used?

CARE PLAN CRITICAL-THINKING ACTIVITY

Please refer to the case study and nursing care plan exercise: A Patient with Folic Acid Deficiency Anemia (page 1080 in your textbook) to answer the following questions.

1. Why was an ice bag and manual pressure applied to Mr. Cruise's nose in the emergency department?

2. Why is it important for Mr. Cruise to avoid contact sports?

3. What information is available on a medical alert bracelet?

SHORT ANSWERS

List three conditions that may result in disseminated intravascular coagulation (DIC).

Tissue Damage	Vessel Damage	Infections
1.	1.	1.
2.	2.	2.
3.	3.	3.

NCLEX-RN® REVIEW QUESTIONS

1. Which of the following statements by a student nurse reflects an adequate understanding about iron deficiency anemia?
   1. "Iron deficiency anemia is the least common type of anemia."
   2. "The body can synthesize hemoglobin even without iron."
   3. "Inadequate dietary iron intake also contributes to anemia in the older adult."
   4. "Iron deficiency anemia results in increased numbers of RBCs."

2. During discharge planning, the nurse is teaching the patient about the sources of heme iron. Which of the following is a source of nonheme iron?
   1. veal
   2. clams
   3. egg yolk
   4. dried fruits

3. The spouse of a patient who has leukemia is providing care for the patient at home. Which of the following indicates the spouse's need for further teaching?
   1. Provide rest periods before meals.
   2. Provide prescribed medications for pain or nausea 10 minutes before meals.
   3. Provide liquids with different textures and tastes.
   4. Provide mouth care before and after meals.

4. The Ann Arbor Staging System is used to assess the extent and severity of lymphomas. Which of the following stages is used to describe the patient who has involvement of lymph node regions or structures on both sides of the diaphragm?
   1. stage I
   2. stage II
   3. stage III
   4. stage IV

5. During discharge planning, the nurse is teaching the patient how to prevent or relieve nausea or vomiting. Which of the following instructions would be unexpected?
   1. Eat soda crackers.
   2. Avoid unpleasant odors and get fresh air.
   3. Eat warm, spicy foods.
   4. Suck on hard candy.

6. A nurse is preparing an educational seminar about aplastic anemia. Which of the following statements should not be included because it is inaccurate?
   1. Manifestations of aplastic anemia include fatigue, pallor, progressive weakness, exertional dyspnea, headache, and ultimately tachycardia and heart failure.
   2. In aplastic anemia, the bone marrow fails to produce red blood cells and platelets.
   3. Aplastic anemia also may occur with viral infections such as mononucleosis, hepatitis C, and HIV disease.
   4. Aplastic anemia is rare.

7. Which of the following statements by a student nurse reflects an adequate understanding about polycythemia?
   1. "In primary polycythemia, RBC production is decreased."
   2. "Secondary polycythemia occurs when erythropoietin levels are elevated."
   3. "In relative polycythemia, the total RBC count is high."
   4. "In relative polycythemia, the hematocrit is abnormally low."

8. The patient has been diagnosed with acute lymphocytic leukemia. Which of the following nursing interventions would be unexpected?
   1. Encourage visitors to visit with the patient to help provide emotional support.
   2. Provide oral hygiene after every meal.
   3. Ensure meticulous handwashing among all people who come in contact with the patient.
   4. Maintain protective isolation as indicated.

Assessing the
Respiratory System

34 CHAPTER

LEARNING OUTCOMES

1. Describe the anatomy, physiology, and functions of the respiratory system.
2. Compare and contrast factors affecting respiration.
3. Identify specific topics for consideration during a health history interview of the patient with health problems involving the respiratory system.
4. Give examples of genetic disorders of the respiratory system.
5. Describe normal variations in assessment findings for the older adult.
6. Identify abnormal findings that may indicate alterations in respiratory function.

MediaLink

Pearson Nursing Student Resources
Audio Glossary
NCLEX-RN® Review
- Care Plan Activity
  - Occupational Respiratory Disorders
- Case Study
  - The Patient with Respiratory Disorders
- MediaLink Applications
- Links to Resources

CLINICAL COMPETENCIES

1. Conduct and document a health history for patients having or at risk for alterations in the respiratory system.
2. Conduct and document a physical assessment of respiratory structures and functions.
3. Monitor the results of diagnostic tests and report abnormal findings.

TERMS MATCHING

Place the letter of the correct definition in the space next to each term.

1. ____ Apnea

2. ____ Atelectasis

3. ____ Bradypnea

4. ____ Crackles

5. ____ Friction rub

6. ____ Lung compliance

7. ____ Oxyhemoglobin

8. ____ Surfactant

9. ____ Tachypnea

10. ____ Tidal volume (TV)

11. ____ Vital capacity (VC)

12. ____ Wheezes

A. The combination of oxygen and hemoglobin in the blood.

B. A loud, dry, creaking, adventitious breath sound that indicates pleural inflammation; auscultated during lung assessment.

C. The collapse of lung tissue following obstruction of the bronchus or bronchioles.

D. The volume inhaled and exhaled with normal quiet breathing.

E. The patient's respiratory rate is abnormally slow.

F. A continuous musical adventitious breath sound that may be heard in patients with bronchitis, emphysema, and asthma.

G. The patient's respiratory rate is abnormally fast.

H. This interferes with the adhesiveness of water molecules, reduces surface tension, and helps to expand the lungs; it is a lipoprotein produced by the alveolar cells.

I. The term that refers to the ability of the lungs to distend under pressure.

J. The total amount of air that can be exhaled after a maximal inspiration.

K. Short, discrete crackling or bubbling sounds; may be auscultated in a patient with pneumonia, bronchitis, or congestive heart failure.

L. Breathing cessation.

FOCUSED STUDY

1. Identify the functions of the pharynx and the larynx.

_____

_____

_____

_____

2. List at least two disorders of the respiratory system that have genetic influences.

_____

_____

3. List three age-related changes that occur in the respiratory system and the significance of each change.

_____

_____

_____

4. Describe the purpose of a bronchoscopy and the associated nursing interventions.

_____

_____

_____

_____

_____

CASE STUDY

Drake Strattman has been working as a registered nurse for 11 years. He is the nursing manager of a unit in a local hospital that admits many patients with respiratory disorders. He has been asked to teach a class to nurses at the hospital today about the respiratory system and respiratory disorders. Answer the following questions based on your understanding of the respiratory system.

1. What are some factors that affect ventilation and respiration?

2. Where are the sinuses, and what is the purpose of sinuses?

3. What is the difference between inspiratory reserve volume (IRV) and expiratory reserve volume (ERV)?

4. What are some implications of changes in the patient's breathing pattern?

5. What are the different characteristics of vesicular, bronchovesicular, and bronchial breath sounds?

6. How does the patient's trachea location change when the patient has a pleural effusion, pneumothorax, or atelectasis?

SHORT ANSWERS

1. Identify the following structures: lungs, mediastinum, visceral pleura, and parietal pleura.

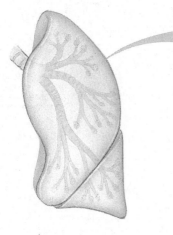
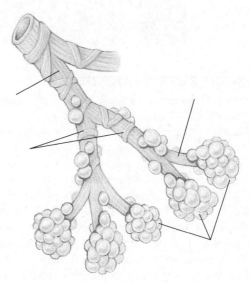

2. Identify the following structures: bronchi, bronchioles, alveolar ducts, and alveoli.

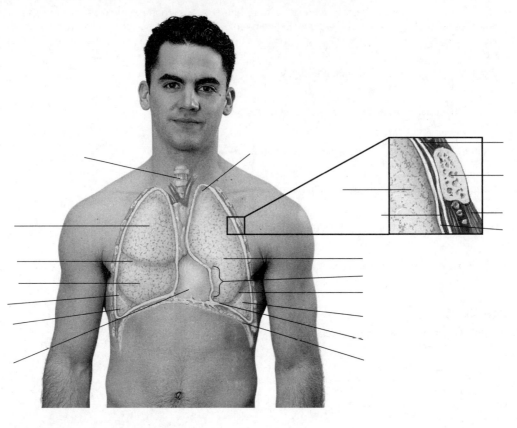

NCLEX-RN® REVIEW QUESTIONS

1. A nurse is planning an educational program about the respiratory system. Which of the following statements needs to be corrected?
    1. The laryngopharynx extends from the hyoid bone to the larynx.
    2. The right lung is smaller and has two lobes, whereas the left lung has three lobes.
    3. The parietal pleura lines the thoracic wall and mediastinum.
    4. During expiration, carbon dioxide is expelled.

2. Which of the following statements made by a student nurse is correct?
    1. "There are 12 pairs of ribs, and all of them articulate with the thoracic vertebrae."
    2. "Posteriorly, the first seven ribs articulate with the body of the sternum."
    3. "The seventh, eighth, and ninth ribs articulate with the cartilage immediately above the ribs."
    4. "The tenth, eleventh, and twelfth ribs are called floating ribs because they are unattached."

3. A nurse is evaluating a nursing student's understanding of inspiration and expiration. Which of the following statements indicates the need for further education?
    1. "During inspiration, the diaphragm contracts and flattens out to increase the vertical diameter of the thoracic cavity."
    2. "Expiration is primarily a passive process that occurs as a result of the elasticity of the lungs."
    3. "During expiration, the inspiratory muscles contract, the diaphragm descends, the ribs expand, and the lungs recoil."
    4. "A single inspiration lasts for about 1–1.5 seconds; whereas expiration lasts for about 2–3 seconds."

4. A nurse is evaluating a patient's understanding of some diagnostic tests that he had while in the hospital. Which of the following statements by the patient indicates a need for further education?
    1. "Arterial blood gases are conducted to evaluate alterations in acid–base balances."
    2. "Pulse oximetry is used to evaluate or monitor the oxygen saturation of the blood."
    3. "A pulmonary angiography provides direct visualization of the larynx, trachea, and bronchi."
    4. "A thoracentesis, when done for diagnostic purposes, is conducted to obtain a specimen of pleural fluid."

5. Two nurses are discussing a patient's respiratory condition. Which of the following statements by one of the nurses is correct?
   1. "Dullness is heard in patients with atelectasis, lobar pneumonia, and pleural effusion."
   2. "Retraction of intercostal spaces may be seen in pneumothorax."
   3. "Bulging of intercostal spaces may be seen in asthma."
   4. "Bilateral chest expansion is increased in emphysema."

6. Which of the following structures is part of the lower respiratory tract?
   1. nose
   2. trachea
   3. pleura
   4. sinuses

7. Which of the following structures is part of the upper respiratory tract?
   1. larynx
   2. lungs
   3. bronchi
   4. rib cage

CHAPTER 35

Nursing Care of Patients with Upper Respiratory Disorders

LEARNING OUTCOMES

1. Relate anatomy and physiology of the upper respiratory tract to commonly occurring disorders and risk factors for these disorders.

2. Describe the pathophysiology of common upper respiratory tract disorders, relating their manifestations to the pathophysiologic process.

3. Discuss nursing implications for medications and other interdisciplinary care measures to treat upper respiratory disorders.

4. Describe surgical procedures used to treat upper respiratory disorders and their implications for patient care and recovery.

5. Identify health promotion actitivities related to reducing the incidence of upper respiratory disorders, describing the appropriate population and setting for implementing identified measures.

6. Discuss treatment options for oral and laryngeal cancers and their implications for the patient's body image and functional health.

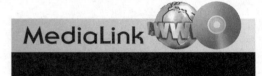

MediaLink

Pearson Nursing Student Resources
Audio Glossary
NCLEX-RN® Review
- Care Plan Activity
  - Upper Respiratory
- Case Study
  - The Patient with an Upper Respiratory Disorder
- Animations/Videos
  - Influenza (Includes H1N1)
  - Pertussis
- MediaLink Applications
- Links to Resources

CLINICAL COMPETENCIES

1. Assess functional health status of patients with upper respiratory disorders, using data to identify and prioritize holistic nursing care needs.

2. Use nursing research and evidence-based practice to plan and implement nursing care for patients with upper respiratory disorders.

3. Provide safe and effective nursing care for patients having surgery involving the upper respiratory system and/or with a tracheostomy.

4. Safely administer medications and prescribed treatments for patients with disorders of the upper respiratory tract.

5. Provide appropriate teaching for the patient and family affected by upper respiratory tract disorders.

6. Evaluate the effectiveness of care, reassessing and modifying the plan of care as needed to achieve desired patient outcomes.

TERMS MATCHING

Place the letter of the correct definition in the space next to each term.

1. ____ Coryza

2. ____ Epistaxis

3. ____ Group A beta-hemolytic streptooccus

4. ____ Influenza

5. ____ Laryngectomy

6. ____ Laryngitis

7. ____ Pertussis

8. ____ Pharyngitis

9. ____ Rhinitis

10. ____ Rhinoplasty

11. ____ Sinusitis

12. ____ Sleep apnea

13. ____ Tonsillitis

A. Inflammation of the nasal cavities; the most common upper respiratory disorder.

B. Inflammation of the pharynx.

C. Profuse nasal discharge.

D. A highly contagious acute upper respiratory infection caused by the bacterium *Bordetella pertussis*; also known as whooping cough.

E. Surgical reconstruction of the nose.

F. Surgical removal of the larynx.

G. Inflammation of the mucous membranes of one or more of the sinuses.

H. A nosebleed.

I. The intermittent absence of airflow through the mouth and nose during sleep; a serious and potentially life-threatening disorder.

J. A highly contagious viral respiratory disease characterized by coryza, fever, cough, and systemic symptoms such as headache and malaise.

K. Acute inflammation of the palatine tonsils.

L. The bacteria that is the most common cause of bacterial pharyngitis; strep throat.

M. Inflammation of the larynx.

FOCUSED STUDY

1. List four clinical manifestations associated with the common cold.

_____

_____

_____

2. List some common decongestants. Discuss health education that should be included for the patient who is taking decongestants.

_____

_____

_____

_____

_____

3. Discuss Reye's syndrome and how it relates to influenza.

_____

_____

_____

_____

4. Identify three risk factors associated with the development of laryngeal cancer.

_____

_____

_____

CASE STUDY

Nathaniel Smith is a 37-year-old male patient who has been diagnosed with obstructive sleep apnea. Part of the nursing responsibilities is to provide Nathaniel with education about sleep apnea before he leaves the clinic. Answer the following questions based on your knowledge of sleep apnea.

1. Explain the pathophysiology of sleep apnea.

2. List the manifestations of obstructive sleep apnea.

3. Review the risk factors associated with obstructive sleep apnea.

4. How is obstructive sleep apnea typically diagnosed?

5. Review the nonsurgical methods used to treat obstructive sleep apnea.

6. Review the surgical methods for treating obstructive sleep apnea.

7. Identify some common nursing diagnoses that may be used in the plan of care for Mr. Smith.

CARE PLAN CRITICAL-THINKING ACTIVITY

Please refer to the case study and nursing care plan exercise: A Patient with Peritonsillar Abscess (page 1152 in your textbook) to answer the following questions.

1. Why is it important for Ms. Wunderman to drink ice-cold fluids?

2. List the types of beverages and foods that Ms. Wunderman should avoid.

SHORT ANSWERS

Identify how laryngeal tumors are staged.

Stage 0	
Stage I	
Stage II	
Stage III	
Stage IV	

NCLEX-RN® REVIEW QUESTIONS

1. A nurse is evaluating a patient's understanding of preventing the spread of acute viral upper respiratory infection. Which of the following patient statements indicates the need for further education?
  1. "I'll use tissues to cover my mouth and nose when I sneeze and cough so I won't spread my infection to other people."
  2. "I'll blow my nose with one nostril open to prevent infected matter from being forced into the eustachian tubes."
  3. "I'll wash my hands after I sneeze or cough."
  4. "I'll limit my use of nasal decongestants to prevent a rebound effect."

2. Which of the following choices is accurate regarding the type(s) of influenza that can be found in humans?
  1. A only
  2. A and C
  3. B and C
  4. A, B, and C

3. A nurse is teaching a patient about home care following a polypectomy. Which of the following statements by the nurse is correct?
   1. "Apply hot compresses to the nose to decrease swelling, promote comfort, and prevent bleeding."
   2. "Avoid blowing the nose for one hour after nasal packing is removed."
   3. "Avoid straining during bowel movements, vigorous coughing, and strenuous exercise."
   4. "Rest for one day after surgery to reduce the risk of bleeding."

4. A nurse is providing a patient's discharge teaching about tracheostomy stoma care and ways to prevent the development of respiratory infections. Which of the following statements indicates that the nurse requires further education?
   1. The patient may safely participate in water sports.
   2. The patient should increase fluid intake to maintain mucosal moisture and loosen secretions.
   3. The patient should shield the stoma with a stoma guard to prevent particulate matter from entering the lower respiratory tract.
   4. The patient should use a humidifier or vaporizer to add humidity to inspired air.

5. A nurse is planning an educational program about nasal polyps. Which of the following statements indicates that the nurse requires further education?
   1. "Polyps form in areas of dependent mucous membrane and present as pale, edematous masses that are covered with mucous membrane."
   2. "Nasal polyps are benign grapelike growths of the mucous membrane that lines the nose."
   3. "Polyps are unilateral and have a broad, firm base, which makes them rigid."
   4. "Polyps may be asymptomatic, although large polyps may cause nasal obstruction, rhinorrhea, and loss of sense of smell."

6. When discussing the management of sleep apnea with the nurse, the patient asks, "What are some methods I can use to manage my sleep apnea?" Which of the following should not be included?
   1. The nurse should discuss the relationship of alcohol and sedatives to sleep apnea and refer the patient to an alcohol treatment program or Alcoholics Anonymous as indicated.
   2. The nurse should recommend the use of the CPAP intermittently throughout the night.
   3. The nurse should discuss the relationship between obesity and sleep apnea.
   4. The nurse should recommend adequate fluid intake by the patient to maintain moist mucous membranes.

CHAPTER 36

Nursing Care of Patients with Ventilation Disorders

LEARNING OUTCOMES

1. Relate the pathophysiology and manifestations of lower respiratory infections and inflammation, lung cancer, chest wall disorders, and trauma to the ability to maintain effective ventilation and respiration (gas exchange).

2. Compare and contrast the etiology, risk factors, and vulnerable populations for lower respiratory infections, lung cancer, chest wall disorders, and trauma.

3. Describe interdisciplinary care and the nursing role in health promotion and caring for patients with lower respiratory infections, lung cancer, chest wall disorders, and trauma.

4. Discuss surgery and other invasive procedures used to treat lung cancer, chest wall disorders, and trauma, and nursing responsibilities in caring for patients undergoing these procedures.

5. Describe the nursing implications for medications used to treat respiratory disorders and oxygen therapy.

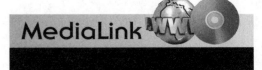

MediaLink

Pearson Nursing Student Resources
Audio Glossary
NCLEX-RN® Review
■ Care Plan Activity
  ■ Pneumonia
■ Case Study
  ■ TB Medication and Compliance
■ Animations/Videos
  ■ Pneumonia
  ■ Tuberculosis: Medication/Drug Administration: Performing a TB Test
  ■ Tuberculosis - Etiology and Pathophysiology
■ MediaLink Applications
■ Links to Resources

CLINICAL COMPETENCIES

1. Assess functional health status and the effects of lower respiratory and chest wall disorders on ventilation and gas exchange.

2. Use assessed data and knowledge of the effects of the disorder and prescribed treatment to identify priority nursing diagnoses and plan care for patients with lower respiratory disorders.

3. Use the nursing process and evidence-based nursing research to plan and implement individualized nursing care, including measures to promote ventilation and gas exchange for patients with lower respiratory disorders.

4. Plan and provide appropriate teaching for health promotion among vulnerable populations and to prepare patients and families for community-based care.

5. Evaluate the effectiveness of nursing interventions and teaching, revising strategies and teaching plans as needed.

6. Knowledgably and safely coordinate interdisciplinary care and administer prescribed medications and treatments for patients with lower respiratory disorders.

TERMS MATCHING

Place the letter of the correct definition in the space next to each term.

1. _____ Asphyxiation
2. _____ Cyanosis
3. _____ Dyspnea
4. _____ Flail chest
5. _____ Hemoptysis
6. _____ Hemothorax
7. _____ Hypoxemia
8. _____ Pleural effusion
9. _____ Pleuritis
10. _____ Pneumonia
11. _____ Pneumothorax
12. _____ Severe acute respiratory syndrome (SARS)
13. _____ Thoracentesis
14. _____ Tuberculosis (TB)

A. Difficult or labored breathing.

B. Low levels of oxygen in the blood.

C. Inflammation of the pleura.

D. The presence of blood in the pleural cavity.

E. Inflammation of the respiratory bronchioles and alveoli.

F. Oxygen deprivation.

G. The accumulation of air in the pleural space.

H. Bloody sputum.

I. A lower respiratory illness; the infective agent is a type of coronavirus; first described in people in Asia in February 2003.

J. The collection of excess fluid in the pleural space.

K. When two or more consecutive ribs are fractured in multiple places, a free-floating segment of the chest wall is produced.

L. A gray, blue, or purple skin color that is caused by deoxygenated hemoglobin.

M. A chronic, recurrent infectious disease that usually affects the lungs, although any organ can be affected; caused by *Mycobacterium tuberculosis*.

N. An invasive procedure in which fluid or air is removed from the pleural space with a needle.

FOCUSED STUDY

1. Discuss the nursing interventions that should be used for the patient with acute bronchitis.

_____

_____

_____

2. The lower respiratory tract is normally sterile. List the body's defense mechanisms used to maintain sterility in this area.

_____

_____

_____

_____

3. Identify the clinical manifestations associated with a lung abscess.

_____

_____

_____

4. Identify risk factors for developing tuberculosis.

_____

_____

_____

_____

CASE STUDY

Mimi Sutter is a 37-year-old female patient who is in the emergency department with complaints of shaking chills, fever, productive cough with yellow sputum, and pleuritic chest pain. The physician diagnoses her with acute bacterial pneumonia. Answer the following questions based on your knowledge of acute bacterial pneumonia.

1. What are some other clinical manifestations of acute bacterial pneumonia?

2. What are some differences in the way Ms. Sutter might present if she were older?

3. Ms. Sutter is diagnosed with pneumococcal pneumonia. What is the pathophysiology of this infection?

4. What are some diagnostic tests that were likely used to determine that Ms. Sutter has pneumococcal pneumonia?

5. Who should receive the pneumococcal pneumonia vaccine?

6. Who should not receive the influenza vaccine?

CARE PLAN CRITICAL-THINKING ACTIVITY

Please refer to the case study and nursing care plan exercise: A Patient with Pneumonia (page 1187 in your textbook) to answer the following questions.

1. Mr. Mueller has small cell carcinoma. When measuring his fluid balance each shift, what does the nurse expect to find?

2. What methods are available to assist Mr. Mueller to stop smoking?

SHORT ANSWERS

Fill in the blanks regarding the surgeries used to treat lung cancer.

Procedure	Description of Procedure	Used for
Laser bronchoscopy		
Mediastinoscopy		
Thoracotomy		
Wedge resection		
Segmental resection		
Sleeve resection (bronchoplastic reconstruction)		
Lobectomy		
Pneumonectomy		

NCLEX-RN® REVIEW QUESTIONS

1. Which of the following statements by a student nurse reflects an accurate understanding about pneumonia?
   1. "Inflammation of the bronchi is known as pneumonia."
   2. "Bacteria, viruses, fungi, protozoa, and other microbes can lead to infectious pneumonia."
   3. "Infectious causes of pneumonia include aspiration of gastric contents and inhalation of toxic or irritating gases."
   4. "The most common causative organism for community-acquired pneumonia is *Staphylococcus aureus*, a gram-negative bacterium."

2. Which of the following statements by a student nurse is accurate?
   1. "The incubation period for SARS is generally one day."
   2. "A low-grade fever below 98.2°F is typically the initial manifestation of the disease."
   3. "The primary population affected by SARS is previously healthy children from 5–10 years of age."
   4. "The infective agent responsible for SARS is a coronavirus not previously identified in humans."

3. A nurse is planning an educational program regarding tuberculosis. Which of the following statements needs to be corrected prior to the presentation?
   1. Primary or secondary tuberculosis lesions may affect other body systems such as the kidneys, the genitalia, bone, and the brain.
   2. Worldwide, TB continues to be a significant health problem.
   3. A previously healed tuberculosis lesion is unable to be reactivated.
   4. *Mycobacterium tuberculosis* is a relatively slow-growing, slender, rod-shaped, acid-fast organism with a waxy outer capsule that increases its resistance to destruction.

4. During discharge teaching, the nurse is teaching the patient who has tuberculosis about some ways to prevent transmitting the disease to others. Which of the following actions by the patient indicates that the patient requires further education?
   1. The patient always coughs and expectorates into tissues.
   2. The patient is placing the used tissues in a closed bag.
   3. The patient is wearing a mask when outside the negative air pressure room.
   4. The patient is using disposable silverware.

5. A nurse is evaluating a patient's understanding of histoplasmosis. Which of the following statements by the patient indicates the need for further education?
   1. "The *Histoplasma capsulatum* organism is found in the soil and is linked to exposure to bird droppings and bats."
   2. "Initial chest x-rays are nonspecific; later ones show areas of calcification."
   3. "Histoplasmosis is the most common bacterial lung infection in the United States."
   4. "Infection occurs when the spores are inhaled and reach the alveoli."

6. A patient is scheduled for a thoracentesis. Which of the following actions by the nurse would be unexpected?
   1. Verify the presence of a signed informed consent for the procedure.
   2. Ensure that the patient has been fasting for 8–12 hours.
   3. Position the patient upright and leaning forward with arms and head supported on an anchored overbed table.
   4. Administer a cough suppressant if indicated.

37 Nursing Care of Patients with Gas Exchange Disorders

LEARNING OUTCOMES

1. Relate the pathophysiology and manifestations of obstructive, pulmonary vascular, and critical respiratory disorders to their effects on ventilation and respiration (gas exchange).

2. Compare and contrast the etiology, risk factors, and vulnerable populations for disorders affecting ventilation and gas exchange within the lungs.

3. Describe interdisciplinary care and the nursing role in health promotion and caring for patients with disorders that affect the ability to ventilate the lungs and exchange gases with the environment.

4. Discuss interdisciplinary interventions to provide airway and ventilatory support for the patient with respiratory failure, and nursing responsibilities in caring for patients with airway and ventilatory support.

5. Describe the nursing implications for medications used to promote ventilation and gas exchange.

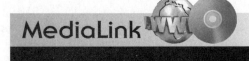

Pearson Nursing Student Resources
Audio Glossary
NCLEX-RN® Review
- Care Plan Activity
  - The Patient with Asthma
- Case Study
  - Acute Asthma Attack
- Animations/Videos
  - COPD
  - Acute Respiratory Distress Syndrome
  - Asthma
- MediaLink Application
- Links to Resources

CLINICAL COMPETENCIES

1. Assess functional health status of patients with disorders affecting ventilation and gas exchange.

2. Use assessed data and knowledge of the effects of the disorder and prescribed treatment to identify priority nursing diagnoses and plan care for patients with disorders affecting ventilation and gas exchange.

3. Use the nursing process and evidence-based nursing research to plan and implement individualized nursing care for patients, including measures to promote ventilation and gas exchange.

4. Plan and provide appropriate teaching for health promotion among vulnerable populations and to prepare patients and families for community-based care.

5. Evaluate the effectiveness of nursing interventions and teaching, revising strategies and teaching plans as needed.

6. Knowledgably and safely coordinate interdisciplinary care and administer prescribed medications and treatments for patients with disorders affecting ventilation and gas exchange.

TERMS MATCHING

Place the letter of the correct definition in the space next to each term.

1. _____ Acute respiratory distress syndrome (ARDS)
2. _____ Asthma
3. _____ Atelectasis
4. _____ Bronchiectasis
5. _____ Chronic bronchitis
6. _____ Chronic obstructive pulmonary disease (COPD)
7. _____ Cor pulmonale
8. _____ Cystic fibrosis (CF)
9. _____ Emphysema
10. _____ Pulmonary embolism
11. _____ Pulmonary hypertension
12. _____ Respiratory failure
13. _____ Reversibility
14. _____ Sarcoidosis
15. _____ Status asthmaticus
16. _____ Weaning

A. A chronic multisystem disease characterized by an exaggerated cellular immune response in involved tissues.

B. A condition characterized by permanent abnormal dilation of one or more large bronchi and destruction of bronchial walls; initiated by inflammation, usually due to recurrent airway infections.

C. A disorder characterized by noncardiac pulmonary edema and progressive refractory hypoxemia; also known as shock lung and adult hyaline membrane disease.

D. A disorder of excessive bronchial mucus secretion; characterized by a productive cough lasting three or more months in two consecutive years.

E. A chronic inflammatory disorder of the airways characterized by recurrent episodes of wheezing, breathlessness, chest tightness, and coughing.

F. Severe, prolonged asthma that does not respond to routine treatment.

G. The process of removing ventilator support and reestablishing spontaneous, independent respirations.

H. Chronic airflow obstruction due to chronic bronchitis and/or emphysema.

I. An abnormal elevation of the pulmonary arterial pressure.

J. A condition associated with many respiratory disorders; a state of partial or total lung collapse and airlessness.

K. An autosomal recessive disorder that affects epithelial cells of the respiratory, gastrointestinal, and reproductive tracts and leads to abnormal exocrine gland secretions.

L. The lungs are unable to oxygenate the blood and remove carbon dioxide adequately to meet the body's needs, even while the patient is resting.

M. An obstruction of blood flow in part of the pulmonary vascular system by an embolus.

N. A condition of right ventricular hypertrophy and failure resulting from long-standing pulmonary hypertension.

O. The patient's ability to breathe returns to normal following an intervention.

P. A disorder characterized by destruction of the walls of the alveoli, with resulting enlargement of abnormal air spaces.

FOCUSED STUDY

1. Identify two age-related changes of the pulmonary system.

2. Provide two examples of medications that are classified as methylxanthines. Identify clinical manifestations that may indicate that the patient has developed toxicity.

3. Identify the patient population that should be prescribed leukotriene modifiers. List three examples of medications that are classified as leukotriene modifiers.

_____

_____

_____

_____

_____

4. Explain how to perform pursed-lip breathing, diaphragmatic breathing, and coughing exercises.

_____

_____

_____

_____

CASE STUDY

Isabella Hitt is a 12-year-old patient who has been brought to the clinic by her mother, Anne. Isabella is coughing, wheezing, and stating that her chest hurts. Anne is very agitated and tells the nurse, "My daughter is having an asthma attack and needs an inhaler right away." Answer the following questions based on your knowledge of asthma.

1. Summarize the triggers of asthma.

2. List the clinical manifestations associated with acute asthma.

3. Explain how to use a metered-dose inhaler and a dry powder inhaler.

4. Discuss methods that can be used to prevent asthma attacks.

5. What is the underlying pathophysiology of asthma?

6. What is status asthmaticus?

7. What diagnostic tests can be used to diagnose asthma?

CARE PLAN CRITICAL-THINKING ACTIVITY

Please refer to the case study and nursing care plan exercise: A Patient with COPD (page 1248 in your textbook) to answer the following question.

1. Why is it important to monitor Ms. Adamson's urine output hourly and to report output of less than 30 mL per hour?

SHORT ANSWERS

Fill in the blanks regarding the stepwise approach to asthma management in adults.

Step/Disease Severity	Preferred Treatment	Alternative or As-Needed Treatment
Step 1 Mild Intermittent		
Step 2 Mild Persistent		
Step 3 Moderated Persistent		
Step 4 Severe Persistent		

NCLEX-RN® REVIEW QUESTIONS

1. Which of the following set of clinical manifestations is an unexpected finding in a patient with cystic fibrosis?
   1. secretions in affected organs becoming very thin and runny
   2. excess mucus production in the respiratory tract with impaired ability to clear secretions and progressive chronic obstructive pulmonary disease
   3. pancreatic enzyme deficiency and impaired digestion
   4. abnormal elevation of sodium and chloride concentrations in sweat

2. Which of the following statements by a student nurse reflects an accurate understanding about atelectasis?
   1. "The least common cause of atelectasis is obstruction of the bronchus that ventilates a segment of lung tissue."
   2. "It is a state of partial or total lung collapse and airlessness."
   3. "It is only a chronic condition."
   4. "The secondary therapy for atelectasis is prevention."

3. Which of the following actions is appropriate for the nurse when teaching a patient how to use a metered-dose inhaler?
   1. Firmly insert a charged metered-dose inhaler canister into the mouthpiece unit or spacer.
   2. When a spacer is being used, hold the canister upright, place the mouthpiece in the mouth, and close the lips around it.
   3. Press and hold the canister down while inhaling deeply and slowly for three to five seconds.
   4. Remove mouthpiece cap. Do not shake canister.

4. A nurse is evaluating a patient's ability to use a dry powder inhaler. Which of the following patient actions indicates the need for further education?
   1. The patient removed the cap and held the inhaler upright.
   2. The patient held the inhaler level, with the mouthpiece end facing up.
   3. The patient removed the inhaler from his mouth and held his breath for 10 seconds.
   4. The patient exhaled slowly through pursed lips.

5. Which nursing intervention for a patient with chronic obstructive pulmonary disease (COPD) is correct?
   1. Restrict fluid intake to 1500 mL per day and provide a bedside dehumidifier.
   2. Keep head of the bed elevated to at least 10 degrees at all times.
   3. Teach the "huff" coughing technique.
   4. Assess respiratory status and level of consciousness every 6 hours until stable, then every 12 hours.

CHAPTER 38
Assessing Patients with
Musculoskeletal Disorders

LEARNING OUTCOMES

1. Describe the anatomy, physiology, and functions of the musculoskeletal system.
2. Identify specific topics for consideration during a health history interview of the patient with health problems involving the musculoskeletal system.
3. Describe normal variations in assessment findings for the older adult.
4. Give examples of genetic disorders of the musculoskeletal system.
5. Identify manifestations of impairment of the musculoskeletal system.

CLINICAL COMPETENCIES

1. Conduct and document a health history for patients at risk for or having alterations in the musculoskeletal system.
2. Conduct and document a physical assessment of musculoskeletal structures and functions.
3. Monitor the results of diagnostic tests and report abnormal findings.

EQUIPMENT NEEDED

- Tape measure
- Goniometer

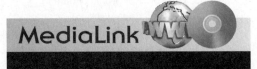

MediaLink

Pearson Nursing Student Resources
Audio Glossary
NCLEX-RN® Review

- Care Plan Activity
  - Impaired Mobility
- Case Study
  - Assessing Patients with Musculoskeletal Disorders
- MediaLink Application
- Links to Resources

TERMS MATCHING

Place the letter of the correct definition in the space next to each term.

1. _____ Bursitis

2. _____ Crepitation

3. _____ Hematopoiesis

4. _____ Kyphosis

5. _____ Lordosis

6. _____ Ossification

7. _____ Scoliosis

8. _____ Synovitis

9. _____ Tendonitis

A. A lateral, S-shaped curvature of the spine.

B. Blood cell formation.

C. An increased lumbar curve.

D. Inflammation of a bursa.

E. The development of bone.

F. Inflammation of the synovial membrane lining the articular capsule of a joint.

G. A grating sound.

H. Inflammation of a tendon.

I. An exaggerated thoracic curvature of the spine common in older adults.

FOCUSED STUDY

1. List manifestations of impairment of the musculoskeletal system.

_____

_____

_____

2. List specific topics for consideration during a health history interview of the patient with health problems that involve the musculoskeletal system.

_____

_____

_____

3. Summarize the anatomy, physiology, and functions of the musculoskeletal system.

_____

_____

_____

4. Describe the normal movements allowed by synovial joints.

_____

_____

_____

CASE STUDY

Michael Baldwin, RN, is preparing for a seminar about the musculoskeletal system. To assess the participants' understanding of the material he is presenting, Michael decides to develop a series of questions. Answer the following questions based on your knowledge of the musculoskeletal system.

1. Bones are classified by which shapes?

2. Summarize bone remodeling in adults.

3. What are the different types of joints?

SHORT ANSWERS

Complete the chart regarding the functional classification of joints.

Type	Description	Examples
Synarthrosis		
Amphiarthrosis		
Diarthrosis		

NCLEX-RN® REVIEW QUESTIONS

1. A nurse is evaluating a patient's understanding of the musculoskeletal system. Which of the following statements by the patient indicates a need for further teaching?
   1. "The musculoskeletal system is composed of bones of the skeletal system, cartilage, ligaments, tendons, and skeletal muscles and joints."
   2. "The bones serve as the framework for the body and for the attachment of muscles, tendons, and ligaments."
   3. "The musculoskeletal system has two subsystems: (1) the bones and joints of the skeleton and (2) the skeletal muscles."
   4. "The tissues and structures of the musculoskeletal system perform one function, which is movement."

2. Which of the following statements about bones is false?
   1. Bones store minerals.
   2. The human skeleton is made up of 226 bones.
   3. Bones of the skeletal system are divided into the axial and the appendicular skeleton.
   4. Bones protect vital organs from injury and serve to move body parts by providing points of attachment for muscles.

3. Which type of bone is longer than it is wide?
   1. short
   2. long
   3. irregular
   4. flat

4. The bones of the wrist and ankle are considered which type of bone?
   1. irregular
   2. long
   3. flat
   4. short

5. Which of the following is not a type of muscle tissue in the body?
   1. rough muscle
   2. skeletal muscle
   3. smooth muscle
   4. cardiac muscle

6. The body has approximately how many muscles?
   1. 200
   2. 400
   3. 600
   4. 800

7. Which type of joint is freely moveable, allows many kinds of movements, and is found at all articulations of the limbs?
   1. amphiarthrosis
   2. cartilaginous
   3. fibrous
   4. synovial

8. During a patient assessment, which of the following instructions by the nurse assesses abduction?
   1. "Make a fist."
   2. "Open your hand."
   3. "Spread your fingers."
   4. "Close your fingers."
9. What is the term for a lateral, S-shaped curvature of the spine?
   1. lordosis
   2. scoliosis
   3. kyphosis
   4. synovitis
10. Numbness and burning in the fingers during which of the following tests may indicate carpal tunnel syndrome?
    1. bulge
    2. Thomas
    3. Phalen's
    4. McMurray's

39 Nursing Care of Patients with Musculoskeletal Trauma

LEARNING OUTCOMES

1. Compare and contrast the causes, risk factors, pathophysiology, manifestations, interdisciplinary care, and nursing care of contusions, strains, sprains, joint dislocations, and fractures.

2. Describe the pathophysiology, interdisciplinary care, and nursing care for repetitive use injuries: carpal tunnel syndrome, bursitis, and epicondylitis.

3. Describe the stages of bone healing.

4. Explain the pathophysiology, manifestations, and related treatment for complications of bone fractures: compartment syndrome, fat embolism syndrome, deep venous thrombosis, infection, delayed union and nonunion, and complex regional pain syndrome.

5. Discuss the purposes and related nursing interventions for casts, fixation devices, traction, and stump care.

6. Explain the causes, levels, types, and potential complications (infection, delayed healing, chronic stump pain, phantom pain, and contractures) of an amputation.

MediaLink

Pearson Nursing Student Resources
Audio Glossary
NCLEX-RN® Review
■ Care Plan Activity
 ■ Below-the-Knee Amputation
■ Case Study
 ■ A Patient with Fractures
■ Animations/Videos
 ■ Hip fractures
 ■ Steps in the Repair of a Fracture
 ■ Amputation
■ MediaLink Applications
■ Links to Resources

CLINICAL COMPETENCIES

1. Assess functional health status of patients with musculoskeletal injuries, and recognize, monitor, document, and report abnormal or unexpected findings.

2. Use evidence-based research to plan and implement nursing care for patients who have experienced musculoskeletal trauma.

3. Determine priority nursing diagnoses, based on assessed data, to plan and implement individualized nursing interventions for patients with musculoskeletal injuries.

4. Provide skilled care for patients with a cast, fixation device, traction, or amputation, maintaining patient and caregiver safety at all times.

5. Coordinate and integrate interdisciplinary care into care of patients with musculoskeletal trauma.

6. Provide teaching appropriate for prevention and self-care of traumatic injuries of the musculoskeletal system.

7. Revise plan of care as needed to provide effective interventions to promote, maintain, or restore functional health status to patients with traumatic injuries of the musculoskeletal system.

TERMS MATCHING

Place the letter of the correct definition in the space next to each term.

1. _____ Amputation
2. _____ Bursitis
3. _____ Compartment syndrome
4. _____ Contracture
5. _____ Contusion
6. _____ Dislocation
7. _____ Fat embolism syndrome (FES)
8. _____ Flail chest
9. _____ Fracture
10. _____ Nonunion
11. _____ Phantom limb pain
12. _____ Sprain
13. _____ Strain
14. _____ Subluxation
15. _____ Volkmann's contracture

A. Bleeding into soft tissue resulting from a blunt force.

B. Causes persistent pain and movement at the fracture site.

C. A stretch and/or tear of one or more ligaments surrounding a joint.

D. An uncommon complication of elbow or forearm fractures that may result from unresolved compartment syndrome.

E. The partial or total removal of an extremity.

F. The fracture of two or more adjacent ribs in two or more places and the formation of a free-floating segment that moves in the opposite direction of the rib cage.

G. Pressure in the fascia constricts and entraps the structures within it.

H. A partial dislocation in which the bones of the joint remain in partial contact.

I. A stretching injury to a muscle or a muscle-tendon unit caused by mechanical overloading.

J. Any break in the continuity of a bone.

K. Inflammation of a bursa.

L. Painful phantom limb sensation.

M. An injury in which the ends of bones are displaced out of their normal position and joint articulation is lost.

N. Characterized by neurologic dysfunction; pulmonary insufficiency; and a petechial rash on the chest, axilla, and upper arms.

O. An abnormal flexion and fixation of a joint caused by muscle atrophy and shortening.

FOCUSED STUDY

1. Explain the interdisciplinary care and nursing care for repetitive use injuries: carpal tunnel syndrome, bursitis, and epicondylitis.

_____
_____
_____
_____
_____

2. Describe the nursing interventions for casts, traction, and internal fixation.

_____
_____
_____
_____

3. Summarize the stages of bone healing.

_____
_____
_____

4. List the potential complications of an amputation.

_____
_____
_____

CASE STUDY

Georgene Smith, a 12-year-old female patient, presented at the clinic after experiencing an injury while ice skating. Georgene states that she heard her right knee "pop" after she landed from an axle jump. Her knee is swollen with slight discoloration. Her pain assessment score is 9 out of 10. Answer the following questions based on your knowledge of sprains and strains.

1. Define *strain* and *sprain*.

2. Give examples of how a strain or sprain could occur.

3. What are the manifestations of a strain and a sprain?

4. Explain RICE therapy.

SHORT ANSWERS

Fill in the table regarding the manifestations of fractures.

Manifestation	Pathophysiology
	Abnormal position of bones secondary to fracture and muscles pulling on fractured bone
	Edema from localization of serous fluid and bleeding
	Muscle spasm, direct tissue trauma, nerve pressure, movement of fractured bone
	Nerve damage or nerve entrapment
	Pain
	Grating of bones or entrance of air into an open fracture. *Note:* Do not manipulate the extremity to elicit crepitus; doing so may cause additional damage.
	Blood loss or associated injuries
	Muscle contraction near the fracture
	Extravasation of blood into the subcutaneous tissue

NCLEX-RN® REVIEW QUESTIONS

1. Which of the following statements about a strain is correct?
   1. The most common sites for a muscle strain are the wrist and ankle.
   2. The manifestations of a strain include pain, limited motion, muscle spasms, swelling, and possible muscle weakness.
   3. Severe strains that partially or completely tear the ligament are very painful but are not disabling.
   4. A strain is a stretch and/or tear of one or more ligaments that surround a joint.
2. What is the meaning of *R* in RICE therapy for musculoskeletal injuries?
   1. rest
   2. relax
   3. raise
   4. rub

3. Which of the following is an injury of a joint in which the ends of bones are forced from their normal position?
   1. dislocation
   2. strain
   3. sprain
   4. fracture

4. Which of the following statements about fractures is correct?
   1. Fractures do not vary in severity.
   2. A fracture occurs when the bone is subjected to less kinetic energy than it can absorb.
   3. Not all of the 206 bones in the body can be fractured.
   4. Two basic mechanisms produce fractures: direct force and indirect force.

5. A nurse is evaluating a student's understanding of compartment syndrome. Which of the following statements by the student indicates a need for further teaching?
   1. "Compartment syndrome usually develops within the first 24 hours of injury, when edema is at its peak."
   2. "Compartment syndrome occurs when excess pressure in a limited space constricts the structures in a compartment, which reduces circulation to muscles and nerves."
   3. "Acute compartment syndrome may result from hemorrhage and edema in the compartment after a fracture or from a crush injury or from external compression of the limb by a cast that is too tight."
   4. "The fascia, which is nonexpendable, supports these tissues."

6. Which of the following types of traction is the application of a pulling force through placement of pins into the bone?
   1. skin
   2. skeletal
   3. balanced suspension
   4. manual

7. Which of the following statements by a student nurse reflects correct understanding about casts?
   1. "The cast is applied to immobilize the joint above and the joint below the fractured bone so that the bone will not move during healing."
   2. "A plaster cast may require up to 24 hours to dry, whereas a fiberglass cast dries in 2 hours."
   3. "Casts are applied on patients who have unstable fractures."
   4. "The cast must be allowed to partially dry before any pressure is applied to it."

8. During discharge planning, the nurse is teaching the patient about cast care. Which of the following statements is correct?
   1. "Scratch under a cast with a dull object."
   2. "Cover the cast while it is drying."
   3. "A cold sensation is normal during drying."
   4. "Use a blow dryer on the cool setting to relieve itching by blowing cool air into the cast."

9. All of the following guidelines except which one may help preserve an amputated part until it can be surgically reattached?
   1. Put the amputated part in direct contact with ice or water.
   2. Apply firm pressure to the bleeding area with a towel or an article of clothing.
   3. Send the amputated part to the emergency department with the injured person and make sure the emergency personnel know what it is.
   4. Wrap the amputated part in a clean cloth.

CHAPTER 40

Nursing Care of Patients with Musculoskeletal Disorders

LEARNING OUTCOMES

1. Explain the etiology, pathophysiology, manifestations, complications, interdisciplinary care, and nursing care of musculoskeletal disorders.

2. Compare and contrast the pathophysiology, manifestations, diagnosis, and management of osteoporosis, osteoarthritis, Paget's disease, and rheumatoid arthritis.

3. Discuss the purposes, nursing implications, and health education for the patient and family for medications used to prevent and treat specific musculoskeletal disorders.

4. Describe the surgical procedures used to treat patients with arthritis.

CLINICAL COMPETENCIES

1. Assess functional status of patients with musculoskeletal disorders, and recognize, monitor, document, and report abnormal or unanticipated manifestations.

2. Use evidence-based research and practice guidelines to plan and provide safe and effective individualized care for patients with musculoskeletal disorders.

3. Determine priority nursing diagnoses, based on assessed data, to select and implement patient-centered nursing interventions for patients with musculoskeletal disorders.

4. Administer medications used to treat musculoskeletal disorders knowledgeably and safely, monitoring for desired and adverse effects of prescribed medications.

5. Provide skilled care of patients having a surgical debridement for osteomyelitis and a total joint replacement.

6. Integrate and coordinate interdisciplinary care into care of patients with musculoskeletal disorders.

7. Provide teaching appropriate for community-based care of patients with musculoskeletal disorders.

8. Revise plan of care as needed to provide effective interventions to promote, maintain, or restore functional health status to patients with musculoskeletal disorders.

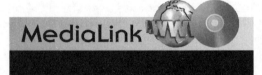

MediaLink

Pearson Nursing Student Resources
Audio Glossary
NCLEX-RN® Review
- Care Plan Activity
  - Lower Back Pain
- Case Studies
  - The Patient with Gout
  - The Patient Having Total Hip Replacement
  - The Patient with Musculoskeletal Disorders
- Animations/Videos
  - Osteoporosis
  - Osteoarthritis
- MediaLink Applications
- Links to Resources

TERMS MATCHING

Place the letter of the correct definition in the space next to each term.

1. _____ Ankylosing spondylitis
2. _____ Arthritis
3. _____ Fibromyalgia
4. _____ Gout
5. _____ Lyme disease
6. _____ Muscular dystrophy (MD)
7. _____ Osteoarthritis (OA)
8. _____ Osteomalacia
9. _____ Osteomyelitis
10. _____ Osteoporosis
11. _____ Paget's disease
12. _____ Polymyositis
13. _____ Reactive arthritis (ReA)
14. _____ Rheumatic disorders
15. _____ Rheumatoid arthritis (RA)
16. _____ Scleroderma
17. _____ Septic arthritis
18. _____ Sjögren's syndrome
19. _____ Systemic lupus erythematosus (SLE)
20. _____ Tophi

A. Adult rickets.

B. "Hardening of the skin."

C. A chronic inflammatory arthritis that affects primarily the axial skeleton, leading to pain and progressive stiffening and fusion of the spine.

D. An inflammatory disorder caused by the spirochete *Borrelia burgdorferi*, which is transmitted primarily by ticks.

E. Also called osteitis deformans, it is a progressive metabolic skeletal disorder that results from localized excessive metabolic activity in bone, with excessive bone resorption followed by excessive bone formation.

F. A chronic systemic autoimmune disease that causes inflammation of connective tissue, primarily in the joints.

G. Inflammation of the joints.

H. A group of inherited muscle diseases that cause progressive muscle degeneration and wasting.

I. A common rheumatic syndrome characterized by musculoskeletal pain, stiffness, and tenderness.

J. Porous bones.

K. A term used to refer to diseases of the muscles and bones as well as the joints.

L. Infection of the bone.

M. Known to manifest a characteristic rash on the face.

N. Urate crystal deposits.

O. A metabolic disorder characterized by an acute inflammatory arthritis triggered by crystallization of urate in the joints.

P. An acute, nonpurulent inflammatory arthritis that is believed to be a response to an exposure or infection with certain types of bacteria, including *Chlamydia*.

Q. An infectious musculoskeletal disorder that requires immediate treatment.

R. A systemic connective tissue disorder characterized by inflammation of connective tissue and muscle fibers, leading to muscle weakness and atrophy.

S. Also called degenerative joint disease.

T. A chronic, progressive autoimmune disorder that causes inflammation and dysfunction of exocrine glands throughout the body.

FOCUSED STUDY

1. Discuss the surgical procedures used to treat patients with arthritis.

_____

_____

_____

2. Summarize the treatments for osteoporosis, osteoarthritis, Paget's disease, and rheumatoid arthritis.

_____

_____

_____

3. Describe the health education for the patient and family for medications used to treat osteoporosis, Paget's disease, gout, osteomalacia, osteoarthritis, rheumatoid arthritis, systemic lupus erythematosus, osteomyelitis, bone tumors, scleroderma, and low back pain.

_____

_____

_____

_____

_____

_____

_____

_____

_____

_____

4. Briefly discuss treatments and diagnostics associated with muscular dystrophy (MD).

_____

_____

_____

_____

_____

_____

CASE STUDY

Christine Scott is a 37-year-old patient in today for her yearly physical. She tells the nurse that her mother was diagnosed with osteoporosis two weeks ago. Christine then asks a few questions. Answer the following questions based on your knowledge of musculoskeletal disorders.

1. "What are the unmodifiable risk factors for osteoporosis?"

2. "What are the modifiable risk factors for osteoporosis?"

3. "What are the most common signs and symptoms of osteoporosis?"

4. "Are there complications of osteoporosis? Explain."

CARE PLAN CRITICAL-THINKING ACTIVITY

Please refer to the case study and nursing care plan exercise: A Patient with Rheumatoid Arthritis (page 1372 of your textbook) to answer the following questions.

1. Ms. James is diagnosed with rheumatoid arthritis at age 42. At what age does rheumatoid arthritis typically occur?

2. List the causes of rheumatoid arthritis.

3. Where can Ms. James obtain information about rheumatoid arthritis?

SHORT ANSWERS

Fill in the table differentiating between the features of osteoporosis and osteomalacia.

Differentiating Features	Osteoporosis	Osteomalacia
Pathophysiology		
Calcium level (serum)		
Phosphate level (serum)		
Parathyroid hormone level (serum)		
Alkaline phosphatase level (serum)		
Hydroxyproline (urine)		
Radiographic findings		

NCLEX-RN® REVIEW QUESTIONS

1. During discharge planning, the nurse is teaching the patient about osteoporosis. Which of the following statements is correct?
   1. Calcitonin (Miacalcin®) is a hormone that decreases bone formation and increases bone resorption.
   2. The most common manifestations of osteoporosis are loss of height; progressive curvature of the spine; low back pain; and fractures of the forearm, spine, or hip.
   3. Fractures are not the most common complication of osteoporosis.
   4. Osteoporosis is not preventable or treatable.
2. Which of the following statements by a student nurse reflects correct understanding about Paget's disease?
   1. "The most common manifestation of Paget's disease is localized pain of the short bones."
   2. "Paget's disease is a progressive metabolic skeletal disorder of the osteoclast that results from excessive metabolic activity in bone, with excessive bone resorption followed by excessive bone formation."
   3. "The bones decrease in size and thickness in Paget's disease."
   4. "Paget's disease is also called osteoporosis."
3. A nurse is evaluating a nursing student's understanding of gout. Which of the following statements by the nursing student indicates a need for further teaching?
   1. "Over time, urate deposits in subcutaneous tissues cause the formation of small white nodules called tophi."
   2. "Gout has an acute onset, usually at night, and often involves the fifth metatarsophalangeal joint."
   3. "Kidney disease may occur in patients with untreated gout, particularly when hypertension is present."
   4. "Serum uric acid is nearly always elevated (usually above 7.5 mg/dL)."
4. A nurse is planning a seminar about osteomalacia. Which of the following statements on a handout needs to be corrected?
   1. Hyperphosphatemia can result from insufficient dietary intake, excessive losses through the urine or stool, or a shift into the cells.
   2. The manifestations of osteomalacia include bone pain and tenderness.
   3. The primary causes of osteomalacia are calcium deficiency and hyperphosphatemia.
   4. Osteomalacia is a metabolic bone disorder characterized by inadequate or delayed mineralization of bone matrix in mature compact and spongy bone, which results in softening of bones.

5. A nurse is evaluating a nursing student's understanding of osteoarthritis. Which of the following statements by the nursing student demonstrates a need for further teaching?
    1. "The onset of osteoarthritis (OA) is usually gradual and insidious, and the course is slowly progressive."
    2. "Osteoarthritis is the most common form of arthritis and is a leading cause of pain and disability in older adults."
    3. "Increasing age is the primary risk factor for OA."
    4. "Women are affected more often than men and at an earlier age, but the rate of osteoarthritis in men exceeds women by the middle adult years."
6. Which of the following is not a manifestation of systemic lupus erythematosus (SLE)?
    1. unexplained fever
    2. white skin discoloration, especially on the face
    3. extreme fatigue
    4. painful or swollen joints
7. Hallux valgus is the enlargement and lateral displacement of the first metatarsal (the great toe). What is another word for *hallux valgus*?
    1. bunion
    2. hammertoe
    3. claw toe
    4. Morton's neuroma
8. Which of the following is a lateral curvature of the spine?
    1. scoliosis
    2. kyphosis
    3. hunchback
    4. lordosis

Assessing the Nervous System

LEARNING OUTCOMES

1. Describe the anatomy, physiology, and functions of the nervous system.
2. Explain manifestations of impairment of neurologic function.
3. Give examples of genetic disorders of the nervous system.
4. Describe normal variations in assessment findings for the older adult.

CLINICAL COMPETENCIES

1. Conduct and document a health history for patients who have or are at risk for alterations in the neurologic system.
2. Conduct and document a physical assessment of neurologic structures and functions.
3. Perform specific neurologic assessments for patients with suspected meningeal irritation and for disoriented or comatose patients.
4. Monitor the results of diagnostic tests and report abnormal findings.

MediaLink

Pearson Nursing Student Resources
Audio Glossary
NCLEX-RN® Review
- Care Plan Activity
  - Neurologic Disorders
- Case Study
  - Assessing an Unconscious Patient
- MediaLink Application
- Links to Resources

EQUIPMENT NEEDED

- Cotton balls
- Safety pin
- Tongue depressor
- Tuning fork
- Reflex hammer
- Pencil and paper
- Penlight
- Printed materials
- Substances to use in testing the senses of smell and taste

TERMS MATCHING

Place the letter of the correct definition in the space next to each term.

1. ____ Anosmia	A.	Difficulty speaking.
2. ____ Aphasia	B.	Drooping eyelids.
3. ____ Ataxia	C.	Loss of voluntary muscle coordination.
4. ____ Decerebrate posturing	D.	Irregular movements.
5. ____ Decorticate posturing	E.	Increased muscle tone.
6. ____ Diaphoresis	F.	An inability to smell.
7. ____ Dysarthria	G.	Occurs with lesions of the corticospinal tracts.
8. ____ Dysphagia	H.	The ability to assess movement or sense of position.
9. ____ Dysphonia	I.	Change in the tone of the voice.
10. ____ Fasciculations	J.	Rhythmic movements.
11. ____ Flaccidity	K.	Defective or absent language function.
12. ____ Kinesthesia	L.	Occurs with lesions of the midbrain, pons, or diencephalon.
13. ____ Nystagmus	M.	Copious production of sweat.
14. ____ Ptosis	N.	Decreased muscle tone.
15. ____ Spasticity	O.	Involuntary eye movement.
16. ____ Tremors	P.	Difficulty swallowing.

FOCUSED STUDY

1. Summarize the assessment of neurologic function.

_____

_____

_____

_____

2. List specific topics to consider during a health history assessment interview of the patient with neurologic disorders.

_____

_____

_____

_____

3. Discuss the anatomy, physiology, and functions of the nervous system.

_____

_____

_____

_____

_____

4. Discuss age-related changes in the nervous system.

_____

_____

_____

_____

CASE STUDY

James Smith is a new nursing student who is attending a seminar today about the central nervous system. At the end of the seminar, he asks a few questions. Answer the following questions based on your knowledge of the central nervous system.

1. "What are the four major regions of the brain?"

2. "What does the brainstem consist of?"

3. "What protects and surrounds the spinal cord?"

4. "How many pairs of spinal nerves are there? Where are they located?"

SHORT ANSWERS

Fill in the table regarding the functions of the cranial nerves.

Name	Function
I Olfactory	
II Optic	
III Oculomotor	
IV Trochlear	
V Trigeminal	
VI Abducens	
VII Facial	
VIII Acoustic	
IX Glossopharyngeal	
X Vagus	
XI Accessory	
XII Hypoglossal	

NCLEX-RN® REVIEW QUESTIONS

1. Which of the following is not a part of a neuron?
   1. dendrite
   2. cell body
   3. axon
   4. nucleus

2. Which of the following statements by a student nurse reflects correct understanding about neurons?
   1. "The dendrite is a short projection from the cell body that conducts impulses away (efferent) from the cell body."
   2. "Many axons are covered with a myelin sheath, which is a thick gray substance."
   3. "Cell bodies, most of which are located in the CNS, are clustered in ganglia or nuclei."
   4. "The myelin sheath serves to decrease the speed of nerve impulse conduction in axons and is essential for the survival of larger nerve processes."

3. Which of the following statements about neurotransmitters is false?
   1. The neurotransmitter may be either inhibitory or excitatory.
   2. The inhibitory neurotransmitter is usually acetylcholine (ACh).
   3. Norepinephrine (NE), which may be either excitatory or inhibitory, is another major neurotransmitter.
   4. Neurotransmitters are the chemical messengers of the nervous system.

4. A nurse is evaluating a patient's understanding of the brain. Which of the following statements by the patient indicates a need for further teaching?
   1. "The brain is the control center of the nervous system, generating thoughts, emotions, and speech."
   2. "The left hemisphere has greater control over nonverbal perceptual functions."
   3. "The brain has four major regions: the cerebrum, the diencephalon, the brainstem, and the cerebellum."
   4. "The brain contains four ventricles, which are chambers filled with cerebrospinal fluid (CSF)."

5. Which of the following is not part of the brainstem?
   1. midbrain
   2. pons
   3. medulla oblongata
   4. ventricles

6. The brain contains ventricles, which are chambers filled with cerebrospinal fluid (CSF). How many ventricles are in the brain?
   1. two
   2. three
   3. four
   4. five

7. Which statement about cerebrospinal fluid (CSF) is false?
   1. CFS is a clear and colorless liquid.
   2. CSF forms a cushion for the brain tissue, protects the brain and spinal cord from trauma, helps provide nourishment for the brain, and removes waste products of cerebrospinal cellular metabolism.
   3. The usual amount of cerebrospinal fluid ranges from 20–80 mL and averages about 40 mL.
   4. Cerebrospinal fluid is normally produced and absorbed in equal amounts.

8. Which metabolic factor does not affect cerebral blood flow?
   1. carbon dioxide
   2. hydrogen ion
   3. oxygen concentrations
   4. potassium

9. The spinal cord is surrounded and protected by how many vertebrae?
   1. 13
   2. 23
   3. 33
   4. 43

10. During a patient assessment, the nurse notes that the patient can smile, frown, wrinkle his forehead, show his teeth, puff out his cheek, purse his lips, raise his eyebrows, and close his eyes against resistance. Which cranial nerve is the nurse assessing?
   1. II
   2. III
   3. V
   4. VII

Nursing Care of Patients with **Intracranial Disorders**

42 CHAPTER

LEARNING OUTCOMES

1. Compare and contrast the pathophysiology, manifestations, interdisciplinary care, and nursing care of patients with alterations in level of consciousness and increased intracranial pressure (IICP).

2. Describe criteria for diagnosing persistent vegetative state and brain death.

3. Explain the pathophysiology, manifestations, complications, interdisciplinary care, and nursing care of intracranial disorders, including seizures, stroke, aneurysms, traumatic brain injury, tumors, and headaches.

4. Discuss the purposes, nursing implications, and health education for the patient and family for medications used to treat intracranial disorders.

5. Discuss surgical options for the treatment of increased intracranial pressure, epilepsy, traumatic brain injury, and brain tumors.

MediaLink

Pearson Nursing Student Resources
Audio Glossary
NCLEX-RN® Review
- Care Plan Activity
  - Migraine Headache
- Case Study
  - The Patient with a Stroke
- Animations/Videos
  - Neurological: Seizure - Absence Seizure
  - Neurological: Seizure - Complex Partial
  - Neurological: Seizure - Tonic Clonic
  - Thrombotic Stroke
  - Traumatic Brain Injury
- MediaLink Applications
- Links to Resources

CLINICAL COMPETENCIES

1. Assess functional status of patients with intracranial disorders and monitor, document, and report abnormal manifestations.

2. Use assessed data, individual and cultural patient values and variations, expressed patient needs and preferences, clinical expertise, and evidence to determine priority nursing diagnoses, and select and implement individualized nursing interventions for patients with intracranial disorders.

3. Administer medications used to treat intracranial disorders knowledgeably and safely.

4. Provide appropriate interventions to patients having intracranial pressure monitoring, tonic-clonic seizures, and intracranial surgery.

5. Effectively communicate with and function within the interdisciplinary team to plan and care of patients with intracranial disorders.

6. Use evidence-based practice to provide care for patients undergoing awake craniotomy.

7. Provide appropriate teaching to facilitate safety and to provide information and support necessary for long-term care of patients with intracranial disorders.

8. Revise plan of care as needed to provide effective interventions to promote, maintain, or restore functional health status to patients with intracranial disorders.

TERMS MATCHING

Place the letter of the correct definition in the space next to each term.

1. _____ Agnosia

2. _____ Aphasia

3. _____ Apraxia

4. _____ Aura

5. _____ Autonomic dysreflexia

6. _____ Brain death

7. _____ Cerebral edema

8. _____ Concussion

9. _____ Consciousness

10. _____ Contralateral deficit

11. _____ Epidural hematoma

12. _____ Epilepsy

13. _____ Hemianopia

14. _____ Hemiparesis

15. _____ Hemiplegia

16. _____ Hydrocephalus

17. _____ Increased intracranial pressure

18. _____ Locked in syndrome

19. _____ Neglect syndrome

20. _____ Persistent vegetative state

21. _____ Seizure

22. _____ Stroke

23. _____ Subdural hematoma

24. _____ Transient ischemic attack (TIA)

25. _____ Traumatic brain injury (TBI)

A. Paralysis of the left or right half of the body.

B. Swelling that displaces normal structures and causes direct or indirect pressure on the opposite hemisphere or brainstem can also affect LOC.

C. The cessation and irreversibility of all brain functions, including the brainstem.

D. A possible warning signal of an ischemic thrombotic stroke.

E. A sustained elevated pressure ($\geq$ 10 mmHg) in the cranial cavity.

F. Any injury of the scalp, skull (cranium or facial bones), or brain.

G. The inability to recognize one or more subjects that were previously familiar.

H. A momentary interruption of brain function involving temporary axonal disturbances.

I. An exaggerated sympathetic response that occurs in patients with SCIs at or above the T_6 level.

J. A stroke in the right hemisphere of the brain that is manifested by deficits in the left side of the body.

K. A syndrome in which an abnormality of overproduction, circulation, or reabsorption of CSF occurs.

L. The inability to carry out some motor pattern.

M. A sensory-perceptual deficit in which the patient has a disorder of attention.

N. A state of awareness.

O. Recurring seizures accompanied by some type of change in behavior.

P. A warning sign of an impending seizure, such as an unusual smell, a sense of déjà vu, or a sudden intense emotion.

Q. A condition in which neurologic deficits result from a sudden decrease in blood flow to a localized area of the brain.

R. A single event of abnormal electrical discharge.

S. Weakness of the left or right half of the body.

T. The loss of half of the visual field of one or both eyes.

U. A hematoma that collects between the dura mater and the arachnoid mater.

V. A hematoma that develops in the potential space between the dura and the skull.

W. A permanent condition of complete unawareness of self and the environment and loss of all cognitive functions.

X. To be alert and fully aware of the environment and have intact cognitive abilities but to be unable to communicate through speech or movement because of blocked efferent pathways from the brain.

Y. The inability to use or understand language.

FOCUSED STUDY

1. Discuss medication usage for the treatment of epilepsy. Include discussion about the goals of medication therapy. Also include the action and nursing considerations associated with medications used in the treatment of epilepsy.

_____

_____

_____

_____

_____

2. Discuss the definition of and criteria used for diagnosing brain death.

_____

_____

_____

_____

3. List the stroke indicators provided by the Stroke Collaborative (2008).

_____

_____

_____

_____

_____

4. Summarize the purpose and criteria for ICP monitoring.

_____

_____

_____

CASE STUDY

Ashley Smith is an 18-year-old female patient in the emergency room. Ashley's mother tells the nurse that Ashley has been complaining of a headache, nasal congestion, and nausea. Ashley states, "I'm seeing those bright spots again." Answer the following questions based on your knowledge of migraines.

1. Discuss the clinical manifestations of a migraine.

2. What factors are believed to trigger an onset of a migraine?

3. List suggestions to decrease the incidence of migraines.

SHORT ANSWERS

Fill in the table regarding the manifestations of brain tumors by location.

Lobe	Manifestations
Frontal Lobe Tumors	
Parietal Lobe Tumors	
Temporal Lobe Tumors	
Occipital Lobe Tumors	
Cerebellum Tumors	
Pituitary Tumors	

NCLEX-RN® REVIEW QUESTIONS

1. During discharge planning, the nurse is teaching the patient how to decrease incidents of migraine headaches. Which of the following suggestions is incorrect?
   1. Wake up at the same time each morning.
   2. Do not use artificial sweeteners.
   3. Do not consume MSG (monosodium glutamate).
   4. Consume a food source or beverage with caffeine before 6 PM.

2. Doll's eye movements are reflexive movements of the eyes in what direction of head rotation?
   1. opposite
   2. parallel
   3. same
   4. downward

3. Which of the following statements by a student nurse reflects correct understanding about brain death?
   1. "Brain death is the cessation and irreversibility of all brain functions, including the brainstem."
   2. "The exact criteria for establishing brain death do not vary from state to state."
   3. "The electrocardiogram (ECG) may be used to establish the absence of cardiac activity when brain death is suspected."
   4. "It is generally agreed that brain death has occurred when there is no evidence of cerebral or brainstem function for an extended period (usually 48–72 hours) in a patient who has an abnormal body temperature and is not affected by a depressant drug or alcohol poisoning."

4. Cerebral edema _____ ICP, which in turn _____ cerebral blood flow.
   1. increases, decreases
   2. decreases, increases
   3. increases, increases
   4. decreases, decreases

5. A nurse is planning a seminar about headaches. Which of the following statements on a handout for the seminar needs to be corrected?
   1. Migraine headaches affect about 20 million people in the United States and are more common in women than in men.
   2. There are two types of migraine headaches: common migraine (with an aura) and classic migraine (without an aura).
   3. Migraine headache is a recurring vascular headache that lasts from 4–72 hours, often initiated by a triggering event and usually accompanied by a neurologic dysfunction.
   4. A cluster headache is an extremely severe, unilateral, burning pain located behind or around the eyes.

6. The nurse is providing first aid to a patient who is having a seizure. Which of the following actions by the nurse is incorrect?
   1. Turn the patient on his side.
   2. Cushion the patient's head.
   3. Place a tongue blade in the patient's mouth.
   4. Loosen items around the patient's neck.

7. During discharge planning, the nurse is teaching the patient's spouse about when she needs to call for medical assistance when her husband is having a seizure. Which of the following actions is incorrect?
   1. The seizure lasts for less than four minutes.
   2. There is slow recovery from the seizure.
   3. There is a second seizure.
   4. There are signs of injury.

8. Which of the following information about hematomas is false?
   1. An epidural hematoma (also called an extradural hematoma) develops in the potential space between the dura and the skull, which normally adhere to each other.
   2. Acute subdural hematomas develop over weeks or months.
   3. Subdural hematoma is a localized mass of blood that collects between the dura mater and the arachnoid mater.
   4. Intracerebral hematomas, which may be single or multiple, are associated with contusions.

Nursing Care of Patients with Spinal Cord Disorders and CNS Infections

LEARNING OUTCOMES

1. Explain the pathophysiology, manifestations, complications, interdisciplinary care, and nursing care of patients with spinal cord injury, herniated intervertebral disk, spinal cord tumor, and CNS infections.

2. Compare and contrast the pathophysiological effects of injuries and tumors of the spinal cord by level of injury.

3. Discuss the purposes, nursing implications, and health education of the patient and family for medications used to treat spinal cord injury and CNS infections.

4. Explain the methods used to stabilize and immobilize spinal cord injuries.

5. Describe the surgical procedures used to treat spinal cord disorders.

CLINICAL COMPETENCIES

1. Assess functional health status of patients with spinal cord disorders and CNS infections and monitor, document, and report abnormal manifestations.

2. Use assessed data, patient values, clinical expertise and evidence to determine priority nursing diagnoses and select and implement individualized nursing interventions.

3. Adapt individual and cultural values and variations as well as expressed needs and preferences into the plan of care for patients with spinal cord disorders and CNS infections.

4. Administer oral and injectable medications used to treat spinal cord disorders and CNS infections knowledgeably and safely.

5. Provide appropriate and safe care to patients having a carotid endarterectomy, halo fixation, and a posterior laminectomy.

6. Integrate interdisciplinary care into care of patients with spinal cord disorders and CNS infections.

7. Provide teaching to facilitate self-catheterization, self-care of a ruptured intervertebral disk, and community-based self-care of disabilities resulting from spinal cord disorders and CNS infections.

8. Use evidence-based research to prevent ventilator-associated pneumonia in patients in the neurologic ICU.

9. Revise plan of care as needed to provide effective interventions to promote, maintain, or restore functional health status to patients with spinal cord disorders and CNS infections.

MediaLink

Pearson Nursing Student Resources
Audio Glossary
NCLEX-RN® Review

- Care Plan Activity
  - Neurologic Disorders
- Case Studies
  - The Patient with Cerebrovascular and Spinal Cord Disorders
  - The Patient with Bacterial Meningitis
- Animations/Videos
  - Spinal Cord Injury
  - Emergency: Musculoskeletal Immobilization, Spinal Supine: Prehospital First Responder
  - Meningitis
- MediaLink Application
- Links to Resources

TERMS MATCHING

Place the letter of the correct definition in the space next to each term.

1. _____ Autonomic dysreflexia

2. _____ Botulism

3. _____ Creutzfeldt-Jakob disease (CJD)

4. _____ Deformation

5. _____ Encephalitis

6. _____ Meningitis

7. _____ Paresthesia

8. _____ Postpoliomyelitis syndrome

9. _____ Quadriplegia

10. _____ Rabies

11. _____ Radiculopathy

12. _____ Sciatica

13. _____ Spasticity

14. _____ Spinal cord injury (SCI)

15. _____ Spinal shock

16. _____ Tetanus

17. _____ Paraplegia

A. More commonly called *lockjaw*, it is by a neurotoxin disorder elaborated by *Clostridium tetani*.

B. An abnormal sensation of the skin, such as numbness, burning, or prickling.

C. Diagnosed by a previous history of polio and manifestations that persist for at least one year.

D. The temporary loss of reflex function (called *areflexia*) below the level of injury at the cervical and upper thoracic spinal cord.

E. An exaggerated sympathetic response that occurs in patients with SCIs at or above the T_6 level.

F. Hyperactive tendon and muscle reflexes.

G. Characterized by degeneration of the gray matter of the brain.

H. A generalized infection of the parenchyma of the brain or spinal cord.

I. Food poisoning caused by ingestion of food contaminated with a toxin produced by the bacillus *Clostridium botulinum*.

J. A pyogenic (purulent) infection that involves the pia mater, the arachnoid, and the subarachnoid space, including the cerebrospinal fluid.

K. The damage to the neural elements of the spinal cord.

L. Pain.

M. Occurs with damage to the neural structures in the thoracic, lumbar, or sacral area of the cord.

N. A virus carried by both wild and domestic animals, including bats, skunks, foxes, raccoons, cats, and dogs.

O. Occurs with damage to the neural structures in the cervical area of the cord, resulting in loss or impairment of motor and/or sensory function in the arms, trunk, legs, and pelvic organs.

P. Alteration of the spinal cord and soft tissues caused by abnormal head and body movements.

Q. Lumbar back pain that radiates down the posterior leg to the ankle and is increased by sneezing or coughing.

FOCUSED STUDY

1. List the manifestations of spinal shock.

_____

_____

_____

_____

2. Discuss conservative treatment modalities utilized to manage care for a patient with ruptured intervertebral disk.

_____

_____

_____

_____

3. List specific topics to consider during a health history assessment interview of the patient with a spinal cord injury (SCI).

_____

_____

_____

_____

4. Autonomic dysreflexia is an emergency that requires immediate assessment and intervention to prevent complications. Discuss nursing interventions to be implemented should autonomic dysreflexia occur.

_____

_____

_____

_____

_____

CASE STUDY

Sandra Brown is a 25-year-old female who arrived at the emergency room (ER) with a complaint of severe back pain. She has rated her pain a 9/10. Her vital signs were taken upon arrival to the ER and were as follows: B/P=160/90, HR=122, RR=26.

1. In an effort to differentiate the cause of the back injury, what diagnostic tests are anticipated?

2. What medications are used in the management of pain and muscle spasms?

3. What are the goals of conservative treatment?

4. What data is collected in the health history and physical assessment?

CROSSWORD PUZZLE

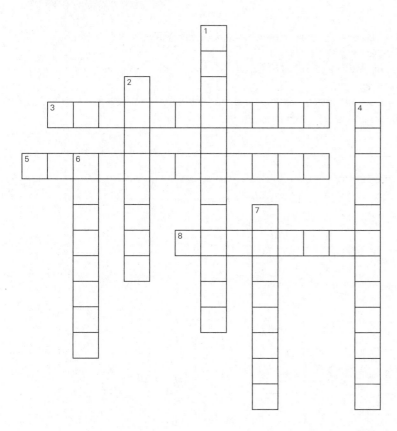

Across

3 Administered to prevent vomiting

5 A forcible bending forward

8 Used to treat bradycardia

Down

1 External force applied in head-on collision

2 A medication used to treat spasticity

4 External force applied in rear-end collision

6 An example of a proton pump inhibitor

7 A medication used to treat hypotension in shock

NCLEX-RN® REVIEW QUESTIONS

1. Which of the following is a priority nursing diagnosis for the nurse caring for a patient diagnosed with a ruptured intervertebral disk?
   1. *Activity Intolerance*
   2. *Self-Care Deficit*
   3. *Impaired Physical Mobility*
   4. *Acute Pain*

2. All of the following except what is considered an intervention when initiating a bowel retraining program?
   1. Assess routine patterns of bowel elimination.
   2. Maintain a high-fluid, low-fiber diet.
   3. Administer stool softeners as prescribed.
   4. Consider implementing digital stimulation or manual removal if patient is unable to evacuate.

3. Which of the following are clinical manifestations of autonomic dysreflexia?
   1. hypertension, bradycardia, and cool skin below the level of injury
   2. hypertension, tachycardia, and cool skin below the level of injury
   3. hypotension, bradycardia, and warm skin above the level of injury
   4. hypotension, tachycardia, and warm skin above the level of injury

4. During assessment, the nurse would consider which of the following to be an expected finding in a patient diagnosed with Creutzfeldt-Jakob disease (CJD)?
   1. hyporeflexia
   2. Battle signs
   3. a positive Babinski
   4. an increased white blood cell count

5. Which of the following is an antifungal agent considered in the treatment of fungal meningitis?
   1. phenytoin (Dilantin®)
   2. amphotericin B (Amphotec®)
   3. rifampin (Rifadin®)
   4. dexamethasone (Decadron®)

6. An emergency room nurse is expected to find which of the following early manifestations in a patient with tetanus?
   1. pain at the site of infection, jaw stiffness, and dysphagia
   2. pain at the site of infection, jaw stiffness, and rigidity of abdominal muscles
   3. pain at the site of infection, hyperreflexia, and dysphagia
   4. pain at the site of infection, jaw and neck stiffness, and spasms of the facial muscles

7. Approximately how much of a fluid loss does a weight loss of 1 lb represent?
   1. 1500 mL
   2. 1000 mL
   3. 500 mL
   4. 100 mL

Nursing Care of Patients with Neurologic Disorders

LEARNING OUTCOMES

1. Identify risk factors for degenerative neurologic, peripheral nervous system, and cranial nerve disorders.

2. Explain the pathophysiology, manifestations, complications, interdisciplinary care, and nursing care of patients with degenerative neurologic disorders (dementia, Alzheimer's disease, multiple sclerosis, Parkinson's disease, Huntington's disease, amyotrophic lateral sclerosis), PNS disorders (myasthenia gravis, Guillian-Barré syndrome), and cranial nerve disorders (trigeminal neuralgia, Bell's palsy).

3. Compare and contrast the manifestations of the progressive stages of Alzheimer's disease.

4. Discuss the purposes, nursing implications, and health education for the patient and family for medications used to treat Alzheimer's disease, multiple sclerosis, Parkinson's disease, and myasthenia gravis.

5. Describe the procedures (thymectomy, percutaneous rhizotomy, plasmapheresis) used to treat selected neurologic disorders.

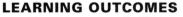

MediaLink

Pearson Nursing Student Resources
Audio Glossary
NCLEX-RN® Review
- Care Plan Activity
  - Guillain-Barré Syndrome
- Case Studies
  - Huntington's Disease
  - Parkinson's Disease
- Animations/Videos
  - Alzheimer's Disease
  - Multiple Sclerosis
  - Parkinson's Disease
- MediaLink Application
- Links to Resources

CLINICAL COMPETENCIES

1. Assess functional status of patients with neurologic disorders and monitor, document, and report abnormal manifestations.

2. Use evidence-based research to design nursing interventions specific to the needs of aging patients with multiple sclerosis.

3. Use assessed data, patient values, clinical expertise and evidence to determine priority nursing diagnoses and select and implement nursing interventions.

4. Administer oral and injectable medications used to treat Alzheimer's disease, multiple sclerosis, Parkinson's disease, and myasthenia gravis accurately and safely.

5. Provide competent care to patients having a thymectomy, percutaneous rhizotomy, or plasmapheresis.

6. Effectively communicate with and function within the interdisciplinary team to plan and provide care of patients with neurologic disorders.

7. Provide appropriate teaching to facilitate safety, communications, and community-based self-care for acute and chronic healthcare needs resulting from neurologic disorders.

8. Adapt individual and cultural values and variations as well as expressed needs and preferences into the plan of care.

9. Revise plan of care as needed to provide effective interventions to promote, maintain, or restore functional health status to patients with neurologic disorders.

TERMS MATCHING

Place the letter of the correct definition in the space next to each term.

1. _____ Alzheimer's disease (AD)

2. _____ Amyotrophic lateral sclerosis (ALS)

3. _____ Bell's palsy

4. _____ Dementia

5. _____ Guillain-Barré syndrome (GBS)

6. _____ Huntington's disease

7. _____ Multiple sclerosis (MS)

8. _____ Myasthenia gravis

9. _____ Neuralgia

10. _____ Parkinson's disease (PD)

11. _____ Sundowning

12. _____ Trigeminal neuralgia

A. A chronic autoimmune peripheral nervous system disorder characterized by fatigue and severe skeletal muscle weakness.

B. Agitation in the evening or night that may include confusion, fearfulness, or panic attacks.

C. An acute inflammatory demyelinating disease of the peripheral nervous system.

D. A progressive degenerative neurologic disease characterized by tremor, muscle rigidity, and bradykinesia.

E. A form of dementia characterized by progressive, irreversible deterioration of general intellectual functioning.

F. A progressive, degenerative inherited neurologic disease characterized by increasing dementia and chorea.

G. A chronic demyelinating neurologic disease of the CNS.

H. A rapidly progressive and fatal degenerative motor neuron disease characterized by weakness and wasting of voluntary control muscles but without sensory or cognitive changes.

I. A chronic disorder of cranial nerve V that causes severe facial pain.

J. A cognitive decline caused by any disorder that permanently damages areas of the brain necessary for memory and learning.

K. Characterized by severe, brief, repetitive attacks of lightening-like or throbbing pain, occurring along the distribution of a spinal or cranial nerve.

L. An acute disorder of cranial nerve VII characterized by unilateral paralysis of the facial muscles.

FOCUSED STUDY

1. Discuss assessment and findings of cranial nerve function.

_____

_____

_____

2. Discuss the criteria that must be met to be diagnosed with dementia and discuss possible risk factors.

_____

_____

_____

_____

3. Summarize the stages of Guillain-Barré syndrome.

_____

_____

_____

_____

4. Describe the following procedures: thymectomy, percutaneous rhizotomy, and plasmapheresis.

_____

_____

_____

_____

_____

CASE STUDY

MiMi Bradley is a 73-year-old female patient in today for a physical examination. Her daughter Christine tells the nurse that her mother has been experiencing memory loss, is having difficulty performing familiar tasks, appears disoriented at times, and is misplacing things and that she sees a change in her mother's personality. Christine then asks the nurse a few questions. Answer the following questions based on your knowledge of Alzheimer's disease.

1. "What are the risk factors of Alzheimer's disease?"

2. "What are the warning signs of Alzheimer's disease?"

3. "What are the stages of Alzheimer's disease?"

WORD SEARCH

C	W	A	S	E	M	D	I	K	G	U	T	P	E	S	H	C	Y	M	J	B
O	E	L	N	O	X	P	O	V	L	D	E	N	B	A	C	L	O	F	E	N
G	S	L	U	N	E	S	A	B	I	R	M	N	M	I	P	W	R	H	T	A
N	Y	Q	B	R	L	F	M	R	W	E	A	V	H	T	A	U	L	F	U	S
L	M	A	T	U	S	T	N	U	L	N	C	E	S	O	I	P	E	I	G	R
A	M	E	R	A	R	A	T	H	P	O	R	N	L	N	A	N	V	N	L	T
I	E	D	M	W	D	L	O	K	Z	A	D	M	M	E	R	I	O	C	Y	M
X	T	U	I	L	S	I	Y	B	F	Q	G	E	T	O	G	V	D	Y	K	H
O	R	S	P	T	S	O	L	A	N	S	A	C	L	S	W	R	O	D	J	C
P	E	I	N	B	W	D	G	V	L	N	C	I	O	D	B	C	P	R	A	T
H	L	X	L	R	E	S	I	R	I	F	K	Y	H	L	F	P	A	Q	L	N
E	M	M	A	U	N	V	M	T	W	A	S	W	O	D	N	S	U	N	C	S
P	R	E	S	J	T	S	N	U	C	L	I	S	M	A	N	Z	E	A	U	J
Z	F	H	Y	O	V	E	T	Y	F	S	E	G	R	D	I	A	D	M	O	A
D	O	N	P	E	G	C	K	A	N	G	H	U	O	L	Y	S	O	N	L	S
E	M	Y	K	O	L	B	T	E	T	D	M	F	S	G	M	B	W	H	R	G
L	M	T	C	N	I	C	M	P	I	I	A	P	R	T	I	O	R	S	Y	O
N	I	U	E	A	P	E	A	R	N	D	E	G	O	Z	A	E	A	J	G	O
J	W	B	S	M	W	K	T	S	O	S	D	I	L	A	N	T	I	N	F	X
Y	D	S	O	A	E	P	K	G	A	Q	Y	N	R	U	W	K	I	C	E	M
S	E	A	C	H	R	I	L	E	H	E	R	W	T	C	L	I	S	N	A	H

DEFINITIONS FOR WORDS IN THE SEARCH

Muscle relaxant

Immunosuppressant

Dopamine precursor

Glutamate antagonist

Dopamine agonist

Anticholinergic

Anticonvulsant

Antiglutamate

Anticancer drug

Glucocorticoid

NCLEX-RN® REVIEW QUESTIONS

1. Which of the following are not warning signs of Alzheimer's disease? **Select all that apply.**
   1. habit of misplacing things
   2. loss of initiative
   3. ability to perform familiar tasks
   4. change in personality
   5. withdrawal from social activities

2. Which of the following statements by a student nurse reflects incorrect understanding about multiple sclerosis (MS)? **Select all that apply.**
   1. "It is a chronic demyelinating neurologic disease of the central nervous system (brain, optic nerves, and spinal cord)."
   2. "The initial onset cannot be followed by a total remission."
   3. "The manifestations of MS do not vary according to the area of the nervous system affected."
   4. "The onset of MS is usually between 40 and 60 years of age."
   5. "It is primarily a disease of northern European ancestry."

3. During discharge planning, the nurse is teaching the patient about Parkinson's disease. Which of the following statements is correct? **Select all that apply.**
   1. "Parkinson's disease is one of the least common neurologic disorders that affects older adults."
   2. "The disorder usually develops after the age of 75, but 25% of those diagnosed are under 50 years of age."
   3. "Women and men are affected equally."
   4. "Women and men are affected equally."
   5. "Drug induced Parkinson's is irreversible."

4. All of the following statements about Parkinson's disease are true except which one?
   1. In Parkinson's disease, neurons in the cerebral cortex atrophy and are lost, the dopaminergic nigrostriatal (pigmented) pathway degenerates, and the number of specific dopamine receptors in the basal ganglia decreases.
   2. Diagnosis is based primarily on a thorough history and physical examination and is made based on having one of the three cardinal manifestations: tremor at rest, bradykinesia, and rigidity.
   3. Surgical treatment of PD may be used for patients who have had the disease for a long time and are no longer able to control manifestations with medications.
   4. Patients with Parkinson's disease commonly have sleep disturbances, although they may experience decreased manifestations during sleep in the early stages.

5. Which of the following is not a complication associated with Parkinson's disease?
   1. falls from balance, posture, and motor changes
   2. depression and social isolation
   3. skin breakdown and pressure ulcers associated with urinary incontinence, malnutrition, and sweat reflex changes
   4. obesity related to dysphagia

6. A nurse is evaluating a patient's understanding of Huntington's disease (HD). Which of the following statements indicates a need for further teaching?
   1. HD is a progressive, degenerative, inherited neurologic disease characterized by increasing dementia and chorea (jerky, rapid, involuntary movements).
   2. Early signs of personality change include severe depression, memory loss with decreased ability to concentrate, emotional lability, and impulsiveness.
   3. HD is a familial disease, and each child of an HD parent has a 25% chance of inheriting the HD gene.
   4. HD causes destruction of cells in the caudate nucleus and putamen areas of the basal ganglia.

7. A nurse is planning a seminar about amyotrophic lateral sclerosis (ALS). Which of the following statements is correct?
   1. ALS is a slow and fatal degenerative neurologic disease characterized by weakness and wasting of tissue with accompanying sensory or cognitive changes.
   2. ALS is also known as Babe Ruth's disease.
   3. There is no cure for ALS.
   4. ALS affects motor neurons in only two locations: the anterior horn cells, which are lower motor neurons (LMNs) of the spinal cord, and the upper motor neurons (UMNs) of the cerebral cortex.

8. The nurse is evaluating a myasthenia gravis class. During the class, she recognizes that further teaching is necessary when which of the following statements is made by a participant?
1. "Myasthenia gravis is an acute inflammatory demyelinating disorder of the peripheral nervous system characterized by an acute onset of motor paralysis that is usually ascending."
2. "The manifestations of myasthenia gravis correspond to the muscles involved. Initially, the eye muscles are affected and the patient experiences either diplopia (unilateral or bilateral double vision) or ptosis (drooping of the eyelid)."
3. "In myasthenia gravis, antibodies destroy or block neuromuscular junction receptor sites, which results in a decreased number of acetylcholine receptors."
4. "Myasthenia gravis is sometimes associated with a tumor of the thymus, thyrotoxicosis (hyperthyroidism), rheumatoid arthritis, and lupus erythematosus."

9. Which of the following statements by a student nurse reflects incorrect understanding about trigeminal neuralgia?
Select all that apply.
1. "Trigeminal neuralgia occurs more commonly in younger adults and affects men more often than women."
2. "Trigeminal neuralgia, is a chronic disease of the trigeminal cranial nerve (V) that causes severe facial pain."
3. "There are three specific diagnostic tests for trigeminal neuralgia."
4. "Trigeminal neuralgia is characterized by brief repetitive episodes of sudden severe facial pain."
5. "Trigeminal neuralgia goes into spontaneous remission for periods lasting from days to years."

45 Assessing the **Eye** and **Ear**

LEARNING OUTCOMES

1. Describe the anatomy, physiology, and functions of the eye and the ear.
2. Identify specific topics for consideration during a health history interview of the patient with health problems involving the eye or ear.
3. Give examples of genetic disorders in vision and hearing.
4. Describe normal variations in assessment findings for the older adult.
5. Identify abnormal findings that may indicate impairment in the function of the eye and the ear.

CLINICAL COMPETENCIES

1. Conduct and document a health history for patients who have or are at risk for alterations in the structure or functions of the eye and ear.
2. Conduct and document a physical assessment of the structure and functions of the eye and ear.
3. Monitor the results of diagnostic tests and report abnormal findings.

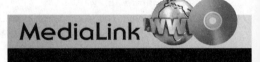

MediaLink

Pearson Nursing Student Resources
Audio Glossary
NCLEX-RN® Review
■ Care Plan Activity
  ■ Ear Disorder
■ Case Studies
  ■ The Patient with Conjunctivitis
  ■ Assessing Patients with Eye or Ear Disorders
■ MediaLink Applications
■ Links to Resources

TERMS MATCHING

Place the letter of the correct definition in the space next to each term.

1. ____ Accommodation

2. ____ Cerumen

3. ____ Convergence

4. ____ Corneal reflex

5. ____ Hyperopia

6. ____ Myopia

7. ____ Nystagmus

8. ____ Presbyopia

9. ____ Ptosis

10. ____ Pupillary light reflex

11. ____ Refraction

A. Farsightedness; the patient is unable to clearly see objects that are near him or her.

B. The eyelids blink when the cornea is touched.

C. Nearsightedness; the patient is unable to see distant objects well.

D. In response to intense light, the pupil normally constricts rapidly.

E. The patient's eyes will constrict and converge to focus on an object that is close to him or her.

F. The bending of light rays as they pass from one medium to another medium of different optical density.

G. The medial rotation of the eyeballs so that each is directed toward the viewed object.

H. Age-related changes resulting in decreased lens elasticity; the decreased ability to focus and accommodate to view objects that are at close range.

I. The brown or yellow waxy substance that is secreted in the ear canal.

J. Drooping of one eyelid.

K. An involuntary rhythmic movement of the eyes; associated with neurologic disorders and the use of some medications.

FOCUSED STUDY

1. Identify two nonverbal cues that may indicate that a patient has a problem with his or her eyes.

_____

_____

2. Discuss some age-related changes that can occur in the eye. Discuss some age-related changes that can occur in the ear.

_____

_____

_____

_____

_____

3. Provide three examples of eye disorders that have a genetic influence. Provide three examples of ear disorders that have a genetic influence.

_____

_____

_____

_____

4. Discuss tests that are used to diagnose eye disorders. Discuss tests used to diagnose ear disorders.

_____

_____

_____

_____

_____

_____

CASE STUDY

Michael Scott RN, BSN, is teaching a nursing course. He is preparing a presentation about eye and ear disorders. He has developed the following questions to ask the nursing students after his lecture to evaluate their level of understanding.

1. What is the colored part of the eye? What is its function?

2. Where is the lens located? What is its function?

3. What is the best way to assess the central visual field?

4. How are sound waves transmitted through the ear so that the patient can perceive and interpret the sounds?

5. Explain equilibrium.

6. What is a tympanogram? What does an abnormal tympanogram indicate?

SHORT ANSWERS

Label the following figures.

Figure 1: Eyebrows, eyelids, eyelashes, conjunctiva, lacrimal apparatus, extrinsic eye muscles

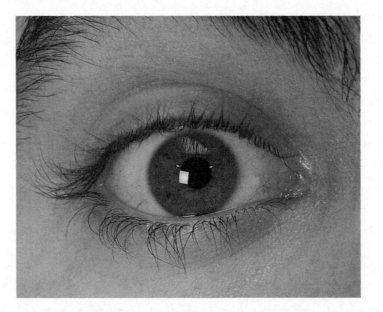

Figure 2: Sclera, cornea, iris, pupil, anterior cavity

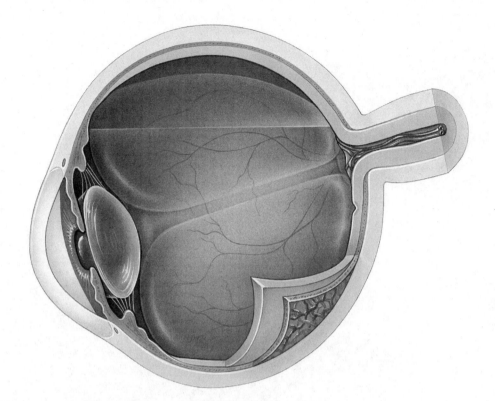

Figure 3: External ear, middle ear, inner ear

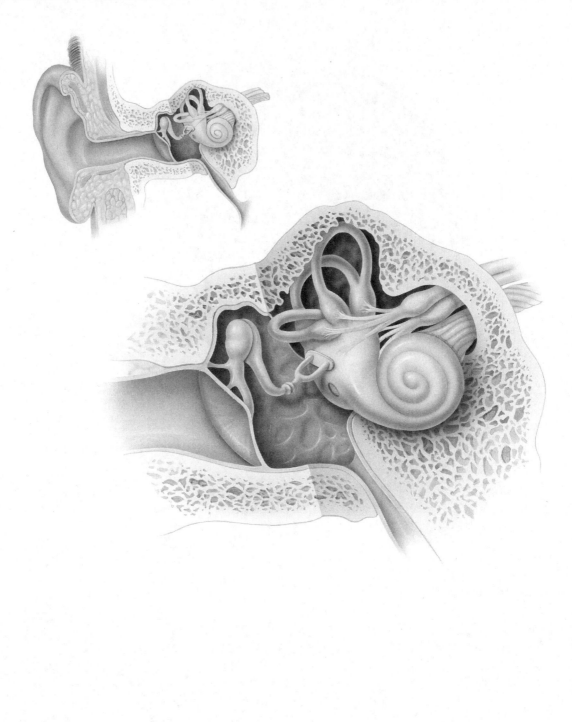

NCLEX-RN® REVIEW QUESTIONS

1. The_____ gives the eye its color and regulates light entry by controlling the size of the_____.
   1. iris, pupil
   2. pupil, iris
   3. iris, sclera
   4. sclera, cornea

2. Which of the following statements about aqueous humor is accurate?
   1. "Aqueous humor is a cloudy fluid."
   2. "Aqueous humor provides nutrients and oxygen to the pupil and the iris."
   3. "Aqueous humor is constantly formed and drained to maintain a relatively constant pressure of 25–30 mmHg in the eye."
   4. "Aqueous humor fills the anterior cavity."

3. What is it called when the eye focuses on an image?
   1. accommodation
   2. refraction
   3. convergence
   4. pupillary light reflex

4. Which of the following actions is correct for the nurse who is measuring a patient's visual fields?
   1. Move the penlight from the periphery toward the center from right to left, above and below, and from the middle of each of these directions.
   2. Ask the patient to look directly at a point behind and to the side of you.
   3. Ask the patient to cover one eye with an opaque cover while you cover your own eye corresponding to the patient's.
   4. Sit directly opposite the patient at a distance of 36–48 inches.

5. Which of the following can be found in the external ear?
   1. incus
   2. stapes
   3. malleus
   4. tympanic membrane

6. Which of the following statements about sound conduction indicates the need for further education?
   1. Hearing is the perception and interpretation of sound.
   2. Sound is produced when the molecules of a medium are compressed, which results in a pressure disturbance evidenced as a sound wave.
   3. Sound waves enter the external auditory canal and cause the tympanic membrane to vibrate at the same frequency.
   4. The human ear is most sensitive to sound waves with frequencies between 100 and 400 cycles per second, but it can detect sound waves with frequencies between 2 and 200 cycles per second."

7. Which of the following assessment findings of the tympanic membrane should be reported to the patient's physician?
   1. It appears shiny.
   2. The color is pearly gray.
   3. It is translucent.
   4. It is bulging.

46 Nursing Care of Patients with Eye and Ear Disorders

LEARNING OUTCOMES

1. Relate knowledge of normal anatomy, physiology, and sensory functions of the eye and ear to the effects of disorders of these organs on the cognitive/perceptual functional health pattern.

2. Describe the pathophysiology of commonly occurring disorders of the eyes and ears, relating their manifestations to the pathophysiological process.

3. Explain the risk factors for selected disorders of the eyes and ears, identifying the nursing implications for these risk factors.

4. Identify diagnostic tests used for specific eye and ear disorders.

5. Discuss the effects of and nursing implications for medications prescribed to treat eye and ear disorders.

6. Describe surgical and other invasive procedures used to treat eye and ear disorders, identifying their implications for nursing care.

7. Discuss the nurse's role in caring for patients with impaired vision or hearing loss.

CLINICAL COMPETENCIES

1. Assess vision, hearing, and functional health of patients with eye and ear disorders.

2. Using assessed data, determine priority nursing diagnoses and interventions for patients with eye and ear disorders.

3. Collaborate with other members of the healthcare team to provide safe, effective care for patients with eye and ear disorders.

4. Plan and implement appropriate and individualized evidence-based nursing interventions and teaching for the patient with an eye or ear disorder.

5. Safely and effectively administer eye and ear medications and prescribed treatments.

6. Provide appropriate care and teaching for the patient having eye or ear surgery.

7. Evaluate the effectiveness of nursing care provided for patients with eye and ear disorders, revising plan of care as indicated.

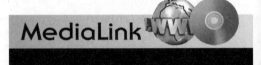
MediaLink

Pearson Nursing Student Resources
Audio Glossary
NCLEX-RN® Review
■ Care Plan Activity
  ■ The Patient with Hearing Loss
■ Case Study
  ■ The Patient with Eye and Ear Disorders
■ Animations/Videos
  ■ Cataract - Etiology and Pathophysiology
  ■ Disease Focus: Glaucoma
  ■ Otitis Media - Geriatric Sensations
■ MediaLink Application
■ Links to Resources

TERMS MATCHING

Place the letter of the correct definition in the space next to each term.

1. _____ Acoustic neuroma

2. _____ Astigmatism

3. _____ Cataract

4. _____ Chalazion

5. _____ Conjunctivitis

6. _____ Corneal ulcer

7. _____ Diabetic retinopathy

8. _____ Enophthalmos

9. _____ Enucleation

10. _____ Glaucoma

11. _____ Hordeolum (sty)

12. _____ Hyperopia

13. _____ Hyphema

14. _____ Keratitis

15. _____ Labyrinthitis

16. _____ Macular degeneration

17. _____ Mastoiditis

18. _____ Ménière's disease

19. _____ Myopia

20. _____ Myringotomy

21. _____ Nystagmus

22. _____ Otitis externa

23. _____ Otitis media

24. _____ Otosclerosis

25. _____ Presbycusis

26. _____ Ptosis

27. _____ Retinal detachment

28. _____ Tinnitus

29. _____ Tympanoplasty

30. _____ Vertigo

A. The patient is unable to see objects that are in close proximity.

B. Inflammation of the inner ear; also known as otitis interna.

C. Local necrosis of the cornea.

D. A condition that is the result of damage to the retina; affects the patient's central vision.

E. A benign tumor of cranial nerve VIII; also known as a schwannoma.

F. A bacterial infection of the mastoid process.

G. The surgical reconstruction of the middle ear.

H. The perception of a sound such as ringing, buzzing, or roaring in the ears.

I. Inflammation of the conjunctiva; the most common eye disease.

J. The sensation of movement when there is none; a disorder of equilibrium.

K. A condition where there is a separation of the retina from the choroid.

L. A term used to describe an eye that appears sunken.

M. Drooping of the eyelid.

N. This develops due to an irregular or abnormal curvature of the cornea; distorts both near and distance vision.

O. Inflammation of the ear canal.

P. Bleeding in the anterior chamber of the eye.

Q. An incision into the tympanic membrane.

R. The surgical removal of an eye.

S. The patient is unable to see distant objects well.

T. A staphylococcal abscess that may occur on either the external or internal margin of the eyelid.

U. Inflammation of the middle ear.

V. An opacification, or clouding, of the lens of the eye.

W. A condition that occurs when there is abnormal bone formation in the osseous labyrinth of the temporal bone; the footplate of the stapes become fixed or immobile in the oval window.

X. Rapid involuntary eye movements.

Y. A chronic disorder characterized by recurrent attacks of vertigo with tinnitus and a progressive unilateral hearing loss; also known as endolymphatic hydrops.

Z. Inflammation of the cornea.

AA. A vascular disorder that affects the capillaries of the retina.

BB. Gradual age-related loss of hearing.

CC. A granulomatous cyst or nodule of the eyelid.

DD. A condition characterized by optic neuropathy with gradual loss of peripheral vision; often associated with increased intraocular pressure.

FOCUSED STUDY

1. Identify the various ways that a patient may develop acute conjunctivitis.

_____

_____

_____

_____

2. Explain the difference between nonulcerative and ulcerative keratitis.

_____

_____

_____

3. Briefly describe the tests that can be used to diagnose an inner ear disorder.

_____

_____

_____

4. Discuss the different surgeries that can be performed to correct problems in the patient's ear.

_____

_____

_____

CASE STUDY

Drake Smith is a 21-year-old male patient who is complaining of an itchy right eye. His right eye is red and is draining a small amount of purulent fluid. He was diagnosed with bacterial conjunctivitis. He asks the nurse several questions. Answer the following questions based on your knowledge of eye disorders.

1. "Is bacterial conjunctivitis the same as pink eye?"

2. "Is pink eye contagious?"

3. "What do most people with pink eye experience?"

4. "How is it normally treated?"

5. "What are some things I need to know so that I don't give this to my girlfriend?"

6. "My eyes are really sensitive to the sunlight right now. Should I just wear sunglasses until this gets better?"

CARE PLAN CRITICAL-THINKING ACTIVITY

Please refer to the case study and nursing care plan exercise: A Patient with Glaucoma and Cataracts (page 1598) to answer the following questions.

1. Why is it important for Mrs. Rainey to avoid shutting her eyelids tightly, sneezing, coughing, laughing, bending over, lifting, or straining to have a bowel movement?

2. Due to Mrs. Rainey's glaucoma, what are some things the nurse can instruct her about regarding her diet?

SHORT ANSWER

Fill in the table regarding the differences between open-angle and angle-closure glaucoma.

	Open-Angle Glaucoma	Angle-Closure Glaucoma
Incidence		
Risk Factors		
Pathophysiology		
Manifestations		
Management		

NCLEX-RN® REVIEW QUESTIONS

1. A patient tells the nurse that he is nearsighted. What does the nurse realize about the patient?
    1. The patient is having rapid involuntary eye movements.
    2. The patient has an opacification of the lens of the eye.
    3. The patient sees objects well at close range but those at a distant are blurred.
    4. The patient sees objects better at a distance than objects that are closer.

2. What is a granulomatous cyst or nodule of the lid?
    1. hordeolum
    2. chalazion
    3. hyphema
    4. cataract

3. A student nurse is discussing the stages of diabetic retinopathy with an experienced nurse who works with diabetic patients. Which of the following terms used by the student nurse indicates that he requires further education?
    1. mild nonproliferative or background retinopathy
    2. moderate nonproliferative retinopathy
    3. severe nonproliferative retinopathy
    4. critical proliferative retinopathy

4. A nurse is evaluating a patient's understanding of otitis externa. Which of the following statements indicates the need for further education?
    1. "It is inflammation of the ear canal."
    2. "It is commonly known as diver's ear."
    3. "It is most prevalent in people who spend significant time in the water."
    4. "Wearing a hearing aid or ear plugs, which hold moisture in the ear canal, is an additional risk factor."

5. Which of the following statements by a student nurse reflects an adequate level of understanding about otosclerosis?
    1. "Otosclerosis occurs most commonly in males."
    2. "Otosclerosis is not a cause of conductive hearing loss."
    3. "Otosclerosis has no genetic influences."
    4. "Otosclerosis is a hearing loss that typically begins in older patients."

6. Which of the following is a chronic disorder characterized by recurrent attacks of vertigo with tinnitus and a progressive unilateral hearing loss?
    1. acoustic neuroma
    2. labyrinthitis
    3. Ménière's disease
    4. otitis externa

7. A nurse is planning an educational program about presbycusis. Which of the following statements on the handout for the seminar needs to be corrected?
    1. Hearing loss of presbycusis is gradual.
    2. Lower-pitched tones and conversational speech are lost initially.
    3. It is associated with aging.
    4. Hearing aids and other amplification devices are useful for most patients with presbycusis.

47 Assessing the **Male** and **Female Reproductive** Systems

LEARNING OUTCOMES

1. Describe the anatomy, physiology, and functions of the male and female reproductive systems, including the breasts.
2. Identify specific topics for consideration during a health history interview of the patient with health problems of the reproductive system and breasts.
3. Give examples of genetic disorders of the male and female reproductive system and breasts.
4. Describe normal variations in reproductive assessment findings for the older adult.
5. Identify manifestations of impairment in the male and female reproductive system and breasts.

CLINICAL COMPETENCIES

1. Conduct and document a health history for men and women who are having or are at risk for alterations of the reproductive system and breasts.
2. Conduct and document a physical assessment of the male and female reproductive system and breasts.
3. Monitor the results of diagnostic tests and report abnormal findings.

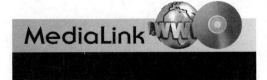

MediaLink

Pearson Nursing Student Resources
Audio Glossary
NCLEX-RN® Review
■ Care Plan Activity
  ■ STDs
■ Case Studies
  ■ Assessing Sexual Function
  ■ The Patient with Reproductive and Breast Disorders
■ MediaLink Applications
■ Links to Resources

TERMS MATCHING

Place the letter of the correct definition in the space next to each term.

1. _____ Androgens
2. _____ Anorgasmia
3. _____ Dyspareunia
4. _____ Estrogen
5. _____ Gynecomastia
6. _____ Impotence
7. _____ Menstrual cycle
8. _____ Menstruation
9. _____ Ovarian cycle
10. _____ Phimosis
11. _____ Progesterone
12. _____ Semen
13. _____ Testosterone

A. Abnormal enlargement of the breast(s) in men.

B. The male sex hormone that is produced primarily in the testes, although the adrenal cortex also produces a small amount.

C. The primary androgen produced by the testes that is essential in maintenance of sexual organs and secondary sex characteristics and for spermatogenesis; it also promotes metabolism, growth of muscles and bone, and libido (sexual desire).

D. The periodic shedding of the uterine lining in a woman of childbearing age who is not pregnant.

E. The inability to achieve or maintain an erection.

F. A body fluid produced in the male that consists of sperm and secretions from the accessory sex organs, the epididymis, the prostate gland, and Cowper's glands; this fluid nourishes the sperm, provides bulk, and increases its alkalinity.

G. The responses of the endometrium of the uterus to changes in estrogen and progesterone.

H. The biological cycle that begins with menstruation.

I. A tightness of the prepuce that prevents retraction of the foreskin.

J. Failure to achieve an orgasm by intercourse.

K. Painful sexual intercourse.

L. A female hormone produced by the ovaries to support the endometrium in the event of a pregnancy.

M. A female hormone produced by the ovaries that is responsible for the normal structure of skin and blood vessels; it also decreases the rate of bone resorption, promotes increased high-density lipoproteins, reduces cholesterol levels, and enhances the clotting of blood.

FOCUSED STUDY

1. Discuss the specific topics for consideration during a health history interview of the patient with health problems involving reproductive and breast structures or functions.

_____

_____

_____

_____

_____

2. Summarize the anatomy and physiology of the female and male reproductive systems.

_____

_____

_____

3. List and explain the functions of the male and female sex hormones.

_____

_____

_____

_____

CASE STUDY

Holly Anne is a 15-year-old female patient. She attended a class about the female reproductive system a few days ago and asks the nurse the following questions.

1. "What is the ovarian cycle?"

2. "Why do I need estrogen?"

3. "What is the difference between the vagina and the cervix?"

NCLEX REVIEW-RN® QUESTIONS

1. The school nurse is providing a presentation to a group of preteen boys. Which of the following statements about the testes indicates the need for further instruction?
   1. The testes are surrounded by two coverings: an outer tunica albuginea and an inner tunica vaginalis.
   2. The testes produce sperm and testosterone.
   3. The testes develop in the abdominal cavity of the fetus and then descend through the inguinal canal into the scrotum.
   4. The testes are homologous to the female's ovaries.
2. Which of the following statements by a student nurse reflects correct understanding about the prostate gland?
   1. "The prostate gland is about the size of a pea."
   2. "The prostate encircles the urethra just above the urinary bladder."
   3. "The prostate is made up of 40–50 tubuloalveolar glands surrounded by smooth muscle."
   4. "Secretions from the prostate gland make up about one-third the volume of semen."
3. A student nurse is preparing a presentation about the scrotum. Which of the following statements needs to be corrected?
   1. The scrotum is a sac or pouch made of two layers.
   2. When the testicular temperature is too low, the scrotum contracts to bring the testes up against the body.
   3. The optimum temperature for sperm production is about 4–5 degrees below body temperature.
   4. The scrotum hangs at the base of the penis, anterior to the anus, and regulates the temperature of the testes.
4. Which of the following statements by a student nurse reflects correct understanding about female external genitalia?
   1. "The female internal genitalia include the mons pubis, the labia, the clitoris, the vaginal and urethral openings, and glands."
   2. "The clitoris is an erectile organ that is analogous to the penis in the male."
   3. "The labia minora, which are folds of skin and adipose tissue covered with hair, are outermost; they begin at the base of the mons pubis and end at the anus."
   4. "After puberty, the mons is covered with hair in a square-shaped distribution."
5. A patient has reported to the physician's office with concerns related to an inability to maintain an erection. The nurse is reviewing the patient's health history. Which of the following medications may be linked to the erectile dysfunction?
   1. antibiotic
   2. oral hypoglycemic agent
   3. antispasmotic
   4. iron supplement
6. Which of the following is a blood test used to diagnose prostate cancer and to monitor treatment of prostate cancer?
   1. PSA
   2. VDRL
   3. RPR
   4. FTA-ABS
7. Which female organ(s) is (are) homologous to the male's testes?
   1. fallopian tubes
   2. ovaries
   3. mons pubis
   4. labia minora
8. A pregnant patient asks the nurse where the hormones to sustain her pregnancy will come from until the placenta begins to function. What response is most appropriate?
   1. the ovaries
   2. the corpus luteum
   3. the anterior pituitary gland
   4. the uterus

Nursing Care of **Men** with **Reproductive System** and **Breast Disorders**

LEARNING OUTCOMES

1. Explain the pathophysiology, manifestations, complications, interdisciplinary care, and nursing care of disorders of the male reproductive system, including disorders of sexual function, the penis, the testes and scrotum, the prostate gland, and the breast.

2. Compare and contrast the risk factors for cancer of the penis, testes, and prostate gland.

3. Discuss the purposes, nursing implications, and health education for medications and treatments used to treat disorders of sexual function, the penis, the testes and scrotum, the prostate gland, and the breast.

4. Describe the various surgical procedures used to treat disorders of the male reproductive system.

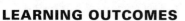

MediaLink

Pearson Nursing Student Resources
Audio Glossary
NCLEX-RN® Review
- Care Plan Activity
  - Prostate Cancer
- Case Studies
  - The Patient with Reproductive and Breast Disorders
  - Prostatitis
- Animations/Videos
  - Prostate Cancer
  - Testicular Cancer
- MediaLink
- Links to Resources

CLINICAL COMPETENCIES

1. Assess functional health status of men with reproductive system and breast disorders and monitor, document, and report abnormal manifestations.

2. Use evidence-based research to provide appropriate pre- and postoperative teaching to men having a laparoscopic radical prostatectomy.

3. Use assessed data, patient values, clinical expertise, and evidence to determine priority nursing diagnoses and, select and implement individualized nursing interventions.

4. Administer and/or teach patients how to administer medications used to treat disorders of the male reproductive system knowledgeably and safely.

5. Provide safe and knowledgeable care to men having prostate surgery.

6. Effectively communicate with and function within the interdisciplinary team to plan and provide patient care.

7. Adapt individual and cultural values and variations as well as expressed needs and preferences into the plan of care.

8. Revise plan of care as needed to provide effective interventions to promote, maintain, or restore functional health status to men with disorders of the reproductive system and breast.

TERMS MATCHING

Place the letter of the correct definition in the space next to each term.

1. _____ Benign prostatic hyperplasia (BPH)
2. _____ Epididymitis
3. _____ Erectile dysfunction (ED)
4. _____ Gynecomastia
5. _____ Hydrocele
6. _____ Impotence
7. _____ Libido
8. _____ Orchitis
9. _____ Phimosis
10. _____ Premature ejaculation
11. _____ Priapism
12. _____ Prostatitis
13. _____ Retrograde ejaculation
14. _____ Spermatocele
15. _____ Testicular torsion
16. _____ Varicocele

A. The inability of the male to attain and maintain an erection sufficient to permit satisfactory sexual intercourse.

B. The total inability to achieve erection, an inconsistent ability to achieve erection, or the ability to sustain only brief erections.

C. A term used to describe sexual desire.

D. An age-related, nonmalignant enlargement of the prostate gland that begins at 40–45 years of age and continues slowly through the rest of life.

E. An abnormal and often painful dilation of a vein in the spermatic cord caused by incompetent or congenitally missing valves that allow blood to pool in the spermatic cord veins.

F. An involuntary, sustained, painful erection not associated with sexual arousal that may result in ischemia and fibrosis of the erectile tissue with high risk of subsequent impotence.

G. Constriction of the foreskin so that it cannot be retracted over the glans penis.

H. The discharge of seminal fluid into the urinary bladder that may develop in aging men but is usually related to treatment of prostate conditions or testicular cancer.

I. A term used to refer to different types of inflammatory disorders of the prostate gland.

J. An infection or inflammation of the epididymis, the structure that lies along the posterior border of the testis.

K. The twisting of the spermatic cord resulting in sudden onset of scrotal swelling, pain, and nausea and vomiting; it occurs most often between birth and age 20 but can occur at any age.

L. A mobile, usually painless mass that forms when efferent ducts in the epididymis dilate and form a cyst.

M. The abnormal enlargement of the male breast thought to result from a high ratio of estradiol to testosterone.

N. A common ejaculatory disorder in which semen is ejaculated before completion of sexual intercourse.

O. The collection of fluid in the tunica vaginalis.

P. An acute inflammation or infection of the testes.

FOCUSED STUDY

1. List the risk factors for cancer of the penis, testes, and prostate gland.

_____

_____

_____

2. Summarize the various surgical procedures used to treat disorders of the male reproductive system.

_____

_____

_____

3. List the diagnostic tests that may be utilized to assess the patient who is reporting erectile dysfunction. Once the testing is completed what treatment options are available to manage this condition?

_____

_____

_____

CASE STUDY

Nathaniel Obermark is a 22-year-old male patient who states, "I have slight enlargement of my right testicle with some discomfort, and I have a feeling of heaviness in the scrotum." He then asks the nurse the following questions.

1. "What is the cause of testicular cancer?"

2. "What are the risk factors for testicular cancer?"

3. "What are the manifestations of testicular cancer?"

SHORT ANSWERS

Complete the chart by indicating the appropriate cause of erectile dysfunction for each category.

Medications	Procedures	Inflammatory Causes	Neurogenic Causes	Arterial Causes
1.	1.	1.	1.	1.
2.	2.	2.	2.	2.
3.	3.		3.	3.
4.	4.		4.	4.
5.			5.	

NCLEX-RN® REVIEW QUESTIONS

1. The nurse is providing a program about erectile dysfunction. When he is assessing the knowledge level of the participants, which of the following statements indicates the need for further education?
   1. Erectile dysfunction is the male's inability to attain and maintain an erection sufficient to permit satisfactory sexual intercourse.
   2. *Impotence* is a term often used synonymously with *erectile dysfunction*.
   3. Erectile dysfunction has many possible causes.
   4. Erectile dysfunction can be treated only with oral medications.

2. Which condition is constriction of the foreskin so that it cannot be retracted over the glans penis?
   1. paraphimosis
   2. phimosis
   3. priapism
   4. hydrocele

3. What is a collection of fluid in the tunica vaginalis and is the most common cause of scrotal swelling?
   1. testicular torsion
   2. spermatocele
   3. hydrocele
   4. varicocele

4. Which of the following statements by a student nurse reflects correct understanding about orchitis?
   1. "Orchitis is a chronic infection of the testes."
   2. "Orchitis most commonly occurs as a complication of a systemic illness or as an extension of epididymitis."
   3. "The most common infectious cause of orchitis in postpubertal men is measles."
   4. "The manifestations of orchitis have a gradual onset, usually within three to four weeks after the swelling of the parotid glands."

5. A nurse is evaluating a patient's understanding of testicular cancer. Which of the following statements indicates a need for further teaching?
   1. "Testicular cancer is more common on the left side, which parallels the incidence of cryptorchidism."
   2. "Testicular cancer is the most common cancer in men between the ages of 15 and 40."
   3. "The first sign of testicular cancer may be a slight enlargement of one testicle with some discomfort."
   4. "Testicular cancer is more common on the right side, which parallels the incidence of cryptorchidism."

6. A nurse is planning a seminar about benign prostatic hyperplasia (BPH). Which of the following statements on an educational handout needs to be corrected?
   1. The two necessary preconditions for BPH are age of 50 and older and the presence of testes.
   2. BPH, which is the twisting of the spermatic cord with scrotal swelling and pain, is a potential medical emergency.
   3. The exact cause of BPH is unknown.
   4. Risk factors of BPH include age, family history, race (highest in African Americans and lowest in native Japanese), and a diet high in meat and fats.

7. What is a mobile, usually painless mass that forms when efferent ducts in the epididymis dilate and form a cyst?
   1. spermatocele
   2. testicular torsion
   3. hydrocele
   4. varicocele

8. A patient has reported to the clinic with manifestations consistent with epididymitis. When assisting the physician, the nurse recognizes that the condition will likely be diagnosed using which of the following tests?
   1. urethral swab culture
   2. blood cultures
   3. ultrasound
   4. urinalysis

Nursing Care of **Women** with **Reproductive System** and **Breast Disorders**

LEARNING OUTCOMES

1. Explain the pathophysiology, manifestations, complications, interdisciplinary care, and nursing care of disorders of female sexual function, menstrual disorders, structural disorders, reproductive tissue disorders, and breast disorders.

2. Describe the physiologic process of perimenopause.

3. Compare and contrast the incidence, risk factors, pathophysiology, manifestations, diagnosis, treatment, and nursing care for cancer of the cervix, endometrium, ovary, vulva, and breast.

4. Explain the purposes, nursing implications, and health education for women and their families for cancer screening, medications, and treatments for disorders of the reproductive system and breast.

5. Discuss alternative and complementary therapies used by women to relieve manifestations associated with menopause and menstrual disorders.

6. Describe the surgical procedures used to treat female reproductive system and breast disorders.

MediaLink

Pearson Nursing Student Resources
Audio Glossary
NCLEX-RN® Review
- Care Plan Activities
  - Ovarian Cancer
  - Breast Cancer
- Case Studies
  - The Patient with Endometriosis
  - Women with Reproductive and Breast Disorders
- Animations/Videos
  - Cervical Cancer
  - Breast Cancer
- MediaLink Applications
- Links to Resources

CLINICAL COMPETENCIES

1. Assess functional status of women with reproductive system and breast disorders and monitor, document, and report abnormal manifestations.

2. Use evidence-based research to design interventions to promote early diagnosis and treatment of African American women with breast cancer.

3. Use assessed data, patient values, clinical expertise and evidence to determine priority nursing diagnoses and, select and implement individualized nursing interventions.

4. Administer medications used to treat female reproductive system and breast disorders knowledgeably and safely.

5. Provide individualized care for the woman having a D&C, a laparoscopy, a hysterectomy, a mastectomy, and breast reconstruction.

6. Effectively communicate with and function within the interdisciplinary team to plan and provide care.

7. Provide teaching appropriate for community-based self-care of female reproductive and breast disorders.

8. Adapt individual and cultural values and variations as well as expressed needs and preferences into the plan of care as needed.

9. Revise plan of care as needed to provide effective interventions to promote, maintain, or restore functional health status to women with reproductive system and breast disorders.

TERMS MATCHING

Place the letter of the correct definition in the space next to each term.

1. _____ Amenorrhea
2. _____ Anorgasmia
3. _____ Dysfunctional uterine bleeding (DUB)
4. _____ Dysmenorrhea
5. _____ Dyspareunia
6. _____ Endometriosis
7. _____ Fibrocystic changes (FCC)
8. _____ Leiomyoma
9. _____ Lymphedema
10. _____ Menopause
11. _____ Menorrhagia
12. _____ Metrorrhagia
13. _____ Premenstrual syndrome (PMS)

A. A condition in which a woman has never experienced an orgasm during the waking state, either through self-stimulation or intercourse.

B. Bleeding between menstrual periods that may be caused by hormonal imbalances, pelvic inflammatory disease, cervical or uterine polyps, uterine fibroids, or cervical or uterine cancer.

C. Benign tumors that originate from smooth muscle of the uterus and are referred to as fibroid tumors.

D. The permanent cessation of menses as a result of aging, surgical removal of the ovaries, or chemotherapy.

E. Painful sexual intercourse.

F. The accumulation of fluid in the soft tissues that is caused by removal of lymph channels in the arm on the operated side, nerve damage, and adhesions and that is due to the role of the lymph nodes in immune system function.

G. The absence of menstruation.

H. The physiological nodularity and breast tenderness that increases and decreases with the menstrual cycle and is experienced by an estimated 50%–80% of all women.

I. A complex of manifestations (for example, mood swings, breast tenderness, fatigue, irritability, food cravings, and depression) that are limited to 3–14 days before menstruation and relieved by the onset of menses.

J. Vaginal bleeding that is usually painless but abnormal in amount, duration, or time of occurrence.

K. Excessive or prolonged menstruation that may result from thyroid disorders, endometriosis, pelvic inflammatory disease, functional ovarian cysts, or uterine fibroids or polyps.

L. Pain or discomfort associated with menstruation that is estimated to occur in 46%–95% of menstruating women.

M. The growth of endometrial tissue outside the uterus.

FOCUSED STUDY

1. List alternative and complementary therapies used by women to relieve manifestations associated with menopause and menstrual disorders.

_____

_____

_____

_____

2. Summarize the surgical procedures used to treat female reproductive system disorders.

_____

_____

_____

3. Discuss the physiological process of menopause.

_____

_____

_____

4. List the risk factors, manifestations, and treatment for cancer of the cervix.

_____

_____

_____

_____

CASE STUDY

Elizabeth Baldwin is a 21-year-old female patient. She is in today to have her first Pap test and breast examination. Answer the following questions based on your knowledge of Pap tests and breast examinations.

1. How often does the American Cancer Society recommend that women have Pap tests?

2. Is Elizabeth a good candidate to receive Gardasil®? Why or why not?

3. What are the instructions for performing a breast self-examination?

CROSSWORD PUZZLE

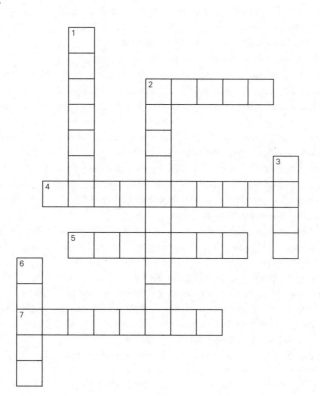

Across

2   Vascular solid tumor attached by a pedicle
4   Tumor removal leaving the uterus intact
5   Abnormal opening between two organs
7   Vaccine administered to prevent cervical cancer as a result of HPV

Down

1   Removable devise used to support the uterus
2   Progesterone-like medications
3   Fluid-filled sac
6   Exercises used to strengthen pelvic muscles

NCLEX-RN® REVIEW QUESTIONS

1. A nurse is planning a seminar about menopause. Which of the following statements made by a participant is correct?

1. Menopause is a disease and is not a normal physiological process.
2. Menopause is the permanent cessation of menses.
3. Late menopause is associated with genetics, smoking, higher altitude, and obesity.
4. The average woman will live one-fourth of her life after menopause.

2. The nurse is taking the health history of a woman who has come to the physician's office with reproductive-related concerns. During the health history, the woman reveals that she has been experiencing bleeding between menstrual periods. What term should be documented by the nurse?

1. menorrhagia
2. metrorrhagia
3. oligomenorrhea
4. amenorrhea

3. During a pelvic examination, the physician explains to the nurse that the patient's uterus is tilting forward in an exaggerated manner. What term can the nurse expect the physician to use to refer to this condition?

1. retroversion
2. retroflexion
3. anteversion
4. anteflexion

4. A nurse is evaluating a patient's understanding of breast self-examination (BSE). Which of the following statements indicates a need for further teaching?

1. "Lie down on your back and place your right arm behind your head."
2. "Use three different levels of pressure to feel all of the breast tissue."
3. "Use overlapping quarter-sized circular motions of the finger pads to feel the breast tissue."
4. "Look at your breasts for any changes in size, shape, contour, or dimpling."

5. A nurse is planning a seminar about ovarian cancer. Which of the following statements by a participant indicates understanding?

1. "Ovarian cancer is the most common gynecologic cancer in women in the United States."
2. "An enlarged abdomen with ascites signals early-stage disease."
3. "There are several types of ovarian cancers: epithelial tumors, germ cell tumors, and gonadal stromal tumors."
4. "In early stages, ovarian cancer generally causes several warning signs or manifestations."

6. A nurse is evaluating a patient's understanding of fibrocystic changes (FCC), or fibrocystic breast disease. Which of the following statements indicates a need for further teaching?

1. "FCC is the physiological nodularity and breast tenderness that increases and decreases with the menstrual cycle."
2. "FCC is most common in women 20–30 years of age and is common in postmenopausal women who are not taking hormone replacement."
3. "FCC includes many different lesions and breast changes."
4. "Women with fibrocystic changes experience bilateral or unilateral pain or tenderness in the upper, outer quadrants of their breasts and report that their breasts feel particularly thick and lumpy the week prior to menses."

7. A nurse is planning an educational program about premenstrual syndrome (PMS). When preparing the handout, which of the following statements may be correctly included?

1. PMS is never a factor in absenteeism at school or work, decreased productivity, difficulties in interpersonal relationships, and disruption in lifestyle.
2. Manifestations of PMS occur during the follicular phase of the menstrual cycle (three to six days prior to the onset of the menstrual flow) and abate when the menstrual flow begins.
3. The treatment of PMS integrates a self-monitored record of manifestations, regular exercise, caffeine, and a diet low in simple sugars and lean proteins.
4. Alternative and complementary therapies that the woman with PMS may find helpful focus on diet, exercise, relaxation, and stress management.

8. What kind of uterine prolapse is complete prolapse of the uterus outside the body, with inversion of the vaginal canal?

1. mild
2. first-degree
3. second-degree
4. third-degree

Nursing Care of Patients with Sexually Transmitted Infections

LEARNING OUTCOMES

1. Explain the incidence, prevalence, characteristics, and prevention/control of sexually transmitted infections (STIs).
2. Compare and contrast the pathophysiology, manifestations, interdisciplinary care, and nursing care of genital herpes, genital warts, vaginitis, chlamydia, gonorrhea, syphilis, and pelvic inflammatory disease.
3. Explain the risk factors for and complications of STIs.
4. Discuss the effects and nursing implications of medications and treatments used to treat STIs.

CLINICAL COMPETENCIES

1. Assess functional health status of patients with STIs and monitor, document, and report abnormal manifestations.
2. Determine priority nursing diagnoses and select and implement individualized nursing interventions for patients with STIs.
3. Administer topical, oral, and injectable medications knowledgeably and safely.
4. Integrate interdisciplinary care into care of patients with STIs.
5. Provide teaching appropriate for prevention, control, and self-care of STIs.
6. Revise plan of care as needed to provide effective interventions to promote, maintain, or restore functional health status to patients with STIs.

MediaLink

Pearson Nursing Student Resources
Audio Glossary
NCLEX-RN® Review
- Care Plan Activity
  - Gonorrhea
- Case Studies
  - The Patient with Pelvic Inflammatory Disease
  - The Patient with Sexually Transmitted Infections
- Animations/Videos
  - Gonorrhea
  - Herpes Simplex 1 & 2
- MediaLink Applications
- Links to Resources

TERMS MATCHING

Place the letter of the correct definition in the space next to each term.

1. ____ Bacterial vaginosis

2. ____ Candidiasis

3. ____ Chancre

4. ____ Chlamydia

5. ____ Dyspareunia

6. ____ Genital herpes

7. ____ Genital warts

8. ____ Gonorrhea

9. ____ Pelvic inflammatory disease (PID)

10. ____ Sexually transmitted infections (STI)

11. ____ Syphilis

12. ____ Trichmoniasis

A. A painless ulceration that appears after being infected with syphilis.

B. Infections transmitted by vaginal, oral, and anal intimate contact and intercourse.

C. An incurable viral infection caused by the human papillomavirus.

D. A viral infection associated with the presence of painful lesions for which there is no cure; treatment focuses on management of outbreaks.

E. The most common cause of vaginal infection in women of reproductive age that may be caused by a number of causative organisms; the relationship of sexual activity to this infection is not clear; the primary manifestation is a vaginal discharge that is thin and grayish-white with a foul, fishy odor.

F. An infection of the pelvic organs, including the fallopian tubes (salpingitis), ovaries (oophoritis), cervix (cervicitis), endometrium (endometritis), pelvic peritoneum, and pelvic vascular system.

G. The most commonly reported sexually transmitted infection; it is bacterial in nature and often is referred to as the "clap."

H. A complex systemic STI caused by the spirochete *Treponema pallidum*; it can infect almost any body tissue or organ and is transmitted from open lesions during any sexual contact (genital, oral–genital, or anal–genital).

I. A bacterial infection that presents with a malodororus frothy discharge that is yellow or white in color.

J. A fungal infection that presents with a thick, cheesey discharge.

K. A bacterial infection that may be asymptomatic for an extended period of time after infection; it typically involves the cervix in women and the urethra in men.

L. Painful sexual intercourse.

FOCUSED STUDY

1. Explain the nursing implications of medications and treatments used to treat sexually transmitted infections.

_____

_____

2. List the risk factors for and complications associated with sexually transmitted infections.

_____

_____

3. Discuss the interdisciplinary care and nursing care of sexually transmitted infections.

_____

_____

_____

_____

4. Summarize the prevention/control of sexually transmitted infections.

_____

_____

CASE STUDY

A 21-year-old patient is seen at the family planning clinic with complaints consistent with a genital herpes simplex infection. During the nurse's interaction with the patient, the patient asks several questions. Answer the following questions based on your knowledge of sexually transmitted infections.

1. "What causes genital herpes?"

2. "How will this be cured?"

3. "What happens with the virus between outbreaks?

4. "Am I required to provide the names of my sexual contacts to anyone?"

5. "How long will it take for the related symptoms to go away?

SHORT ANSWERS

Fill in the table regarding sexually transmitted diseases.

Infection	Characteristics of Discharge
Candidiasis	
Bacterial vaginosis	
Trichomoniasis	
Gonorrhea	

NCLEX-RN® REVIEW QUESTIONS

1. Sexually transmitted infections (STIs) have reached epidemic proportions in the United States and continue to increase worldwide. Which of the following statements about STIs is incorrect?
   1. Many STIs are more easily transmitted from a woman to a man than from a man to a woman.
   2. The incidence of STIs is highest in young adults aged 15–24.
   3. STIs are caused by bacteria, *Chlamydiae*, viruses, fungi, protozoa, and parasites.
   4. Infections that are transmitted by vaginal, oral, and anal intimate contact and intercourse are referred to as sexually transmitted infections (STIs).

2. What is associated with cold sores but may be transmitted to the genital area by oral intercourse or by self-inoculation through poor handwashing practices?
   1. HSV-2
   2. HPV
   3. HSV-1
   4. GC

3. Which of the following is not a reportable disease?
   1. genital warts
   2. gonorrhea
   3. syphilis
   4. AIDS

4. When preparing to discuss chlamydia with a patient, the nurse recognizes which of the following statements to be incorrect?

1. Because chlamydia is asymptomatic in most women until the uterus and fallopian tubes have been invaded, treatment may be delayed, which results in devastating, long-term complications.
2. Chlamydia may be present for days to weeks without producing noticeable symptoms in women.
3. The infections caused by chlamydia include acute urethral syndrome, nongonococcal urethritis, mucopurulent cervicitis, and pelvic inflammatory disease (PID).
4. Complications of chlamydial infections in men include epididymitis, prostatitis, sterility, and Reiter's syndrome.

5. What stage of syphilis is characterized by the appearance of a chancre and by regional enlargement of lymph nodes with little or no pain accompanying these warning signs?

1. secondary
2. latent
3. primary
4. tertiary

6. A nurse is planning a seminar about pelvic inflammatory disease (PID). Which of the following statements on an educational handout needs to be corrected?

1. PID is a reportable disease in the United States.
2. PID is usually polymicrobial (caused by more than one microbe) in origin; gonorrhea and chlamydia are common causative organisms.
3. Manifestations of PID include fever, purulent vaginal discharge, severe lower abdominal pain, and a painful cervical movement.
4. Complications include pelvic abscess, infertility, ectopic pregnancy, chronic pelvic pain, pelvic adhesions, dyspareunia, and chronic pelvic pain. Abscess formation is common.

7. Which of the following are slightly raised lesions that are often invisible to the naked eye and develop on keratinized skin?

1. keratotic warts
2. papular warts
3. flat warts
4. condyloma acuminata

8. Which of the following statements by a student nurse reflects an accurate understanding of trichomoniasis?

1. "It is caused by *Trichomonas vaginalis,* a protozoan parasite."
2. "It is the least common noncurable STI in young, sexually active women."
3. "Manifestations of trichomoniasis usually appear within one to four days of exposure."
4. "Women with trichomoniasis have a nonfrothy, red-orange vaginal discharge with a strong fishy odor that is often accompanied by itching and irritation of the genitalia."

Answer Key

Chapter 1

Terms Matching
1. E
2. H
3. A
4. F
5. J
6. G
7. B
8. D
9. I
10. C

Focused Study
1. As you review your state's nurse practice act, you will be better able to determine what kinds of activities can be delegated. Your state's nurse practice act will help you understand your own practice limitations.
2. The nursing process is the cyclical series of critical-thinking activities that nurses use to provide patient care to promote wellness, maintain health, restore health, or facilitate coping with disability or death. The five interrelated phases of the nursing process are assessment, diagnosis, planning, implementation, and evaluation. The nurse assesses the patient to determine what kinds of health issues the patient may be experiencing. The nurse identifies the patient's health issue in the diagnosis phase. The nurse can plan how to assist the patient during the planning phase. The nurse implements various nursing interventions in the implementation phase. The nurse evaluates how well the plan and nursing interventions worked during the evaluation phase.
3. The code of ethics assists the nurse who encounters an ethical dilemma in setting priorities, making judgments, and taking appropriate action. Nurses are responsible for promoting patient health, preventing illness, and helping to alleviate suffering.
4. You should be able to find at least one NANDA nursing diagnosis label that describes your current needs.

Case Study
1. *How may this constitute an ethical dilemma for the nursing staff?* Medical-surgical nurses frequently face ethical dilemmas. This specific issue is related to the nurse's wish to adequately control the patient's pain without inadvertently overdosing the patient with opioid pain medications. The nurse must use ethical and legal guidelines to make decisions. The nurse can give an ordered pain medication, but this nursing intervention may result in respiratory depression and even in the patient's death.
2. *What is one NANDA nursing diagnosis that best applies to this patient?* Impaired Gas Exchange, Acute Pain, Ineffective Breathing Pattern
3. *What role or roles might the nurse play in helping the patient and the family at this time?* The nurse must use critical thinking to guide his or her role as caregiver, educator, and advocate.
4. *How does the code of ethics apply to this patient?* In summary, the Code of Ethics for Nurses (ICN) helps guide the nurse in setting priorities, making judgments, and taking action when he or she faces ethical dilemmas in clinical practice. The philosophical base for the ICN code is that nurses are responsible for promoting health, preventing illness, and alleviating suffering.
5. *Identify two activities the nurse could safely delegate to unlicensed personnel in caring for this patient.* It would be safe to allow an unlicensed staff member to gather vital signs, bathe the patient, and turn the patient. The nurse should provide the unlicensed staff member with clear instructions about care provision and when to notify the nurse. The unlicensed staff member should consider these tasks as routine and should have been adequately trained in how to perform these types of care activities. The nurse should perform activities that require nursing judgment. The nurse is ultimately responsible for the care provided by the unlicensed staff member.
6. *The patient has become confused and lethargic. What are two NANDA nursing diagnoses that may apply to this patient?* Potential for Impaired Skin Integrity, Altered Thought Processes, Acute Confusion, Potential for Infection

Short Answers

1. *Name one type of unit that uses Primary Nursing as its model of care delivery.* intensive care unit
2. *Name one type of unit or facility that uses Team Nursing as its model of care delivery.* long-term care facility
3. *Name one type of unit or agency that uses Case Management as its model of care delivery.* psychiatric nursing, utilization management department, home healthcare service, hospice service

NCLEX-RN® Review Questions

1. Answer: 2

   Rationale: The five phases in the nursing process are assessment, diagnosis, planning, implementation, and evaluation. These phases are interrelated and interdependent. The patient assessment is performed by collecting data about the patient. This includes subjective and objective information. Developing nursing diagnoses is performed during the diagnosis stage. Planning includes developing a patient care plan. Evaluating how well the patient has met his or her goals is called the evaluation stage.

   Nursing Process: Assessment

   Patient Need: Safe, Effective Care Environment

2. Answer: 1, 2, 5

   Rationale: During the evaluation, the nurse needs to determine whether the previous nursing care plan was effective. If the outcome criteria that were previously established are unmet, the nurse can safely modify the nursing diagnosis, modify future outcome criteria, or modify the nursing care plan. Termination of a nursing care plan is usually reserved for the point at which the patient has met his or her outcome criteria. Continuation of the nursing care plan without changes indicates that there is still a potential for the problem to develop but that the nursing interventions established previously are currently working.

   Nursing Process: Evaluation

   Patient Need: Safe, Effective Care Environment

3. Answer: 1

   Rationale: The nurse is ultimately responsible and accountable for the care that was delegated. The nurse should ensure that the staff member has received training about how to perform the task. The task should be something the unlicensed staff member is comfortable performing and he or she considers routine. The nurse should understand that not all tasks are appropriate to delegate to an unlicensed staff member. The nurse should have a working knowledge of his or her state's nurse practice act. The nurse should give specific directions about how the care should be performed. The unlicensed staff member should receive clear instructions about the task. The staff member should feel comfortable asking questions about the task. While the nurse is ultimately responsible for the task

   being completed correctly, the nurse delegates so that he or she can perform other tasks while the delegated task is being completed. The nurse should not feel the need to be present during the task's completion.

   Nursing Process: Implementation

   Patient Need: Safe, Effective Care Environment

4. Answer: 2

   Rationale: Nurses use four major critical-thinking skills to solve problems: divergent thinking, reasoning, clarifying, and reflection. The nurses uses divergent thinking to weigh the importance of patient information. Reasoning is the ability to use known facts to determine why something is happening. The nurse can use reasoning to identify if and why the patient's data is abnormal. Clarifying is when the nurse notes similarities or differences between something that is currently happening and something that has happened in the past. Reflection is when the nurse spends time analyzing a problem. Reflection cannot occur in emergent situations.

   Nursing Process: Implementation

   Patient Need: Safe, Effective Care Environment

5. Answer: 2

   Rationale: Data collected by the nurse about the patient is objective and subjective. Information that can be verified by another person is objective information. Objective information includes vital signs, pupil size, and information about an infection. This information can be seen, heard, touched, or smelled. Only the patient can provide subjective information for the nurse. The nurse cannot merely look at the patient and determine the patient's pain level, but the nurse can note that the patient is acting restless, crying out, and grimacing. The patient can provide subjective information to the nurse regarding pain, dizziness, or anxiety or how the patient feels.

   Nursing Process: Assessment

   Patient Need: Physiological Integrity

6. Answer: 2

   Rationale: When the nurse collects information about the patient, the nurse should interpret the meaning of the data. The data should not be used to judge the patient. The nurse should describe the patient's behavior carefully and objectively.

   Nursing Process: Assessment

   Patient Need: Safe, Effective Care Environment

7. Answers: 2, 4

   Rationale: Nursing diagnoses can be noted as actual, potential, or collaborative problems. An actual nursing diagnosis is used when the health problem has already been identified, such as unilateral neglect. A potential nursing diagnosis is used when the problem is likely to occur if the nurse doesn't intervene in some way. A collaborative problem is a health issue that must be treated with medical and nursing interventions. This patient is less likely to experience problems with an increased caloric intake. This patient is at risk for altered nutrition; less than body requirements based on his need for a gastric tube and his difficulty swallowing.

Nursing Process: Diagnosis

Patient Need: Physiological Integrity

8. Answer: 4

Rationale: Critical pathways are healthcare plans designed to provide care in a multidisciplinary manner. Pathways are developed for patients who have specific diagnoses that are high-volume, high-risk, and associated with a high cost. The pathways include goals that are based on a timeline. Patients with sprained ankles, cataracts, or cholecystitis are less likely to be placed on a critical pathway.

Nursing Process: Planning

Patient Need: Safe, Effective Care Environment

9. Answer: 1

Rationale: The nurse can use guidelines about care provision to help plan and implement nursing interventions. Nurses should use their skills to perform assessments and provide nursing care together. The nurse can provide the patient with a bath while assessing the patient's skin, neurological status, circulatory status, etc. The nurse should examine the patient's skin at the time of the bath. It is important to assist the patient in becoming more independent. The nurse can perform an activity for the patient and then, over a period of time, teach the patient how to perform the activity independently. Sometimes the nurse will need to involve family members in educational activities. It is a legal requirement that interventions be documented. The nurse should set daily goals with the patient. It is very important to monitor the patient's blood pressure and to set a goal of the patient's blood pressure returning to normal by a certain time.

Nursing Process: Planning

Patient Need: Safe, Effective Care Environment

10. Answer: 2

Rationale: The health information privacy rules are often misinterpreted. To ensure that the correct patient receives care, it is appropriate to display the patient's name outside his or her room. Health information can be disclosed in the treatment of patients, even without their documented consent. Laws can override the patient's right to privacy. When a patient is abused, the abuse must be reported. Also, unless the patient objects, it is appropriate to discuss a patient's care with family members.

Nursing Process: Implementation

Patient Need: Safe, Effective Care Environment

Chapter 2

Terms Matching

1. C
2. I
3. K
4. A
5. E
6. F
7. G
8. J
9. H
10. D
11. B
12. L

Focused Study

1. a. Genetic makeup
    b. Cognitive abilities and educational level
    c. Race, ethnicity, and cultural background
    d. Age, gender, and developmental level
    e. Lifestyle and environment
    f. Socioeconomic level
    g. Geographic areas
2. a. Genetic defects
    b. Developmental defects
    c. Biologic agents or toxins (including viruses, bacteria, rickettsia, fungi, protozoa, and helminths
    d. Physical agents such as temperature extremes, radiation, and electricity
    e. Chemical agents such as alcohol, drugs, strong acids or bases, and heavy metals
    f. Generalized response of tissues to injury or irritation
    g. Alterations in the production of antibodies, resulting in allergies or hypersensitivities
    h. Faulty metabolic processes
    i. Continued, unabated stress
3. Acute illness is a short-term ailment that is resolved. Chronic illness does not have a rapid return to health. A chronic illness may be permanent, leave a permanent disability, cause nonreversible pathologic alterations, or require special training of the patient for rehabilitation.
4. a. Primary level of prevention includes generalized health-promotion activities as well as specific actions that prevent or delay the occurrence of a disease.

    Following are examples of primary prevention activities:
    • Protecting oneself against environmental risks such as air and water pollution
    • Eating nutritious foods

    b. Secondary level of prevention involves activities that emphasize early diagnosis and treatment of an illness that is already present to stop the pathologic process and enable the person to return to his or her former state of health as soon as possible.

    Following are examples of secondary prevention activities:
    • Having screenings for diseases such as hypertension, diabetes mellitus, and glaucoma
    • Obtaining physical examinations and diagnostic tests for cancer

    c. Tertiary level of prevention focuses on stopping the disease process and returning the affected individual to a useful place in society within the constraints of any disability. The activities primarily revolve around rehabilitation.

Following are examples of tertiary prevention measures:

- Obtaining medical or surgical treatment for an illness
- Enrolling in specific rehabilitation programs for cardiovascular problems, head injuries, and strokes

Case Study

1. *What alterations in health is Jacob at risk for developing as a middle-aged adult?* Jacob is at risk for alterations in health from obesity, cardiovascular disease, cancer, substance abuse, and physical and psychosocial stressors.
2. *What guidelines are useful in assessing the achievement of significant developmental tasks in the middle adult?* The nurse can use the following guidelines to assess the developmental tasks of the middle adult. Does the middle adult:
   a. Accept the aging body?
   b. Feel comfortable with and respect oneself?
   c. Enjoy the freedom to be independent?
   d. Accept changes in family roles?
   e. Enjoy success and satisfaction from work and/or family roles?
   f. Interact well and share activities with a partner?
   g. Expand or renew previous interests?
   h. Pursue charitable and altruistic activities?
   i. Consider plans for retirement?
   j. Have a meaningful philosophy of life?
   k. Follow preventive healthcare practices?
3. *How can the nurse promote healthy behaviors in Jacob?*

   Healthy Behaviors in the Middle Adult
   - Choose foods from all food groups and eat a variety of foods.
   - Choose a diet low in fat (30% or less of total calories), saturated fat (less than 10% of calories), and cholesterol (less than 300 mg daily).
   - Adjust daily calorie intake to maintain healthy weight.
   - Choose a diet each day that includes at least three servings of vegetables, two servings of fruits, and six servings of grains.
   - Use sugar, salt, and sodium in moderation.
   - Increase calcium intake (in perimenopausal women) to 1200 mg daily.
   - Consume high-fiber foods.
   - Make exercise a part of life, carrying out regular exercise that is moderately strenuous, is consistent, and avoids overexertion. Exercise for 30 minutes at least four or five times a week.
   - Include exercise as part of any weight reduction program.
   - Have an annual vision examination.
   - Have an annual dental checkup.

Short Answers

Fill in the information table for recommended adult immunizations.

Vaccine	Indications	Do not give to:
Measles-mumps-rubella	Anyone born after 1956 and never infected or anyone likely to be exposed, such as someone entering college or the military.	Pregnant women, immunocompromised people, or anyone with a history of anaphylactic reaction to egg protein or neomycin.
Tetanus and diphtheria toxoids	Anyone who has never been vaccinated should have the primary series, followed by a booster every ten years.	None identified.
Hepatitis B	Anyone likely to have repeated exposure (such as healthcare providers or sex partners of a known carrier) or who have been exposed (such as a healthcare worker suffering a needle-stick injury).	People with a history of anaphylactic reaction to common baker's yeast.
Influenza A	Anyone at high risk for complications, healthcare providers, and those wanting immunity.	Those with a high fever or a history of anaphylactic reaction to egg protein.
Pneumoccal pneumonia	Anyone at high risk for pneumonococcal disease and those over 65 years of age.	Pregnant women.
Varicella	Anyone never infected, especially healthcare providers and child care workers.	Pregnant women, immunocompromised people, those who have received an immune globulin or a blood transfusion within five months, or those with a history of anaphylactic reactions to neomycin or gelatin.

NCLEX-RN® Review Questions

1. Answer: 1

    Rationale: Influenza is an acute illness that lasts for a relatively short time and is self-limiting. Cancer, hemophilia, and sickle cell disease are chronic illnesses that are associated with genetic makeup.

    Nursing Process: Assessment

    Patient Need: Physiological Integrity

2. Answer: 3

    Rationale: Examples of altered responses are the relationship of obesity to hypertension, cigarette smoking to chronic obstructive pulmonary disease, a sedentary lifestyle to heart disease, and a high-stress career to alcoholism.

    Nursing Process: Diagnosis

    Patient Need: Health Promotion and Maintenance

3. Answer: 1

    Rationale: Practices that are known to promote health and wellness include exercising moderately and regularly, sleeping seven to eight hours each day, limiting alcohol consumption to a moderate amount and favoring red wine, smoking cessation, keeping sun exposure to a minimum, and maintaining recommended immunizations. Sleeping five to six hours a day is not known to promote health and wellness.

    Nursing Process: Assessment

    Patient Need: Health Promotion and Maintenance

4. Answer: 4

    Rationale: Self-preoccupation is characteristic of assuming the sick role stage, and the person focuses on alterations in function that result from the illness. Experiencing symptoms is the first stage of an acute illness. During this stage, a person experiences one or more manifestations that serve as cues that a change in normal health is occurring. The stage of assuming a dependent role begins when a person accepts the diagnosis and planned treatment of the illness. As the severity of the illness increases, so does the dependent role. The final stage of an acute illness is recovery and rehabilitation. This focus makes patient education and continuity of care a major goal of nursing.

    Nursing Process: Assessment

    Patient Need: Psychosocial Psychologic Integrity

5. Answer: 1

    Rationale: The adult years commonly are divided into three stages: the young adult (aged 18 to 40), the middle adult (aged 40 to 65), and the older adult (over age 65).

    Nursing Process: Assessment

    Patient Need: Health Promotion and Maintenance

6. Answer: 2

    Rationale: Cancers of the breast, colon, lung, and reproductive system are common in the middle years. The middle adult is at risk for cancer as a result of increased length of exposure to environmental carcinogens, as well as alcohol and nicotine use.

    Nursing Process: Diagnosis

    Patient Need: Health Promotion and Maintenance

7. Answer: 4

    Rationale: Obesity is a frequently occurring condition in the middle adult years. The most frequently occurring conditions in the older adult are hypertension, arthritis, heart disease, cancer, sinusitis, and diabetes.

    Nursing Process: Diagnosis

    Patient Need: Health Promotion and Maintenance

8. Answer: 3

    Rationale: The developmental tasks of the family with adolescents and young adults focus on transition. The family with infants and preschoolers must adjust to having and supporting the needs of more than two members. The family with school-age children has the developmental tasks of adjusting to the expanded world of children in school and encouraging educational achievement. The family with middle adults has the developmental tasks of maintaining ties with older and younger generations and planning for retirement.

    Nursing Process: Diagnosis

    Patient Need: Psychosocial Integrity

9. Answer: 4

    Rationale: From age 18 to 25, the healthy young adult is at the peak of physical development and is at risk for alterations in health from sexually transmitted diseases. Certain diseases occur at a higher rate of incidence in some races and ethnic groups than in others. For example, eye disorders are more prevalent in Chinese Americans. Cardiovascular disorders are uncommon in young adults, but the incidence increases after the age of 40. The middle adult often has a problem maintaining a healthy weight.

    Nursing Process: Diagnosis

    Patient Need: Health Promotion and Maintenance

10. Answer: 2

    Rationale: Confronting the inevitability of death is a positive coping skill for patients with chronic illnesses.

    Nursing Process: Assessment

    Patient Need: Psychosocial Integrity

Chapter 3

Terms Matching

1. D
2. H
3. B
4. C
5. E
6. G
7. A
8. I
9. J
10. F

Focused Study

1. The primary predictors of the need for home care services are age and level of disability.
2. The nurse must communicate in an open and honest manner. The nurse must establish a contract and follow through with plans identified in the plan of care.
3. **a.** Individuals who cannot live independently at home because of age, illness, or disability
   b. Individuals having chronic, debilitating illnesses such as congestive heart failure, heart disease, kidney disease, respiratory diseases, diabetes mellitus, or muscle-nerve disorders
   c. Individuals who are terminally ill and want to die with comfort and dignity at home
   d. Individuals who do not need in-patient hospital or nursing home care but require additional assistance
   e. Individuals needing short-term help at home for postoperative care
4. The services provided in the home may include professional nursing care, care provided by home care aides, physical therapy, speech therapy, occupational therapy, medical social worker services, and nutritional services.

Case Study

1. *What distractions limited the nurse's ability to assess and care for Mr. Cohen?* Mr. Cohen's friends are a wonderful support system, but when they interrupt the nurse's visit, they are a distraction. Explaining the importance of focus during the nurse's visit may help Mr. Cohen and his friends to respect that time. Schedule visits so that they are not during a high visitation time.

   Encourage Mr. Cohen to have a support person with him if this would help him understand the information. The nurse should make note of the time the patient is having lunch, ask if this is his normal lunch time, and avoid visits during this time.
2. *What safety concerns do you see in Mr. Cohen's home setting? Would these be expensive to repair? Explain.* Isolation could be a concern. But while Mr. Cohen lives alone, his friends help to prevent social isolation and would find him if he were to fall or have an emergency. There is no expense related to this issue.

   The extension cord, particularly the cord under the rug, increases the risk of fire. It could be expensive to have additional outlets installed, but the nurse needs to check whether the plugged-in item is necessary or whether it could be moved to a safer location. The heavy cookware could be another concern. The patient is able to handle the cookware today, but the risk of dropping the heavy cookware when he is in a hurry, is tired, or becomes weaker increases the risk of fire. The expense of replacing the cookware is small to moderate. The patient may find this real expense to be emotional if the cookware was used by his now-deceased wife.

3. *What can you do to improve Mr. Cohen's safety with regard to his medication administration?* A weekly medication holder designed for the elderly might make it easier for him to get to his medications and to determine whether he took them. Mr. Cohen can organize his medications with the assistance of the nurse.

Care Plan Critical-Thinking Activity

1. Nursing Diagnoses
   a. Physiological needs: *Pain, Acute Related to Injury*
   b. Psychosocial needs: *Social Isolation Related to Living Arrangement*
   c. Teaching needs: *Knowledge Deficit Related to Home Care Services*
   d. Safety needs: *High Risk for Falls Related to Recent History*

NCLEX-RN® Review Questions

1. Answer: 2, 3, 4, 5
   Rationale: A variety of factors impact the health and wellness of a community. Environmental factors such as air and water quality increase or decrease the community members' risk of both acute and chronic illnesses. Access to health care improves preventive care as well as the administration of care during acute situations. The ability to provide care in the home is not related to the actual health of the community.
   Nursing Process: Evaluation
   Patient Need: Health Promotion and Maintenance
2. Answer: 2
   Rationale: Community-based healthcare services often allow patients with early stages of Alzheimer's disease to remain at home while their caregivers work or run errands. These programs are designed to provide for the patient's physical and psychosocial needs in a safe environment. Meals on Wheels is a good example, but it does not describe a community program. Programs such as Meals on Wheels help to promote wellness and early intervention so that, in the long run, they decrease the need for hospitalization; however, that is not the focus of community-based health care.
   Nursing Process: Implementation
   Patient Need: Physical and Psychosocial Integrity
3. Answer: 4
   Rationale: The purpose of home health care is to promote, maintain, or restore the level of independence of the patient, not to promote his or her dependence. Patients who require daily nursing care do best in a more intensive care setting. The largest single source of reimbursement for home health care is Medicare. Patients who do not need inpatient care benefit most from the type of assistance and education that home health care provides.
   Nursing Process: Assessment
   Patient Need: Health Promotion and Maintenance

4. Answer: 2

Rationale: While home health care is less expensive per day than a hospital admission, it is not inexpensive. Contact a local home health agency and find out what the cost would be for a registered nurse to do a dressing change or to administer an IV antibiotic once a day for one week. Some home healthcare agencies receive donations, endowments, or monies from charities to help provide home health care for patients who have limited income and no health insurance. Family members can be one referral source for home health care. Friends and family may see needs or issues the patient does not recognize. A physician's order and management of the patient's care is legally and ethically required for home health care.

Nursing Process: Planning

Patient Need: Health Promotion and Maintenance

5. Answer: 3

Rationale: Evaluation of outcomes established during the hospital stay should occur during that stay. The home health nurse will work with the patient to establish outcomes for the home health experience. A referral and physician order must be obtained prior to the initial visit. The initial visit is similar to the first meeting in any other setting. It focuses on assessing the patient and obtaining data that will allow the nurse and patient to establish the goals of care. The goal for all patients is to be successful in reaching their maximum level of independence.

Nursing Process: Assessment

Patient Need: Health Promotion and Maintenance

6. Answer: 3

Rationale: *Deficient knowledge related to a diagnosis of chronic obstructive pulmonary disease* is a nursing diagnosis that could be used for a home health patient but is not an outcome statement. "Patient will use oxygen" statement is not measurable. *Patient will demonstrate application of oxygen by the second home health visit* identifies the person, the means, and a timeframe for evaluation. *Apply oxygen per physician order* is not measurable.

Nursing Process: Planning

Patient Need: Physiological Integrity

7. Answer: 1

Rationale: The nurse must be able to communicate with all members of the healthcare team to coordinate the care of the patient. Changes in the plan of care may begin with the patient, nurse, or physician, but changes in the plan of care must be approved by the physician. Documentation is a legal requirement and is a necessary part of the nursing process. Documentation supports care for the purpose of reimbursement as well but this is not the most complete response. A fax machine may be used in some organizations to share information, but faxes do not ensure patient confidentiality.

Nursing Process: Planning

Patient Need: Safe, Effective Care Environment

8. Answer: 2

Rationale: The patient should be independent in the home and have ample support to provide for his or her health and safety. The nurse can be seen as an extension of the family, visiting on days off and taking calls after the patient's discharge. To work with the patient and family, a positive rapport must be established. Multiple caregivers who share responsibility for the patient's care help to reduce the risk of caregiver burnout.

Nursing Process: Planning

Patient Need: Safe, Effective Care Environment

9. Answer: 2

Rationale: The patient will have many influential people in his or her life, including family members and friends. Encouraging the patient to be in tune with his or her body and encouraging the patient to ask questions ensures that he or she is an active participant in the learning process. Providing the patient with information that is currently of concern is more effective. Involving an individual in the patient's learning will help provide support, but involving too many people in the process can limit the learning opportunities by creating distractions.

Nursing Process: Implementation

Patient Need: Health Promotion and Maintenance

10. Answer: 4

Rationale: A discussion with social services should come only after a discussion with the patient and failure to correct the safety issues. Ignoring safety issues is considered nursing negligence. These suggestions do not address the medication issue or identify any underlying issues. By talking with the patient, the nurse is able to advocate for the patient.

Nursing Process: Assessment

Patient Need: Safe, Effective Care Environment

Chapter 4

Terms Matching

1. L
2. F
3. B
4. E
5. D
6. G
7. O
8. A
9. I
10. H
11. P
12. J
13. C
14. N
15. K
16. M

Focused Study

1. **a.** Preoperative phase: begins when the decision for surgery is made and ends when the patient is transferred to the operating room
   b. Intraoperative phase: begins with the patient's entry into the operating room and ends with admittance to the postanesthesia care unit (PACU), or recovery room
   c. Postoperative phase: begins with the patient's admittance to the PACU and ends with the patient's complete recovery from the surgical intervention

2. **a.** The surgeon is the physician who performs the surgical procedure. The surgeon is in charge of the medical team.
   b. The circulating nurse is a highly experienced registered nurse who coordinates and manages a wide range of activities before, during, and after the surgical procedure. The circulating nurse oversees the physical aspects of the operating room, including the equipment; assists with transferring and positioning the patient; prepares the patient's skin; ensures that no break in aseptic technique occurs; and counts all sponges and instruments.
   c. The scrub nurse's role primarily involves technical skills, manual dexterity, and in-depth knowledge of the anatomic and mechanical aspects of a particular surgery. The scrub nurse handles sutures, instruments, and other equipment immediately adjacent to the sterile field.
   d. The anesthesiologist is a physician who is responsible for the administration of anesthesia during the operative procedure.
   e. The phlebotomist is responsible for performing blood draws on the patient during the surgical experience.
   f. The x-ray technician is responsible for obtaining the radiologic tests ordered during the surgical experience.
   g. The transporter assists with moving the patient between locations.

3. Describe the differences between general anesthesia, regional anesthesia, and conscious sedation.

Type of Anesthesia	Mode of Administration	State of Consciousness of the Patient	Method of Action
General Anesthesia	IV or Inhalation	Unconscious	Central nervous system depression
Regional Anesthesia	Injection	Awake	Analgesia, relaxation, and reduced reflexes
Conscious Sedation	IV	Awake	Analgesia, amnesia, and moderate sedation

4. Describe the following postoperative complications and their appropriate nursing interventions.
   a. Hemorrhage is an excessive loss of blood. It may result from a blood vessel that is no longer sutured or cauterized or from a drainage tube that has eroded a blood vessel. An obvious hemorrhage occurs externally from a dislodged or ill-formed clot at the wound. Hemorrhage also may result from abnormalities in the blood's ability to clot; these abnormalities may result from a pathologic condition, or they may be a side effect of medications.
   b. Deep venous thrombosis (DVT) is the formation of a thrombus (blood clot) in association with inflammation in deep veins. This complication most often occurs in the lower extremities of the postoperative patient. It may result from a combination of several factors, including trauma during surgery, pressure applied under the knees, and sluggish blood flow during and after surgery.
   c. Pneumonia is an inflammation of lung tissue. Inflammation is caused by a microbial infection or by a foreign substance in the lung, which leads to an infection. Numerous factors may be involved in the development of pneumonia, including aspiration infection, retained pulmonary secretions, failure to cough deeply, impaired cough reflex, and decreased mobility.

Case Study

1. *Mrs. Elvira's informed consent document includes the surgeon's name, the alternatives and risks of treatments, and the date and time she and her surgeon signed the consent. What is missing?* The type of surgery is missing, which is a right radical mastectomy.

2. *What postoperative complication(s) is Mrs. Elvira at most risk of developing based on her history?* Due to her smoking history, she is at risk for developing pneumonia. Her inactivity places her at risk for a deep vein thrombosis (DVT). The patient's aspirin use and herbal diet aids place her at risk for hemorrhage.

3. *What preoperative studies and interventions will Mrs. Elvira undergo to reduce the likelihood of intraoperative and postoperative complications?* She will undergo lab testing, such as blood and urine testing, to determine her blood count, clotting ability, and creatinine levels. Based on her smoking history, she will be given a chest x-ray. Antiembolism stockings will be placed on her preoperatively. Pre- and postoperative teaching will include the need for coughing and deep breathing exercises, as well as the importance of mobility.

4. *Prior to discharge, Mrs. Elvira will be instructed to assess her incision site for signs of infection. What are they?* Signs of incision infection include redness, pain, swelling, an increased temperature, and presence of purulent material.

Short Answers

Classification of Medication	Potential Surgical Complication	Nursing Care
Anticoagulants	May cause intra-operative and postoperative hemorrhage.	Monitor for bleeding. Assess PT/PTT values.
Antidepressants (particularly monoamine oxidase inhibitors)	Increase the hypotensive effects of anesthesia.	Closely monitor blood pressure.
Antihypertensives	Increase the hypotensive effects of anesthesia.	Closely monitor blood pressure.
Antibiotics (particularly the "mycin" group)	May cause apnea and respiratory paralysis.	Monitor respirations.
Diuretics	May lead to fluid and electrolyte imbalances, producing altered cardiovascular response and respiratory depression.	Monitor I&O and electrolytes. Assess cardiovascular and respiratory status.

NCLEX-RN® Review Questions

1. Answer: 1, 2, 4, 5

Rationale: Informed consent does not include the date, time, and location of the planned surgical procedure. This information will be shared with the patient as part of the preoperative surgical instructions. Informed consent must include the proposed surgical procedure, alternative treatments available, the patient's right to refuse or withdraw from treatment, and potential complications.

Nursing Process: Planning

Patient Need: Safe, Effective Care Environment

2. Answer: 3

Rationale: The anesthetized patient loses heat intraoperatively. The nurse must work to prevent further heat loss. Fluids for irrigation and intravenous administration must be warmed to prevent hypothermia. The application of warm blankets upon the patient's arrival in the surgical area and after sterile drapes are removed will prevent the patient from becoming chilled. Warm, humidified air will assist in the prevention of hypothermia. Wet surgical drapes allows cooling of the body through evaporation. Keeping the surgical drapes dry prevents hypothermia in the surgical patient. Although frequent monitoring of the vital signs is important, it is not a preventive intervention.

Nursing Process: Implementation

Patient Need: Physiological Integrity

3. Answer: 4

Rationale: Administration of an epidural blood patch is an effective method for eliminating a spinal headache. Hydration should be increased in a patient suffering from a spinal headache. Intake of caffeine may be increased to help decrease the severity of the headache. The patient's head should remain flat because any elevation will increase the intensity of the headache.

Nursing Process: Implementation

Patient Need: Physiological Integrity

4. Answer: 2

Rationale: The circulating nurse is responsible for documenting intraoperative nursing activities, medications, blood administration, placement of drains and catheters, and length of the procedure. The surgeon is the physician who performs the procedure. The Certified Registered Nurse Anesthetist (CRNA) evaluates the patient preoperatively, administers the anesthesia and other required medications, transfuses blood or other blood products, infuses intravenous fluids, continuously monitors the patient's physiological status, alerts the surgeon to developing problems and treats them as they arise, and supervises the patient's recovery in the Post Anesthesia Care Unit. The role of the surgical scrub primarily involves technical skills, manual dexterity, and in-depth knowledge of the anatomic and mechanical aspects of a particular surgery. The surgical scrub handles sutures, instruments, and other equipment that is immediately adjacent to the sterile field.

Nursing Process: Planning

Patient Need: Safe, Effective Care Environment

5. Answer: 1

Rationale: Improper positioning can lead to sensory and motor dysfunction and result in nerve damage. Improper positioning can cause injury to muscles and joints.

Nursing Process: Evaluation

Patient Need: Physiological Integrity

6. Answer: 3

Rationale: Postoperative testing must be completed as ordered to assess for any physiological contraindication to the proposed surgical intervention. Patients should remove nail polish and contacts before arriving at the hospital. Patients should bring a pair of eyeglasses with a case for pre- and postoperative use. The patient must adhere to the NPO order as directed by the surgeon and reinforced by means of preoperative teaching.

Nursing Process: Evaluation

Patient Need: Safe, Effective Care Environment

7. Answer: 1

Rationale: Nursing care includes keeping the affected extremity at or above heart level, ensuring that the affected area is not rubbed or massaged, recording bilateral calf or thigh circumferences every shift, and teaching and supporting the patient and family.

Nursing Process: Implementation

Patient Need: Physiological Integrity

8. Answer: 3
   Rationale: The respiratory rate of a patient who is experiencing a pulmonary embolism will increase. Other common assessment findings include mild to moderate dyspnea, chest pain, diaphoresis, anxiety, restlessness, rapid pulse, dysrhythmias, cough, and cyanosis.
   Nursing Process: Assessment
   Patient Need: Physiological Integrity

Chapter 5

Terms Matching
1. G
2. N
3. Q
4. A
5. K
6. O
7. L
8. C
9. B
10. H
11. P
12. I
13. D
14. M
15. J
16. E
17. F

Focused Study

1. Hospice is a philosophy of care rather than a program of care. It is comprehensive and coordinated care for patients with limited life expectancy. It is provided at home, hospitals, and long-term care facilities that reaffirm the right of every patient and family to fully participate in the final stages of life. Provided by hospice agency nurses and other members of a healthcare team (including social workers, ministers, home health aides, and volunteers), it is based on a philosophy of death with comfort and dignity, encompassing biomedical, psychosocial, and spiritual aspects of the dying experience. Although most hospice care is provided in the home, it may also be provided in hospitals, long-term care facilities, and other community-based settings. Palliative care is an area of care that has evolved out of the hospice experience, but exists outside hospice programs and is not restricted to the end of life and is used earlier in the disease experience. Palliative care, which can be used in all types of healthcare settings, is focused on the relief of physical, mental, and spiritual distress for individuals who have an incurable illness. The goal of palliative care is to prevent and relieve suffering through early assessment and treatment of pain and other physical, psychosocial, and spiritual needs to improve the patient's quality of life.

Although palliative care may be provided by a single person, it usually involves the combined efforts of an interdisciplinary team, including physicians, nurses, social workers, chaplains, home health aides, and volunteers. Care is provided in the patient's home (or long-term care facility, senior living facility, or hospital). The expected outcomes of care are directed by interventions to manage current manifestations of the illness and to prevent new manifestations from occurring.

2.
   - Difficulty talking or swallowing
   - Nausea, flatus, abdominal distention
   - Urinary and/or bowel incontinence, constipation
   - Decreased sensation, taste, and smell
   - Weak, slow, and/or irregular pulse
   - Decreasing blood pressure
   - Decreased, irregular, or Cheyne-Stokes respirations
   - Changes in level of consciousness
   - Restlessness, agitation
   - Coolness, mottling, and cyanosis of the extremities

3. American Indian: Some tribes prefer not to openly discuss terminal prognosis and DNR decisions because negative thoughts may make inevitable loss occur sooner. Suggest a family meeting to discuss care and end-of-life issues. If the family feels comfortable, all members of the family and close friends may remain 24 hours a day (eating, joking, singing). Mourning is done in private, away from the dying person. After death, the family may hug, touch, sing, and stay close to the deceased.

   Black/African American: Suggest that the family have a family meeting or talk with a minister or family elder. Patient may decide to have an older family member disclose a poor prognosis. Care for the dying family member is often done at home until death is imminent.

   Chinese American: Ensure that the head of the family is present when the terminal illness is discussed. The patient may not want to discuss approaching death. Special amulets or cloths may be brought from home. Family members may prefer to bathe the body after death.

   Iranian: Information about a terminal illness should be presented by a trusted member of the healthcare team to the family and never to the patient when he or she is alone. Most Iranians believe in *tagdir* (will of God) in life and death as a predestined journey. When death occurs, notify the head of the family first. DNR decisions are often made by the family. The family may want to bathe the body.

   Mexican American: Based on the belief that worry may make health worse, the family may want to protect the patient from the seriousness of the illness. The information is often handled by an older daughter or son. Extended family members are obligated to pay respects to the sick and dying, although pregnant women do not care for dying people or attend funerals. The patient may prefer to die at home. Prayers, amulets, and rosary beads are used, and the priest should be notified. Death is seen as an important spiritual event. The family may bathe the body and spend time with the body.

Vietnamese: Consult head of family before telling patient about a terminal illness. Entire family will make DNR decision, often with assistance from a priest or monk. Patients often prefer to die at home. Family should have extra time with the body and may cry loudly and uncontrollably. Spiritual/religious rites are often conducted in the room.

Case Study

1. *Discuss Spiritual assessment, including questions to consider during this assessment process.* Because spiritual beliefs and practices greatly influence people's reaction to loss, it is important to explore them with the patient when assessing a loss. The spiritually healthy patient has inner resources that help in working through the grief process. Faith, prayer, trust in God or a superior being, perception of a purpose in life, or belief in immortality are examples of the inner resources that may sustain the patient during an actual or perceived loss. Patients who had not considered themselves religious before the actual or perceived loss often turn to religion to seek comfort or to cope with feelings of despair, helplessness, hopelessness, or guilt.

Assessing the dying patient's spiritual life and its significance to the patient and family helps identify spiritual support systems. Some nurses are uncomfortable with assessing the patient's spiritual needs; the following questions may be helpful:
- What are the spiritual aspects of the patient's philosophy about life? About death?
- Are the values and beliefs about life and death congruent with those of people who are important to the patient?
- Which spiritual resources and rituals have significance for the patient?

Belief systems that are incompatible with those of family members can be an additional source of stress for patients dealing with a loss. The anger and resentment often observed in families faced with decisions concerning dying members may be avoided if the nurse assesses the potential impact of differing beliefs.

Patients coping with a loss often perceive that it is a punishment from God for their wrongdoing or for their failure to remain faithful to their religious practices. Therefore, it is important to assess the level of guilt the patient or family expresses. Assessing the patient's comments regarding feelings of responsibility for the loss helps determine whether these feelings are an expected phase of grieving or indicate dysfunctional grieving.

2. *Discuss Kübler-Ross's stages of death and dying, including reactions that may occur during the grieving process.*

Kübler-Ross's research on death and dying provided a framework for gaining insight about the stages of coping with an impending or actual loss. According to Kübler-Ross, not all people dealing with a loss go through these stages, and those who do may not experience the stages in the sequence described. In identifying the stages of death and dying, Kübler-Ross stressed the danger of prematurely labeling a "stage" and emphasized that her goal was to describe her observations of how people come to terms with situations of loss.

Some or all of the following reactions may occur during the grieving process and may reappear as the person experiences the loss:
- *Denial.* A person may react with shock and disbelief after receiving word of an actual or potential loss.
- *Anger.* In this stage, the person resists the loss. The anger is often directed toward family and healthcare providers.
- *Bargaining.* The bargaining stage serves as an attempt to postpone the reality of the loss. The person makes a secret bargain with God, expressing a willingness to do anything to postpone the loss or change the prognosis.
- *Depression.* The person enters a stage of depression as the full impact of the actual or perceived loss is realized. The person prepares for the impending loss by working through the struggle of separation.
- *Acceptance.* The person begins to come to terms with the loss and resumes activities with hopefulness for the future. Some dying people reach a stage of acceptance in which they may appear to be almost devoid of emotion. The struggle is past, and the emotional pain is gone.

3. *What factors will affect the parents' ability to grieve their upcoming loss?*
Characteristic factors that can interfere with successful grieving include the following:
- Perceived inability to share the loss
- Lack of social recognition of the loss
- Ambivalent relationships prior to the loss
- Traumatic circumstances of the loss

A well-functioning family usually rallies after the initial shock and disbelief and provides support for each other during all phases of the grieving process. After a loss, the functional family is able to shift roles, levels of responsibility, and ways of communicating. See the Moving Evidence into Action box for research about factors that affect family members' ability to care for a dying family member at home.

The family may experience negative as well as positive effects. For example, the dying patient may request that someone the family perceives as an outsider be near, and the family may respond with anger to the perceived "intrusion." Similarly, certain family members may express hurt feelings or anger if the patient is unresponsive to other family members. Well-meaning family members also may try to shield the patient from the pain of grieving. It is rare for the family and the patient to experience anger, denial, and acceptance in unison. While one member is in denial, another may be angry because "not enough is being done."

Crossword Puzzle

question	term answer
Stage of grief in which the person's behavior becomes disorganized	DESPAIR
Kübler-Ross stage of grief in which individual resists loss	DENIAL
Legal documents that allow a person to plan for health care	LIVINGWILL
A healthcare _____ is an individual selected to make medical decisions when another person is no longer able to do so	SURROGATE
Signify a killing prompted by some humanitarian motive	EUTHANASIA
A combination of intellectual and emotional responses and behaviors by which people adjust their self-concept in the face of an actual or potential loss	GRIEVING

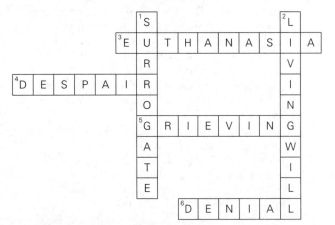

NCLEX-RN® Review Questions

1. Answer: 3

   Rationale: Often when patients initiate conversations about dying, nurses may feel unprepared for their questions. They can take nurses by surprise, and can often lead them to believe that the patient expects a crystal ball response. Nurses must remember that the purpose of all such discussions is to keep the lines of communication open with the patient. The idea is to make the subject of dying discussible and to communicate to the patient that it does not make nurses afraid to do so. An open-ended statement such as "Tell me what concerns you the most" provide a means of encouraging communication.

   Nursing Process: Implementation
   Patient Need: Safe, Effective Care Environment

2. Answer: 4

   Rationale: Grieving is painful and lonely. One's social support system is important because of its potentially positive influence on the successful resolution of grief. Some losses may lead to social isolation, placing affected people at high risk for dysfunctional grief reactions.

   Nursing Process: Evaluation
   Patient Need: Safe, Effective Care Environment

3. Answer: 2

   Rationale: A durable power of attorney can delegate the authority to make health, financial, and/or legal decisions on a person's behalf. It must be in writing and must state that the designated person is authorized to make healthcare decisions.

   Nursing Process: Implementation
   Patient Need: Safe, Effective Care Environment

4. Answer: 1

   Rationale: A common problem for patients at the end of life, pain is what people often say they fear the most. Pain, a subjective experience, is influenced by the patient's emotions, previous experiences with pain, and family and culture. Unfortunately, pain is often undertreated at the end of life because physicians and nurses fear they will cause addiction or cause harm from the high dose of opioids necessary to to control pain. However, nearly all pain at the end of life can be managed without causing addiction or hastening death through respiratory depression. It is of utmost importance to keep the patient comfortable through general comfort measures by administering ordered medications for pain, neuropathic pain (which is rarely relieved by opioids), seizures, and/or anxiety.

   Nursing Process: Implementation
   Patient Need: Safe, Effective Care Environment

5. Answer: 1

   Rationale: In the anger stage, the person resists the loss. The anger is often directed toward family members and healthcare providers.

   Nursing Process: Assessment
   Patient Need: Physiological Integrity

6. Answer: 2

   Rationale: Palliative care is an area of care that has evolved out of the hospice experience, but exists outside hospice programs and is not restricted to the end of life and is used earlier in the disease experience. Palliative care, which can be used in all types of healthcare settings, is focused on the relief of physical, mental, and spiritual distress for individuals who have an incurable illness. The goal of palliative care is to prevent and relieve suffering by early assessment and treatment of pain and other physical, psychosocial, and spiritual needs to improve the patient's quality of life.

   Although palliative care may be provided by a single person, it usually involves the combined efforts of an interdisciplinary team, including physicians, nurses, social workers, chaplains, home health aides, and volunteers. Care is provided in the patient's home (or long-term care facility, senior living facility, or hospital). The expected outcomes of care are directed by interventions to manage current manifestations of the illness and to prevent new manifestations from occurring.

Nursing Process: Implementation

Patient Need: Safe, Effective Care Environment

7. Answer: 3

Rationale: As death nears, respirations often become fast or slow, shallow and labored. The patient may have apnea or Cheyne-Stokes respirations (regular periods of deep, rapid breathing following by no breaths for 5 to 30 seconds). Fluid may accumulate in the lungs, causing crackles, especially in patients who are well hydrated and in those who are having difficulty swallowing or coughing. These sounds are not painful for the patient, but they may be treated with oxygen, opioids (to improve respirations and decrease anxiety), and medications to decrease secretions (atropine, scopolamine, hyoscyamine, or glycopyrrolate). It should be noted that oxygen and suctioning are only temporary measures and (especially with suctioning) may even be traumatic for the patient. Nursing care to improve respirations includes keeping the head of the bed elevated. Keeping the room cool and providing a breeze from a fan often makes the patient more comfortable.

Nursing Process: Implementation

Patient Need: Safe, Effective Care Environment

8. Answer: 4

Rationale: If the patient is conscious and complains of nausea, antiemetics such as prochlorperazine (Compazine) or ondansetron (Zofran) should be administered. Preferred method of administration is IV if patient has intractable vomitting.

Nursing Process: Implementation

Patient Need: Safe, Effective Care Environment

Chapter 6

Terms Matching

1. H
2. K
3. N
4. J
5. C
6. B
7. F
8. G
9. E
10. L
11. I
12. D
13. M
14. A
15. O
16. R

Focused Study

1. a. Research has been done that supports an apparent hereditary factor, especially with alcohol use and dependence. Evidence supports the D2 dopamine receptor gene (DRD2 A1 allele) as a genetic marker in adolescent males with increased risk for developing substance use problems (Conner et al., 2005). The discovery that the DRD2 A1 allele gene appeared to be associated with alcoholism has led to a growing body of genetic research into substance abuse disorders.

   b. Scientists have hypothesized that addiction to alcohol may have a biochemical basis and have identified specific phases of the disease. Research has implicated low levels of dopamine and serotonin in the development of alcohol dependence. Dopamine and dopamine receptor sites are intricately involved in the complex workings between the nervous system and abusive substances. Any drug's ability to have an impact on the biochemical mechanism of the brain must be able to do so at a receptor site or at a number of receptor sites. Most abused substances either mimic or block the brain's most important neurotransmitters at their respective receptor sites.

   c. Researchers have attempted to explain substance abuse through a combination of psychoanalytic, behavioral, and family system theories. Psychoanalytic theorists view substance abuse as a fixation at the oral stage of development, while behavioral theorists see addiction as a learned, maladaptive behavior. Family system theory focuses on the pattern of family relationships throughout several generations. No addictive personality type has been identified; however, several common factors seem to exist among alcoholics and drug users.

   Many substance abusers have experienced sexual or physical abuse in their childhood and, as a result, have low self-esteem and difficulty expressing emotions. A link also exists between substance abuse and psychiatric disorders such as depression, anxiety, and antisocial and dependent personalities. The habit of using a substance becomes a form of self-medication to cope with day-to-day problems and, over time, develops into an addiction.

   d. Social variables and norms often influence individuals' decisions as to when they use substances, what substances they use, and how they use substances. Ethnic differences in the way alcohol is metabolized may explain why some individuals choose not to drink.

2.

Addictive Substance	Effect
Caffeine	A stimulant that increases the heart rate and acts as a diuretic.
Nicotine	Low doses cause vasoconstriction, heart rate acceleration, increase in gastric acid secretion, tone and motility of GI smooth muscle, and promotion of vomiting.
	Initially, nicotine increases respiration, mental alertness, and cognitive ability, but eventually it depresses these responses.
	Moderate doses of nicotine can cause tremors.
	High doses of nicotine found in some insecticides can cause acute poisoning, resulting in convulsions and death.
Cannabis	Short-term use increases heart rate and bronchodilation.
	Chronic long-term use results in airway constriction, bronchitis, sinusitis, asthma, and increased risk for respiratory cancer.
	Decreased spermatogenesis and testosterone levels are found in males, and cannabis suppresses follicle-stimulating, luteinizing, and prolactin hormones in females, making breast-feeding for new mothers impossible.
	Birth defects may also be associated with cannabis use.
Alcohol	Alteration in the sleep cycle, intensified obstructive sleep apnea, and reduced total sleeping time may occur.
	Heavy drinkers have a higher mortality rate, and many fatalities occur from alcohol-related accidents.
	Euphoria, reduced inhibitions, impaired judgment, and increased confidence are also seen.
CNS Depressants	Impact ranges from mild sedation to coma.
Psychostimulants	Euphoria is common.
	Birth defects, preterm labor, or miscarriage may occur.
Amphetamines	Arousal, mood elevation, a sense of increased strength, mental capacity, self-confidence, and a decreased need for food and sleep may occur. Physical symptoms include weight loss, tachycardia, tachypnea, hyperthermia, insomnia, and muscular tremors.
	Behavioral and psychiatric symptoms reported most often include violent behavior, repetitive activity, memory loss, paranoia, delusions of reference, auditory hallucinations, and confusion or fright.
Opiates	Use of opiates may cause CNS depression.
	Some substances may promote a sense of euphoria.
	Tolerance may result in respiratory depression, nausea, and constipation.
	Physical dependence occurs with long-term use of opiates. Initial withdrawal symptoms such as drug craving, lacrimation, rhinorrhea, yawning, and diaphoresis usually take ten days to run their course, with the second phase of opiate withdrawal lasting for months with insomnia, irritability, and fatigue and potential GI hyperactivity and premature ejaculation as problems.
Hallucinogens	Use of hallucinogens results in thoughts, perceptions, and feelings that occur in dreams.
Inhalants	Effects are similar to those for alcohol use.

3. **a.** This ten-question, dichotomous, self-administered questionnaire takes 10 to 15 minutes to complete. An answer of yes to three or more questions indicates a potentially dangerous pattern of alcohol abuse.
   b. This tool is useful when the patient may not recognize that he or she has an alcohol problem or is uncomfortable acknowledging it. The questionnaire is designed to be a self-report of drinking behavior, or it may be administered by a professional. One affirmative response indicates the need for further discussion and follow-up. Two or more yes answers signifies a problem with alcohol that may require treatment.
   c. This yes/no self-administered questionnaire is useful in identifying people who may be addicted to drugs other than alcohol. A positive response to one or more questions suggests significant drug abuse problems and warrants further evaluation.

4.
- Hospitals, psychiatric units, special substance abuse units, methadone clinics, or outpatient settings for medical detoxification
- Residential rehabilitation programs, halfway houses, and partial hospitalization programs
- Alcoholics Anonymous, Narcotics Anonymous, and other self-help groups
- Employee assistance programs
- Individual, group, and/or family counseling
- Community rehabilitation programs
- National Alliance for the Mentally Ill

Case Study

1. *How long does Ryan need to have had excessive drinking behaviors to be considered substance-dependent?* Three months or more
2. *What factors affect the rate of alcohol absorption?* Factors such as body mass, food intake, and liver function can affect the rate of alcohol absorption.
3. *What vitamin deficiency is associated with alcoholism?* Thiamine. *How will the nurse assist Ryan in meeting his nutritional needs?* The nurse will perform the following interventions:
   a. Administer vitamins and dietary supplements as ordered by the physician.
   b. Monitor lab work and report significant changes to the physician.
   c. Collaborate with a dietitian to determine the number of calories needed to provide adequate nutrition and ensure realistic weight gain.
   d. Teach the importance of adequate nutrition by explaining the Food Guide Pyramid and relating the physical effects of malnutrition on body systems.
4. *The nurse will teach Ryan HALT. What is HALT?* HALT is a method used to identify relapsing behavior. The acronym HALT stands for hungry, angry, lonely, and tired.

Crossword Puzzle

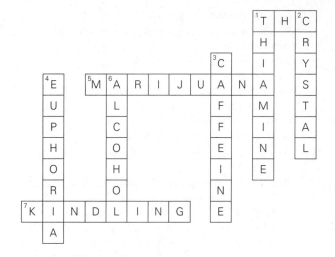

question	term answer
Substance referred to as hash	MARIJUANA
Vitamin deficiency commonly seen in alcoholics	THIAMINE
Most commonly abused legal drug in the United States	ALCOHOL
Long-term changes in brain neurotransmission that occur after repeated detoxifications	KINDLING
Stimulant found in food and beverages that causes heart rate increases	CAFFEINE
The psychoactive component of marijuana	THC
The primary subjective effect associated with cocaine and amphetamines	EUPHORIA
Street term commonly used to refer to methamphetamine	CRYSTAL

NCLEX-RN® Review Questions

1. Answer: 1
   Rationale: Dopamine and dopamine receptor sites are intricately involved in the complex workings between the nervous system and abusive substances. Studies show that dopamine D(1) and D(2) receptors sustain the addictive danger of drugs. Recent studies have also shown that the dopamine D(3) receptor is involved in drug-seeking behavior.
   Nursing Process: Diagnosis
   Patient Need: Comprehension
2. Answer: 4
   Rationale: Compared to other ethnic groups, Asian Americans report the lowest prevalence of family history of alcoholism (Ebberhart, Luczak, Avenecy, & Wall, 2003). Caucasians, Hispanics, and African Americans, on the other hand, have insufficient amounts of the enzyme aldehyde dehydrogenase for metabolizing alcohol and report higher alcoholism rates (Bersamin, Paschall, & Flewelling, 2005).
   Nursing Process: Diagnosis
   Patient Need: Health Maintenance and Promotion
3. Answer: 3
   Rationale: Marijuana use can trigger psychosis in schizophrenic patients, and according to recent research, cannabis use may be a risk factor in developing future psychotic symptoms (Ferdinand et al., 2005).
   Nursing Process: Diagnosis
   Patient Need: Health Promotion and Maintenance
4. Answer: 1
   Rationale: Methamphetamine is a powerful stimulant drug that is commonly referred to as "speed"; "crystal"; "crank"; "go"; and, most recently, "ice." Examples of common opiate brand names include Vicodin®, Percocet®, OxyContin®, and Darvon®. Hallucinogens are called psychedelics and include phencyclidine (PCP), 3,4-methylenedioxy-methamphetamine (MDMA), d-lysergic acid diethylamide (LSD), mescaline, dimethyltryptamine (DMT), and psilocin.

Nursing Process: Diagnosis

Patient Need: Health Promotion and Maintenance

5. Answer: 3, 4

Rationale: Tears are not tested for drug content. Stool may be used for newborns, but it is not frequently used for adult drug testing. The body fluids most often tested for drug content are blood and urine, although saliva, perspiration, and even hair can be tested.

Nursing Process: Assessment

Patient Need: Health Promotion and Maintenance

6. Answer: 3

Rationale: Ask questions in a nonthreatening, matter-of-fact manner phrased to avoid implying wrongdoing. The appropriate question from those listed is, "Have you ever been treated in an alcohol or drug abuse clinic?" This is an open-ended, nonthreatening question. The other questions are closed-ended and imply wrongdoing.

Nursing Process: Assessment

Patient Need: Health Promotion and Maintenance

7. Answer: 2

Rationale: The CAGE questionnaire is most useful when the patient may not recognize he or she has an alcohol problem or is uncomfortable acknowledging it. This questionnaire is designed to be a self-report of drinking behavior, although it may be administered by a professional. Because self-report tools are not always answered truthfully, patients who screen positive for drug addiction should be evaluated according to other diagnostic criteria. HALT is a tool used to identify addictive relapse behavior.

Nursing Process: Implementation

Patient Need: Health Promotion and Maintenance

8. Answer: 1

Rational: Nursing interventions employed for a patient with a substance abuse addiction includes assessing the patient's level of disorientation, providing a private room but never leaving the patient alone without monitoring, not accepting the use of defense mechanisms as an attempt to blame others for his or her actions, and encouraging the patient to verbalize anxieties.

Nursing Process: Implementation

Patient Need: Psychosocial Integrity

9. Answer: 3

Rationale: Healthcare professionals have a higher risk for opiate abuse than other professionals due to the high accessibility of opiates in their line of work (Trinkoff et al., 2000).

Nursing Process: Diagnosis

Patient Need: Health Promotion and Maintenance

Chapter 7

Terms Matching

1. P
2. Q
3. M
4. H
5. C
6. F
7. A
8. O
9. J
10. T
11. I
12. R
13. K
14. B
15. L
16. G
17. E
18. D
19. N
20. U
21. S

Focused Study

1. Emergencies can be handled through a local emergency management system. Disasters usually involve multiple victims. Disasters are more complex emergencies that can overwhelm local hospitals, healthcare facilities, and local emergency medical resources.

2. Conventional weapons include all types of bombs and guns (hand grenades, handguns, semiautomatic rifles, rocket-propelled devices, missiles). Nonconventional terrorist weapons include chemical, radiologic, and biologic weapons. Terrorists may release a toxin, which is a form of a chemical attack. A dirty bomb would be classified as a radiologic attack. Anthrax is one form of a biologic attack.

3. Level I disaster—This can be effectively managed by a local emergency response system.

   Level II disaster—The local emergency response system is unable to manage this type of disaster, and the local system requires assistance from surrounding communities and regions.

   Level III disaster—Local and regional resources are overwhelmed and assistance from state and federal government is required.

4. A triage system is used to sort victims. Those victims who require the most assistance are labeled as "red" and these victims are treated first. Victims who require less assistance but still require transfer to an emergency care center are labeled "yellow" and are cared for next. Those victims who do not require assistance are labeled "green" and do not require transport to an emergency care center. Victims who are labeled as "black" are expected to die or have already died. A reverse triage system is used to manage victims during a mass casualty event especially when victims may need to be evacuated from a hot zone and decontaminated. During a reverse triage system, victims who are ambulatory and require the least amount of care are assisted first. Victims who require more assistance and may need to be transferred to an

emergency care center are assisted and evacuated next. Those victims who require the most assistance are assisted and evacuated last.

Case Study

1. *What is a hurricane?* A hurricane is a type of tropical cyclone. It is a low-pressure system that generally forms in the tropics.
2. *What physical effects of a hurricane is Mrs. Deckman at risk for, regardless of her past medical history?* Common physical effects include asphyxia due to drowning; wounds, bone, joint, and muscle injuries; aggravation of chronic illnesses; stress-related symptoms; upper respiratory infections; gastrointestinal illnesses; clean-up injuries; animal, snake, and insect bites; skin irritations and infections; obstetrical complications; and waterborne and insect-borne diseases from contaminated water supplies and insect breeding grounds (Clark, 2003; Smith & Maurer, 2000).
3. *Mrs. Deckman was given a triage level of "red" after she was taken to a local shelter. What does this mean?* Her age and the potential complications of diabetes are the reason for her red triage level. Her blood sugar levels require assessment and monitoring, as does her physical health due to uncontrolled blood sugar levels.
4. *Mrs. Deckman asks the nurse for assistance in developing a disaster box to be used in case of another disaster. What items should the nurse suggest to be kept in the box?* Mrs. Deckman's disaster box should include the following: a current list of medications, doses, and times of administration; names and phone numbers of significant persons; eyeglass prescriptions; style and serial numbers of medical devices; healthcare policies and numbers; identification; list of allergies; blood type; checkbook; credit cards; insurance agent's name and number; copy of driver's license; 72-hour supply of medications; dentures; eyeglasses; list of special dietary needs; sturdy shoes; and warm clothing, blankets, incontinence briefs, prostheses, hearing aids, hearing aid batteries, extra wheelchair batteries, oxygen, and other assistive devices.
5. *What is the role of the nurse who works with the victims of this natural disaster?* The nurse should begin by triaging and assessing victims to provide the best care with available resources. Quick, direct treatment can be provided. The area should be secured by security personnel or the local police. Nurses should follow emergency preparedness plans outlined in their communities and employment agencies.
6. *Of the five stages of disaster preparedness, which stage is being described in this scenario?* The stage that is being described is most likely the emergency stage. The disaster has already occurred and there has been an initial response to the disaster.
7. *What should the triage nurse document on the Mass Trauma Data Instrument?* The CDC created a document called the Mass Trauma Data Instrument that is used to document data about victims of disasters. The nurse can record demographic information, circumstances surrounding the Mrs. Deckman's injuries, the condition of the injuries, and any other details. The triage nurse initially documents information about Mrs. Deckman on this form, and it is transferred with her as she moves through the healthcare system.
8. *A crowd has developed at the site of the shelter where Mrs. Deckman is being treated. What is one consequence of poor crowd management?* Security forces or local police forces must control crowds. If the crowd is not adequately controlled, chaos can ensue and healthcare providers will be unable to care for the victims. An area should be secured before healthcare workers enter the area.

Short Answers

1. *List types of injuries that may be seen in victims of chemical and radiologic terrorism. Briefly describe three nursing interventions that should be provided for these two types of terrorism.*

Type of terrorism	Chemical	Radiologic
Types of injuries	1. Wounds on skin	1. Suppression of bone marrow 2. Nausea, vomiting, anorexia, diarrhea (also, blood vessel damage, skin erythema, and nerve cell damage)
Nursing interventions	1. Remove clothing from injury site. 2. Flush chemicals from skin. 3. Cover wounds with sterile dressings.	1. Prevent infection. 2. Treat gastrointestinal symptoms. 3. Protect skin.

NCLEX-RN® Review Questions

1. Answer: 3
   Rationale: Anthrax is a chemical nonconventional terrorist weapon. Conventional weapons include incendiary bombs, guns, missiles, and hand grenades.
   Nursing Process: Planning
   Patient Need: Safe, Effective Care Environment
2. Answer: 1, 2, 3
   Rationale: People are exposed to ionizing radiation frequently, but in small doses. Some of the sources of this everyday exposure are from outer space (including stars and the sun), natural radioactive isotopes, and x-ray machines. Cell phones and fire are not sources of ionizing radiation.

Nursing Process: Planning

Patient Need: Safe, Effective Care Environment

3. Answer: 2

Rationale: A level II disaster requires mutual aid from surrounding communities and regional efforts. A level I disaster can be effectively handled by local emergency response personnel and local organizations. A level III disaster overwhelms local and regional assets, and statewide or federal assistance is required. There is no such thing as a level IV disaster.

Nursing Process: Planning

Patient Need: Safe, Effective Care Environment

4. Answer: 2

Rationale: The pre-disaster stage involves warning, preimpact mobilization, and evacuation, if appropriate. The nondisaster stage is the time for planning and preparation because the threat of a disaster is still in the future. The impact stage is the time when the disaster event has occurred and the community experiences the immediate effects. The emergency stage involves the immediate response to the effects of the disaster.

Nursing Process: Planning

Patient Need: Safe, Effective Care Environment

5. Answer: 2

Rationale: Those victims who are in less critical condition but still in need of transport to emergency centers for care are classified as "yellow." Those requiring the most support and immediate emergency care are classified as "red." Those who are least likely to survive or who are already deceased are classified as "black."

Nursing Process: Assessment

Patient Need: Physiological Integrity

6. Answer: 3

Rationale: The site of the disaster where a weapon was released or where the contamination occurred is called the hot zone. The warm zone (or the hot zone) is adjacent to the hot zone. It is where decontamination of victims or triage and emergency treatment take place. The cold zone is considered to be a safe zone.

Nursing Process: Planning

Patient Need: Safe, Effective Care Environment

7. Answer: 2, 3, 4, 5

Rationale: Nursing diagnoses that may apply during disaster situations include *Anxiety, Impaired Verbal Communication, Ineffective Individual Coping, Powerlessness,* and *Risk for Injury.*

Nursing Process: Diagnosis

Patient Need: Psychosocial Integrity

8. Answer: 2

Rationale: Overexertion and exhaustion are major problems that affect a victim during the snow shoveling that follows a snowstorm. The exertion required to shovel heavy snow in the extreme cold may cause a myocardial infarction. Care for persons injured by blast injuries typically focuses on

abdominal and lung injuries, penetrating wounds, traumatic amputations, and burns. The most common health effects experienced by victims of earthquakes include stress-related symptoms, wounds, traumatic injuries, burns, gastrointestinal problems, and respiratory problems. Flying debris causes most fatalities and injuries in tornadoes.

Nursing Process: Planning

Patient Need: Safe, Effective Care Environment

Chapter 8

Terms Matching

1. F
2. K
3. N
4. R
5. O
6. B
7. C
8. L
9. S
10. D
11. A
12. G
13. E
14. H
15. U
16. I
17. M
18. T
19. Q
20. P
21. J

Focused Study

1. Mitosis and meiosis are the two types of cell division in human cells. Mitosis is the process of making new cells, and it takes place in the somatic, or tissue, cells of the body. Cell division through mitosis heals wounds and replaces cells lost daily on skin surfaces and in the lining of gastrointestinal and respiratory tracts. In addition, mitosis is responsible for human development. The mitotic activity of the zygote and its daughter cells is the foundation for a human's growth and development. The zygote undergoes mitosis to form a multicellular embryo, then fetus, then infant. Cell division through mitosis results in two cells called daughter cells that are genetically identical to the original cell, or mother cell, and each other.

   Meiosis is also known as the reductional division of a cell. Meiosis occurs only in the sex cells of the testes and ovaries and results in the formation of the sperm and oocyte (gametes). Meiosis is very similar to mitosis in that it is a form of cell division; however, through a series of complex mechanisms, the amount of genetic material is reduced by half (23 chromosomes). This is very important because when the two sex cells combine during fertilization, the total number of chromosomes (46) is present in the offspring's cells. Meiosis has three purpose: (1) to produce gametes, (2) to reduce the number of chromosomes by half, and (3) to make new combinations of genetic material from crossing over and independent assortment processes, which allows for diversity in the human population.

2. Together the total sum of DNA in a human cell is referred to as the human genome, or the complete set of inheritance for an individual. Knowledge of inheritance allows the nurse to provide genetic information to patients and their families, to assist them in managing their care, and in making reproductive decisions. The basic underlying principles of inheritance that nurses can apply to inheritance risk assessment and teaching include the following: (1) All genes are paired; (2) only one gene of each pair is transmitted (passed on) to an offspring; and (3) one copy of each gene in the offspring comes from the mother, and the other copy comes from the father.

3.
   - *Newborn screening* provides a means to identify children who have an increased risk for a genetic disease such as phenylketonuria, sickle cell disease, or maple syrup urine disease.
   - *Carrier testing* is completed on asymptomatic individuals who may be carriers of one copy of a gene alteration that can be transmitted to future children in an autosomal recessive or X-linked pattern of inheritance. This may be part of a couple's premarriage or preconception planning if they belong to a particular ethnic group with known incidence of genetic disorders such as sickle cell anemia and Tay-Sachs disease. It may be necessary to determine the exact gene mutation from an affected family member prior to carrier testing. This is often completed through lineage analysis.
   - *Preimplantation genetic diagnosis (PGD)* involves the detection of disease-causing gene alterations in human embryos just after in vitro fertilization and before implantation in the uterus, thus providing an opportunity for preselection of unaffected embryos for implantation. This type of genetic testing is most often used by both parents who are carriers of a single-gene recessive disorder and who want to implant into the uterus only the embryo(s) without the disease-causing gene alteration. It has also been used to determine tissue type for donation of tissue such as bone marrow to a sibling or parent. PGD is usually not covered by insurance, is very costly, and is available at only a small number of centers and for only a small number of disorders (U.S. National Library of Medicine, 2008).
   - *Predictive genetic testing* is usually made available to the asymptomatic individual and includes both predispositional and presymptomatic testing. A positive predispositional testing result indicates that there is an increased risk that the individual will develop the disease. Common examples include breast cancer and hereditary nonpolyposis

colorectal cancer. A presymptomatic test is performed when development of the disease is certain if the gene alteration is present. These tests are medically indicated when the seriousness and mortality of the disease can be reduced with knowledge of the gene alteration. Examples are hereditary hemochromatosis and familial hypercholesterolemia. Life planning and lifestyle choices can be influenced by predictive testing.
   - Other uses of genetic testing include organ transplantation tissue typing and pharmacogenetic testing, which involves predicting or studying the patient's response to particular medications.

4. Family history has long been a part of nursing assessment, but the relative importance of obtaining a family history has recently increased as knowledge of the interaction of genes and the environment has expanded. In fact, it is an inexpensive first "genetic screen," often underused by healthcare professionals. Yet with the number of genetics professionals being less than the projected need, professionals in primary care and other specialties must share some of the responsibility in obtaining this information and making appropriate referrals.

   A pedigree is a pictorial representation or diagram of the medical history of a family (typically three generations). A pedigree provides the nurse, genetic counselor, or geneticist with a clear visual representation of relationships of affected individuals to the immediate and extended family. It can identify other individuals in the family who might benefit from a genetic consultation. It also can identify a single-gene alteration pattern of inheritance or a cluster of multifactorial conditions; a referral and/or reproductive risk teaching for the individual and family may result. A family's learning can be enhanced by the visual teaching contribution a pedigree provides and can clarify any misunderstandings or misconceptions regarding inheritance.

   By simply integrating into practice the genetic aspects of assessment, observation, and history gathering, the nurse can improve the standard of care delivered and have a positive effect on the patient. The nurse does not need to be a genetics expert, but with heightened awareness, the nurse can make appropriate inquiries and provide referrals to genetic specialists.

Case Studies

Case Study 1

1. *Why did the physician order carrier testing for Mrs. Steinman?* Mrs. Steinman reports that her relatives have a history of Tay-Sachs disease. Carrier testing may be part of a couple's premarital or preconception planning if they belong to a particular ethnic group with known incidence of genetic disorders such as sickle cell anemia and Tay-Sachs disease.

2. *How can the Steinmans be assured of the accuracy of their genetic testing results?* Genetic testing involves the analysis of DNA, RNA, chromosomes, and serum levels of specific enzymes or metabolites. Genetic tests can be classified into two categories: screening and diagnostic. A positive screening genetic test result indicates an increased risk or probability, but it must be confirmed by diagnostic testing. Screening genetic tests are most commonly completed in prenatal, newborn, and carrier circumstances. In contrast, a diagnostic test can definitively validate or eliminate a genetic disorder in the symptomatic patient and then guide clinical management.

3. *Who may obtain the results of the Steinmans' genetic testing?* Those providing the genetic tests must provide the patient with assurance that the results will be handled confidentially and that there will be no access to the genetic information by a third party without written permission of the individual being tested.

Case Study 2

1. *Describe the predictive genetic testing that Ms. Simmons will have performed.* Predictive genetic testing is usually made available to the asymptomatic individual and includes both predispositional and presymptomatic testing. A positive predispositional testing result indicates that there is an increased risk that the individual will develop the disease. Common examples include breast cancer and hereditary nonpolyposis colorectal cancer. A presymptomatic test is performed when development of the disease is certain if the gene alteration is present. These tests are medically indicated when the seriousness and mortality of the disease can be reduced with knowledge of the gene alteration. Examples are hereditary hemochromatosis and familial hypercholesterolemia. Life planning and lifestyle choices can be influenced by predictive testing.

2. *Why is it important to discuss and map Ms. Simmons' family tree in relation to breast cancer?* A pedigree is a pictorial representation or diagram of the medical history of a family (typically three generations). A pedigree provides the nurse, genetic counselor, or geneticist with a clear visual representation of relationships of affected individuals to the immediate and extended family. It can identify other individuals in the family who might benefit from a genetic consultation. It also can identify a single-gene alteration pattern of inheritance or a cluster of multifactorial conditions; a referral and/or reproductive risk teaching for the individual and family may result. A family's learning can be enhanced by the visual teaching contribution a pedigree provides and can clarify any misunderstandings or misconceptions regarding inheritance.

3. *What type of nursing diagnoses will the nurse include in Ms. Simmons' genetic counseling care plan?* Deficient Knowledge—The nurse must be aware of available genetic resources and participate in the education of genetic disorders as well as health promotion and prevention.

4. *How can the testing information obtained by Ms. Simmons be used in the care of her extended family members?* The findings from Ms. Simmons genetic testing will provide information that may be used by other members of the family. Information concerning potential diseases that Ms. Simmons has a genetic predisposition for can be used to promote disease prevention activities in others.

Crossword Puzzle

question	term answer
The loss of a single chromosome from a pair	MONOSOMY
The gain of a single chromosome	TRISOMY
The normal number of 46 chromosomes	EUPLOIDY
The same	HOMO
Different	HETERO
A picture of an individual's chromosomes	KARYOTYPE

NCLEX-RN® Review Questions

1. Answer: 3
   Rationale: Life starts as a single cell, but the developed human body is made up of many cells. These cells share common features (for example, a nucleus that contains 46 chromosomes and organelles such as mitochondria).
   Nursing Process: Assessment
   Patient Need: Physiological Integrity

2. Answer: 1
   Rationale: DNA molecules consist of long sequences of nucleotides or bases represented by the letters A, G, T, and C.
   Nursing Process: Assessment
   Patient Need: Physiological Integrity

3. Answer: 3

Rationale: Down syndrome is better known as Trisomy 21. Trisomy is the gain of a single chromosome, making a total of three copies of a certain chromosome

Nursing Process: Assessment

Patient Need: Physiological Integrity

4. Answer: 1, 2

Rationale: A family history of multiple male miscarriages may be a sign of an X-linked dominant condition. The sex chromosome X is unevenly distributed to males and females. The female has two X chromosomes, and the male has only one. Thus, the family history and pattern of inheritance has a characteristic distribution pattern among the males and females in the family. An individual with a recessive condition has inherited one altered gene from his or her mother and one from his or her father. Homozygous dominant conditions are generally more severe than heterozygous dominant conditions and are often lethal.

Nursing Process: Planning

Patient Need: Health Promotion and Maintenance

5. Answer: 4

Rationale: Newborn screening provides a means to identify children who have an increased risk for having a genetic disease such as phenylketonuria, sickle cell disease, or maple syrup urine disease. Several states now screen for more than 30 conditions (expanded newborn screen) as part of routine newborn care. Predictive genetic testing is usually made available to the asymptomatic individual and includes both predispositional and presymptomatic testing. Common examples include breast cancer and hereditary nonpolyposis colorectal cancer. Pharmacogenetic testing involves predicting or studying a patient's response to particular medications. Carrier testing is completed on asymptomatic individuals who may be carriers of one copy of a gene alteration that can be transmitted to future children in an autosomal recessive or X-linked pattern of inheritance. This may be part of a couple's premarriage or preconception planning

Nursing Process: Assessment

Patient Need: Health Promotion and Maintenance

6. Answer: 4

Rationale: All genetic testing should be voluntary, and the nurse's responsibility is to ensure that the informed consent process includes discussion of the risks and benefits of the test, including any physical harm as well as potential psychologic and societal injury by stigmatization, discrimination, and emotional stress. The nurse should discuss the cost of genetic tests, which may range from hundreds to thousands of dollars depending on the size of the gene being tested. Most insurance companies do not cover genetic tests, but if insurance coverage is available, the individual must weigh the cost of allowing the insurance company to have access to the genetic information (HGPb, 2008).

Nursing Process: Planning

Patient Need: Health Promotion and Maintenance

7. Answer: 1

Rationale: A woman with a strong family history and/or mutations in the BRCA1 and BRCA2 tumor suppressor genes should have screening clinical breast exams and mammographies at an earlier age compared to the general population.

Nursing Process: Evaluation

Patient Need: Health Promotion and Maintenance

8. Answer: 1

Rationale: Mitochondrial genes and any diseases due to DNA alterations on those genes are transmitted through the mother in a matrilineal pattern.

Nursing Process: Assessment

Patient Need: Physiological Integrity

9. Answer: 1

Rationale: A positive test result may lead to feelings of unworthiness, confusion, anger, depression, fear, shame, and self-image disturbance. Survivor guilt may affect adults with negative results if their siblings are positive.

Nursing Process: Assessment

Patient Need: Physiological Integrity

Chapter 9

Terms Matching

1. I
2. D
3. H
4. B
5. C
6. G
7. F
8. A
9. E

Focused Study

1. Acute pain is usually self-limited, has a sudden onset, and is localized. Generally, the cause of the acute pain can be identified. It is most commonly a result of tissue injury from trauma, inflammation, or surgery. The pain is usually localized and sharp, although it may radiate to other parts of the body. Tissue healing results in pain relief. Chronic pain is pain that is prolonged or pain that persists after the condition causing it has already resolved. Although the cause may be identifiable (such as diabetic neuropathy, arthritis, a migraine, cancer, or a headache), this type of pain does not always have an identifiable cause.

2. The individualized response to pain is shaped not only by physiological responses, but also by multiple and interacting factors, including age, gender, sociocultural influences, emotional state, past experiences with pain, the source and meaning of the pain, and knowledge base.

3. Medications can be administered through oral, rectal, transdermal, parenteral, intravenous, and intraspinal routes.

4. The nurse should educate the patient about the following issues: Do not take aspirin when using other types of NSAIDs. NSAIDs can further lower serum glucose levels in patients who require hypoglycemic agents. Take this medication with milk, a full glass of water, or a meal to reduce gastric irritation. NSAIDs increase a patient's risk of bleeding. Report any instance of bleeding. Avoid drinking alcohol.

Case Study

Case Study 1

1. *Which nerve fibers will transmit pain sensations from John Browning's injury to his spinal cord?* Pain will be transmitted through small afferent A-delta and even smaller C nerve fibers to the spinal cord.

2. *What form of acute pain will he experience immediately after the injury?* The patient will experience acute somatic pain. Acute somatic pain arises from nerve receptors originating in the skin; subcutaneous tissues; or deep body structures such as the periosteum, muscles, tendons, joints, and blood vessels.

3. *Which type of pain is Mr. Browning most at risk for developing as a result of his injuries?* He may experience phantom limb pain after the amputation. This type of pain is described as burning, cramping, or shooting.

4. *What strategies will the nurse employ to best assess Mr. Browning's pain?* The nurse should assess his vital signs and ask him to describe his pain using a pain assessment tool.

Case Study 2

1. *What factors will influence Mr. Bowen's perceived level of pain?* Mr. Bowen's perceived level of pain will be influenced by his age, his gender, his emotional state, his sociocultural influences, his past experience with pain, the meaning the pain has for him, and his knowledge base.

2. *What strategies other than medication administration can be used to lessen Mr. Bowen's perceived level of pain?* The following complementary therapies can be used to lessen Mr. Bowen's pain: acupuncture, biofeedback, hypnotism, relaxation techniques, distraction, and cutaneous stimulation.

3. *What types of medications would you expect this patient to be prescribed for pain control at home?* The patient may be placed on one or more of the following medications: nonnarcotic analgesics, nonsteroidal anti-inflammatory drugs (NSAIDs), narcotics, synthetic narcotics, and antidepressants.

4. *Mr. Bowen's doctor has discussed placing a transcutaneous electrical nerve stimulation (TENS) unit on the patient. Explain how this may benefit a patient with chronic pain.* A TENS unit consists of a battery-operated low-voltage transmitter connected to the skin with two or more electrodes. The patient or the physical therapist may place the electrodes. The TENS unit generates a high- or low-frequency electrical pulse. With high-frequency application, pulse intensity is low and does not cause muscle contraction; low-frequency applications produce an intensity that does produce muscle contraction. The patient experiences a gentle tapping or vibrating sensation over the electrodes. The patient can adjust the voltage to achieve maximum pain relief.

Crossword Puzzle

question	term answer
Dull, poorly localized pain arising from body organs	VISCERAL PAIN
A type of pain with associated changes in sensations that is caused by a lesion or damage to the brain or spinal cord	CENTRAL
The amount of pain a person can endure before outwardly responding to the pain	TOLERANCE
A brand name of an analgesic that should be avoided if the patient has a history of alcohol abuse	TYLENOL
Another name for an opioid analgesic	NARCOTIC
A surgery used to remove or destroy a nerve	NEURECTOMY
The dorsal spinal roots are severed during this type of surgery	RHIZOTOMY
The "T" of the PQRST mnemonic	TIMING
The "Q" of the PQRST mnemonic	QUALITY

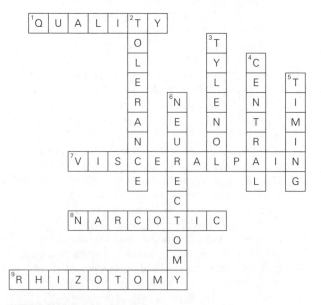

NCLEX-RN® Review Questions

1. Answer: 2
   Rationale: Visceral pain is usually poorly localized because of the low number of nociceptors. Visceral

pain arises from body organs. It can be associated with nausea and is often described as cramping, intermittent pain or colicky pain. Somatic pain arises from nerve receptors that originate in the skin or close to the surface of the body. Somatic pain may be described as sharp and well-localized or dull and diffuse. Referred pain is pain that is perceived in an area distant from the site of the stimuli. Hyperesthesia is a condition of oversensitivity to tactile and painful stimuli.
Nursing Process: Diagnosis
Patient Need: Physiological Integrity

2. Answer: 3
Rationale: Older adult patients may hesitate to ask for pain medication because they fear narcotic addiction and loss of independence. The perception of pain does not decrease with age. Opioids do not cause excessive respiratory depression in older adults. Pain is not a natural part of aging.
Nursing Process: Diagnosis
Patient Need: Physiological Integrity

3. Answer: 4
Rationale: Research about treating pain with analgesics consistently shows no impact on physical assessment findings or diagnosis. Pain can be a health condition and a symptom of a health problem. Very few patients lie about their pain. Narcotic medication is widely used to treat chronic pain. A common misconception that narcotic medications are too risky to be used to treat chronic pain often deprives patients of an effective source of pain relief.
Nursing Process: Assessment
Patient Need: Physiological and Psychologic Integrity

4. Answer: 2
Rationale: Anticonvulsants are useful as initial medications for patients with neuropathic pain, including shingles (herpes zoster). Local anesthetics block the initiation and transmission of nerve impulses in a local area. Narcotics, or opioids, are the pharmacologic treatment of choice for moderate to severe pain. NSAIDs are the treatment of choice for mild to moderate pain.

5. Answer: 1
Rationale: Administering analgesics before the pain occurs allows the patient to spend less time in pain. Frequent analgesic administration may allow for smaller doses and less analgesic administration. The patient's fears and anxiety about pain will be decreased, and his or her physical activity will increase. When a patient's pain is well controlled, he or she experiences less fear and anxiety about the return of pain. Patients may become more physically active when their pain is managed well.
Nursing Process: Implementation
Patient Need: Physiological Integrity and Psychosocial Integrity

6. Answer: 3
Rationale: Exercise and use of electric blankets or heating pads may accelerate absorption of the transdermal medication. The effectiveness of a patch lasts about 72 hours. The patch should not be applied to the same site consecutively; sites should be altered. A therapeutic level of the medication will be achieved within 12–24 hours.
Nursing Process: Evaluation
Patient Need: Physiological Integrity

7. Answer: 4
Rationale: Patients experiencing pain will demonstrate rapid, shallow breathing patterns; an increase in blood pressure and pulse rate; and pupil dilation.
Nursing Process: Assessment
Patient Need: Physiological Integrity

Chapter 10

Terms Matching
1. M
2. F
3. Q
4. J
5. O
6. N
7. C
8. A
9. P
10. G
11. B
12. L
13. D
14. K
15. R
16. H
17. I
18. E

Focused Study
1. ICF refers to the fluid found in cells. ICF is essential for normal cell function because it provides a medium for metabolic processes. ECF refers to the fluid that is located outside cells and can be further classified by its location. Interstitial ECF is located in the spaces between cells in the body. Intravascular ECF is contained in the circulatory system. Transcellular ECF includes urine; cerebrospinal and pericardial fluids; digestive secretions; and synovial, gonadal, intraocular, and pleural fluids. The concentration of specific electrolytes differs significantly between ICF and ECF.

2. a. Osmosis is how water moves across a selectively permeable membrane from an area of lower solute concentration to an area of higher solute concentration.

   b. Diffusion is the process by which solute molecules move from an area of higher solute concentration to an area of lower solute concentration to become more evenly distributed.

   c. Filtration is the process by which water and solutes move from an area of higher hydrostatic pressure to an area of lower hydrostatic pressure. This usually occurs across capillary membranes.

   d. Active transport is a process that allows molecules to move against a concentration gradient across epithelial membranes and cell membranes. This movement requires energy and a carrier mechanism to maintain a higher concentration of a substance on one side of the membrane than on the other.

3. a. Metabolic acidosis is produced when there are excess amounts of nonvolatile acids in the body and a deficiency in the amount of available bicarbonate. Metabolic alkalosis occurs when there is too much bicarbonate in the body.

   b. Respiratory acidosis occurs when the body retains carbon dioxide and there is an excess of carbonic acid. Respiratory alkalosis is a result of a loss of carbonic dioxide and deficient levels of carbonic acid.

4. Answers may include the following: Patient will regain normal arterial blood gas values, patient will be oriented to surroundings or will return to baseline, reflexes will become normal or return to baseline, patient will not develop any dysrhythmias, blood pressure will stabilize, and patient will not develop any signs and symptoms associated with respiratory failure.

Case Study

1. *Which acid–base imbalance is this patient most at risk for developing?* Metabolic acidosis
2. *What is a normal pH?* 7.35–7.45. *What does the nurse expect Mr. Sweeney's pH to be based on his admitting diagnosis and abnormal arterial blood gas values?* Below 7.35
3. *The nurse would expect Mr. Sweeney's respirations to be of what quality and depth?* Respirations will increase in rate and depth. *What is the specific name for this type of breathing?* Kussmaul's respirations
4. *What are the early manifestations of this type of acid–base imbalance?* Fatigue, general malaise, anorexia, nausea, and abdominal pain
5. *As the nurse reviews the results of this patient's laboratory tests, what are some expected changes that may be seen in potassium and magnesium levels?* Elevated serum potassium levels and possible low magnesium levels
6. *What are vital teaching areas for Mr. Sweeney?* Diet and medication management are vital teaching areas to prevent future episodes of acidosis.
7. *How is the heart's ability to function affected by this type of acid–base imbalance?* Metabolic acidosis affects cardiac output by decreasing myocardial contractility, slowing the heart rate, and increasing the patient's risk for developing dysrhythmias.

Short Answers

Condition	Laboratory Values	Short Questions Regarding Clinical Manifestations
Hyponatremia	< 135 mEq/L	*Has this patient's blood pressure increased or decreased?* Decreased
Hypernatremia	> 145 mEq/L	*Has this patient gained or lost weight?* Gained weight
Hypokalemia	< 3.5 mEq/L	*Hypokalemia increases the patient's risk of developing toxicity related to which medication?* Digitalis
Hyperkalemia	> 5.0 mEq/L	*Which medication may be ordered to increase renal potassium excretion?* Lasix (furosemide)
Hypocalcemia	< 8.5 mg/dL	*When should the hypocalcemic patient be instructed to take his or her ordered oral calcium salts?* 1–11/2; hours before bedtime with a full glass of water
Hypercalcemia	> 10.0 mg/dL	*Will the hyperkalemic patient develop muscle weakness or tetany?* Tetany
Hypomagnesemia	< 1.6 mg/dL	*This patient is receiving intravenous magnesium sulfate. The function of which organ should be monitored during this type of therapy?* Kidneys
Hypermagnesemia	> 2.6 mg/dL	*Will deep tendon reflexes be hyperactive or hypoactive in a patient with this condition?* Hypoactive

Hypophosphatemia	< 2.5 mg/dL	*Nursing interventions for this patient should be focused on which types of issues?* Safety, high risk for infection, high risk for bleeding, high risk for falls
Hyperphosphatemia	> 4.5 mg/dL	*Is this patient more likely to suffer from complications related to hypotension or hypertension?* Hypotension

NCLEX-RN® Review Questions

1. Answer: 1

   Rationale: Plasma is an intravascular fluid that can be immediately replaced through venous access. Transcellular fluids cannot be immediately replaced. They include urine; digestive secretions; perspiration; and cerebrospinal, pleural, synovial, intraocular, gonadal, and pericardial fluids.

   Nursing Process: Assessment

   Patient Need: Physiological Integrity

2. Answer: 1

   Rationale: Osmosis is the process that controls body fluid movement between the intracellular fluid (ICF) and extracellular fluid (ECF) compartments from an area of lower solute concentration to an area of higher solute concentration. Diffusion is the process by which solute molecules move from an area of high solute concentration to an area of low solute concentration and become evenly distributed. Active transport allows molecules to move across cell membranes and epithelial membranes against a concentration gradient. Filtration is the process by which water and dissolved substances (solutes) move from an area of high hydrostatic pressure to an area of low hydrostatic pressure.

   Nursing Process: Planning

   Patient Need: Physiological Integrity

3. Answer: 1

   Rationale: Loss of skin elasticity with aging makes skin turgor assessment findings less accurate in older adults. Tongue furrows are not generally affected by age and are a more accurate indicator of fluid volume deficit. Postural or orthostatic hypotension is a sign of hypovolemia. Rapid weight loss is a good indicator of fluid volume deficit.

   Nursing Process: Assessment

   Patient Need: Physiological Integrity

4. Answer: 4

   Rationale: Patients experiencing a fluid volume deficit have increased hematocrit laboratory values due to their dehydrated state. A dehydrated patient's laboratory results demonstrate a decreased potassium with fluid volume deficit, elevated hemoglobin, and increased urine specific gravity.

   Nursing Process: Assessment

   Patient Need: Physiological Integrity

5. Answer: 3

   Rationale: Thirst is the first clinical manifestation associated with hypernatremia. After thirst, the following clinical manifestations develop: lethargy, weakness, and irritability.

   Nursing Process: Assessment

   Patient Need: Physiological Integrity

6. Answer: 1

   Rationale: Buffers are substances that prevent major changes in pH by removing or releasing hydrogen ions. Hydrogen ions control the acid–base balance of the body. Calcium is essential to cardiac function and blood clotting. Sodium affects intracellular and intravascular fluid volumes. Magnesium controls the sedative effects on the neuromuscular junction.

   Nursing Process: Planning

   Patient Need: Physiological Integrity

Chapter 11

Terms Matching

1. G
2. D
3. I
4. B
5. C
6. J
7. A
8. H
9. E
10. F

Focused Study

1. Multiple factors can influence the host's potential for injury: sex, age, economic status, race, preexisting conditions, and use of medications or substances.
2. a. Absence of midline cervical spine tenderness
   b. Normal alertness
   c. Absence of intoxication
   d. Absence of a painful distracting injury
   e. No focal neurological defects
3. Universal receiver: Type AB
   Universal donor: Type O
4. According to this act, consent for organ donation may be given not only by the donor, but also by a spouse, adult children, parents, adult siblings, a guardian, or any other adult authorized to do so.

Case Study

1. *What types of trauma did Mr. Key potentially experience?* Mr. Key may have experienced multiple trauma, which involves injuries to more than one organ system or a major injury to one organ system. Motor vehicle accidents often result in multiple

trauma. Depending on how he fell, he may have experienced blunt and penetrating trauma. The accident occurred on a country road, which may have been covered with gravel or dirt that could have injured or punctured the skin. Also, falling into a fence or mailbox post could result in a penetrating injury.

2. *What method of transportation will most likely be used to transport Mr. Key to the hospital?* Because Mr. Key's accident occurred in a rural area that may be some distance from a hospital, he will most likely be airlifted by helicopter to the trauma center. Unstable patients and those injured in the wilderness or other areas in which ground access is difficult may also be airlifted to the closest trauma center.

3. *As healthcare providers assess Mr. Key, what is their highest priority?* Assessment of the airway is the highest priority in the trauma patient. If the airway is not patent and the patient is unable to deliver oxygen to vital organs, all other interventions are futile.

4. *What diagnostic studies may be performed on Mr. Key once he reaches the trauma center?* Mr. Key may undergo the following diagnostic studies upon arrival at the trauma center: blood type and crossmatch, blood alcohol level, complete blood count (CBC), arterial blood gases (ABGs), urine drug screen, focused assessment by sonography in the trauma department, diagnostic peritoneal lavage (based on FAST finding), and/or a computed tomography (CT) scan and/or magnetic resonance imaging (MRI).

5. *The physician notes that Mr. Key has developed a tension pneumothorax in the right lung. What clinical manifestations are associated with this diagnosis?* The increased intrapleural pressure collapses the injured right lung and shifts the mediastinal contents, compressing the heart, great vessels, trachea, and eventually the uninjured left lung. This causes the following signs and symptoms: severe respiratory distress, hypotension, jugular vein distension, tracheal deviation toward the left side, and cyanosis.

6. *After several days, healthcare providers determine that Mr. Key has experienced brain death. The family wants to donate his organs. Mr. Key is found to be an ineligible donor. What are some possible reasons for this?* Mr. Key may have abused intravenous drugs, or he has an untreated infection, cancer, or active tuberculosis. A primary brain tumor would not exclude Mr. Key's organs from being donated.

7. *What criteria are used to determine that Mr. Key has experienced brain death?* The clinical signs of brain death include the following: Mr. Key's condition is deemed irreversible; he is experiencing apnea with a $PaCO_2$ that is greater than 60 mmHg; he exhibits no responses to deep stimuli, no spontaneous movement, no gag or corneal reflex, no oculocephalic or oculovestibular reflexes; and there is no concurrent diagnosis of a toxic or metabolic disorder. These findings are confirmed by an electroencephalogram and a cerebral blood flow study.

Short Answers

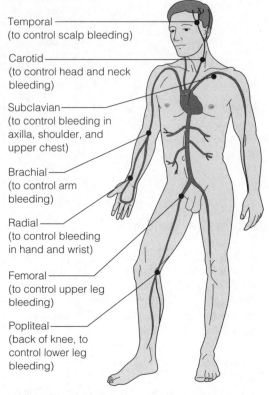

Temporal (to control scalp bleeding)

Carotid (to control head and neck bleeding)

Subclavian (to control bleeding in axilla, shoulder, and upper chest)

Brachial (to control arm bleeding)

Radial (to control bleeding in hand and wrist)

Femoral (to control upper leg bleeding)

Popliteal (back of knee, to control lower leg bleeding)

Figure 11–3 ■ The major pressure points used for the control of bleeding.

NCLEX-RN® Review Questions

1. Answer: 1
   Rationale: Mechanical energy is the most common type of energy transferred to a host in trauma. The most common mechanical source of injury in all adult age groups is the motor vehicle. Gravitational, thermal, and electrical energy do cause trauma, but mechanical energy is a more common cause of injuries.
   Nursing Process: Assessment
   Patient Need: Physiological Integrity

2. Answer: 4
   Rationale: Minor traumas are classified as an injury to a single part or system of the body and are usually treated in a physician's office or in the hospital emergency department. A fracture of the clavicle, a small second-degree burn, and a laceration requiring sutures are examples of minor trauma. A gunshot wound, a compression injury, and a stab wound are classified as multiple trauma. Injuries associated with multiple trauma involve very serious single-system injury or multiple-system injuries.
   Nursing Process: Assessment
   Patient Need: Physiological Integrity

3. Answer: 1
   Rationale: The primary organ systems involved in MODS are respiratory, pulmonary, renal, hepatic,

hematologic, cardiovascular, gastrointestinal, and neurological. The reproductive system is not involved in MODS.

Nursing Process: Planning

Patient Need: Health Promotion and Maintenance

4. Answer: 2

Rationale: Vasodilators are not commonly used to treat the patient who has experienced trauma. Medications used to treat the patient who has experienced trauma depend on the type and severity of the injuries as well as the degree of traumatic shock that is present. The following general categories of medications may be used: blood components and crystalloids, inotropic drugs, vasopressors, opioids, and immunizations.

Nursing Process: Planning

Patient Need: Safe, Effective Care Environment

5. Answer: 3

Rationale: Manifestations of shock do not include increased gastric motility. Manifestations of shock include *decreased* gastric motility, tachycardia, decreased oxygen levels, increased carbon dioxide levels, and cerebral hypoxia.

Nursing Process: Assessment

Patient Need: Physiological Integrity

6. Answer: 2

Rationale: Septic shock is the leading cause of death in intensive care units. It is one part of a progressive syndrome called systemic inflammatory response syndrome (SIRS). Hypovolemic shock is the most common type of shock. It is caused by a decrease in intravascular volume of 15% or more. Distributive shock includes several types of shock that result from widespread vasodilation and decreased peripheral resistance. Neurogenic shock is the result of an imbalance between parasympathetic and sympathetic stimulation of vascular smooth muscle.

Nursing Process: Planning

Patient Need: Physiological Integrity

7. Answer: 2

Rationale: The goal of blood administration is to keep the hematocrit at 30%–35%. A hematocrit below 30% results in clotting dysfunctions. A hematocrit above 35% results in an increase in solids in the circulating blood volume. Obstructions and thrombus may form if the hematocrit rises above 35%.

Nursing Process: Planning

Patient Need: Health Promotion and Maintenance

Chapter 12

Terms Matching

1. H
2. J
3. N
4. Q
5. S
6. B
7. C
8. U
9. P
10. D
11. F
12. O
13. M
14. W
15. K
16. I
17. A
18. T
19. Z
20. G
21. E
22. L
23. V
24. X
25. R
26. Y

Focused Study

1. a. The spleen is the largest lymphoid organ in the body and the only lymphoid organ that can filter blood. It is located in the upper left quadrant of the abdomen. The spleen contains two kinds of tissue—white pulp and red pulp. White pulp is lymphoid tissue that serves as a site for lymphocyte proliferation and immune surveillance. B cells predominate in the white pulp. Blood filtration occurs in the red pulp. In blood-filled venous sinuses, phagocytic cells dispose of damaged or aged RBCs and platelets. Other debris and foreign matter, such as bacteria, viruses, and toxins, are also removed from the blood. The spleen can store blood and the breakdown products of RBCs for future use. The spleen is not essential for life. If it is removed because of disease or trauma, the liver and the bone marrow assume its functions.

   b. The thymus gland is located in the superior anterior mediastinal cavity beneath the sternum. It reaches its maximum size at puberty, then slowly begins to atrophy. By adulthood, it is difficult to differentiate from surrounding adipose tissue even though it remains active. During fetal life and childhood, the thymus serves as a site for the maturation and differentiation of thymic lymphoid cells, the T cells. Thymosin, an immunoregulatory hormone of the thymus, stimulates lymphopoiesis, the formation of lymphocytes or lymphoid tissue.

   c. Bone marrow is soft organic tissue found in the hollow cavity of the long bones, particularly the femur and humerus, as well as the flat bones of the pelvis, ribs, and sternum. Bone marrow produces and stores hematopoietic stem cells, from which all cellular components of the blood are derived.

2. **a.** Acquired immunity: chickenpox, MMR, polio, DPT, hepatitis B vaccines, and hepatitis A

    b. Passive immunity: The transfer of maternal antibodies via the placenta and breast milk to the infant; immunizations: rabies human immune globulin and hepatitis B immune globulin (HBIG)

3. Erythema, heat, pain, loss of function, and edema at the site. The older adult's risk for developing an infection is greater. They do not present in the same manner as younger patients. They may not be able to produce clinical manifestations of inflammation or infection due to changes in their immune system and the inability to adequately increase their body temperature. The only signs and symptoms of an infection that may be present in the older adult are disorientation, restlessness, and an increased respiratory rate.

4. Most antibiotics have little effect on viruses because the virus has no cell wall and no cytoplasm, produces no enzymes, and sequesters itself in a host cell to reproduce.

Case Study

1. *What should the nurse include when educating Sally about taking penicillin?* Sally should not take penicillin if she has a history of a severe allergic reaction to any form of the drug; a cross-reactivity may occur in patients allergic to cephalosporin or carbapenem antibiotics. Sally's parents should notify the physician if they see white patches on the oral mucosa or if vaginitis develops. An antifungal drug may be prescribed and the antibiotic continued. Consuming yogurt or buttermilk may prevent superinfection. Sally shouldn't consume these products within one hour of taking the drug.

2. *What test was performed to identify the organism that is causing Sally's infection?* A culture and sensitivity (C&S) test was ordered. This test helps determine the presence of the infectious organism(s) and to identify antibiotics that can be used to treat the infection.

3. *What are some important nursing diagnoses the nurse should use to create Sally's care plan?* The key nursing diagnoses are *Anxiety*, *Hyperthermia*, and *Pain*. If Sally required hospitalization, another applicable nursing diagnosis would be *Risk for Infection*.

    a. *Risk for Anxiety:* Sally may experience anxiety related to her manifestations, treatment measures, the prognosis, and the expected outcome of the disease. The diagnosis of an infection can be traumatic and cause feelings of uneasiness, isolation, guilt, apprehension, or depression.

    b. *Risk for Hyperthermia:* Hyperthermia is an expected consequence of the infectious disease process. It can be controlled using antipyretics. Sally's temperature will likely increase as a result of the body's response to an infection.

    c. *Risk for Pain:* Pain often accompanies infection as part of the inflammatory process or is secondary to delayed healing. Sally may experience increased pain secondary to the pustules on her tonsils.

4. *While taking penicillin, what types of things should Sally or her parents report to the physician?* If hypersensitivity response occurs, the patient should discontinue the drug immediately, such as skin rashes, urticaria (hives), itching, fever, chills, and anaphylaxis. Monitor Sally for superinfection (vaginitis, stomatitis, or diarrhea) due to elimination of resident bacteria. In this case an antifungal drug may be prescribed and the antibiotic continued.

5. *Sally is presenting to physician's office in which stage of the infectious process?* The initial stage is known as the incubation period, when the pathogen begins active replication but does not yet cause manifestations. The prodromal stage follows with nonspecific manifestations such as general malaise, fever, myalgias, headache, and fatigue. The maximal impact of the infectious process is felt during the acute phase as the pathogen proliferates and disseminates rapidly. Manifestations are more pronounced and specific to the infecting organism and site during the acute stage. Fever and chills may be significant during this phase. If the infectious process is prolonged, manifestations of the continuing immune response may become apparent. Catabolic and anorexic effects of the infection can lead to loss of body fat and muscle wasting. Immune complexes may be deposited at sites other than the primary infection, resulting in an inflammatory process. As the infection is contained and the pathogen eliminated, the convalescent stage of the disease occurs. During this stage, affected tissues are repaired and manifestations resolve.

6. *If this streptococcal throat infection is prolonged, what specific health problems may Sally be at an increased risk for developing?* Glomerulonephritis is a complication that can follow a streptococcal throat infection. Another possible consequence of prolonged infection and the immune response is that an autoimmune disease process may be triggered in the body, such as type 1 diabetes mellitus, rheumatic cardiomyopathy, or celiac disease.

Short Answers

Fill in the table identifying the major chemical mediators of inflammation.

Factor	Source	Effect
Histamine	Mast cells, basophils, and platelets	Vasodilation and increased capillary permeability, producing tissue redness, warmth, and edema
Kinins (bradykinin and others)	Plasma protein factors	Histamine-like effects; chemotaxis and pain inducers

Prostaglandins	Metabolism of arachidonic acid from cell membranes	Histamine-like effects; chemotaxis, pain, and fever inducers
Leukotrienes	Arachidonic acid metabolism	Smooth muscle constriction (especially bronchoconstriction), increased vascular permeability, and chemotaxis

NCLEX-RN® Review Questions

1. Answer: 4

   Rationale: The vascular response localizes invading bacteria and keeps them from spreading. The cellular response involves the margination and emigration of leukocytes into the damaged tissue. Phagocystosis is a process by which a foreign target cell is engulfed, destroyed, and digested. The specific immune response involves the introduction of antigens into the body.

   Nursing Process: Diagnosis

   Patient Need: Physiological Integrity

2. Answer: 4

   Rationale: Vaccines stimulate active immunity by inducing the production of antibodies and antitoxins. Vaccines are suspensions of whole or fractionated bacteria or viruses that have been treated to make them *nonpathogenic*. Vaccines are administered to induce an immune response and subsequent immunity. Although vaccine development has been a major factor in improving public health, no vaccine is completely effective and entirely safe.

   Nursing Process: Implementation

   Patient Need: Health Promotion and Maintenance

3. Answer: 3

   Rationale: A patient with an infectious process is encouraged to rest; to increase fluid intake; and to eat a well-balanced, nutritious diet. Anti-inflammatory medications are administered only when the inflammatory process has become problematic.

   Nursing Process: Evaluation

   Patient Need: Health Promotion and Maintenance

4. Answer: 2

   Rationale: Keep the inflamed area dry and expose it to air as much as possible. This promotes healing and helps prevent infection. Interventions to maintain tissue integrity include cleaning the inflamed tissue gently, balancing rest with a tolerable degree of mobility, and providing protection and support for inflamed tissue.

   Nursing Process: Implementation

   Patient Need: Safe, Effective Care Environment

5. Answer: 1

   Rationale: A urinary tract infection is the most common type of nosocomial infection, which leads to the most frequent cause of gram-negative septicemia in hospitalized patients. Pneumonia is the second most common hospital-acquired infection.

Bacteremia is associated with intravascular and urinary catheters, yet is not the most common type of nosocomial infection. *Clostridium difficile*-associated diarrhea is also a frequently acquired nosocomial infection, but it is not the most common.

Nursing Process: Diagnosis

Patient Need: Safe, Effective Care Environment

6. Answer: 4

   Rationale: Hepatitis has not been used as a biologic weapon. The most likely pathogens to be used as a biologic weapon include anthrax, smallpox, botulism, pneumonic plague, and viral hemorrhagic fevers.

   Nursing Process: Diagnosis

   Patient Need: Safe, Effective Care Environment

7. Answer: 1

   Rationale: Signs of an opportunistic infections include loose, watery, and foul-smelling diarrhea; fuzzy growth or white plaques in mouth or on tongue; vaginal discharge or itching; blood in urine; chills; fever; or an unusual cough.

   Nursing Process: Assessment

   Patient Need: Health Promotion and Maintenance

Chapter 13

Terms Matching

1. E
2. K
3. N
4. P
5. A
6. I
7. D
8. M
9. B
10. F
11. C
12. L
13. G
14. J
15. H

Focused Study

1. **a.** Hyperacute tissue rejection occurs immediately to three days after the transplant of new tissue. This type of rejection is a result of preformed antibodies and sensitized T cells to antigens in the donor organ. It is more likely to occur in someone who has had a previous transplant. This type of rejection also can occur during the transplant surgery.

   b. Acute tissue rejection is the most common and treatable type of rejection. It occurs between four days and three months after the transplant. It is a cellular immune response and results in transplant cell destruction. The patient will demonstrate fever, redness, swelling, and tenderness over the graft site. Without treatment, the transplanted organ will not function adequately during this time.

c. Chronic tissue rejection occurs four months or years after the transplant. It is a result of antibody-mediated immune responses. The transplanted organ will gradually deteriorate.

d. Graft-versus-host disease is a frequent and potentially fatal complication of bone marrow transplants, some types of liver transplants, or transfusions of nonirradiated blood to immuno-compromised patients. It occurs within the first 100 days after the transplant. This type of rejection typically affects primarily the skin, liver, and gastrointestinal tract.

2. a. Example: Allergic asthma, allergic rhinitis, allergic conjunctivitis, hives, and anaphylactic shock
   Type of interaction: Antigen–antibody

   b. Example: Hemolytic transfusion reaction to blood of an incompatible type; hemolytic anemia associated with the administration of medications such as penicillins, cephalosporins, and streptomycin; also, endogenous antigens can stimulate a type II reaction that leads to autoimmune disorders
   Type of interaction: Antigen–antibody

   c. Example: Serum sickness occurring in response to medications such as penicillin and sulfonamides; a streptococcal infection or systemic lupus erythematosus that results in glomerulonephritis; breathing in moldy hay, resulting in an alveolar inflammatory response
   Type of interaction: Antigen–antibody

   d. Example: Contact dermatitis, a positive tuberculin test, episodes of graft rejection
   Type of interaction: Antigen–lymphocyte

3. Administer oxygen at 2–4 liters per minute. Assess the patient's respiratory rate, respiratory pattern, level of consciousness, level of anxiety, presence of nasal flaring, use of accessory muscles of respiration, abnormal chest wall movement, and audible stridor. Palpate for respiratory excursion and auscultate lung fields for any adventitious sounds. Position in Fowler's to high-Fowler's. Insert an artificial airway, administer epinephrine, and provide calm reassurance.

4. Antihistamines block histamine-1 receptors, drying respiratory secretions and reducing tissue edema. Sympathomimetics improve decongestant activity and counteract the sedative effects that are associated with some antihistamines. Glucocorticoids produce an anti-inflammatory effect.

Case Studies

Case Study 1

1. *What are Mr. Jones's specific risk factors for acquiring HIV?* General risk factors for acquring HIV include homosexuality, intravenous drug use, and hemophilia. Gary is a homosexual African American male. These factors increase his risk for acquring HIV.

2. *How long after exposure would the nurse expect seroconversion to occur in Mr. Jones?* Antibodies are produced against the HIV proteins within six weeks to six months postexposure.

3. *A few weeks ago Mr. Jones had nausea, diarrhea, and abdominal cramping. What might this indicate to the nurse?* Mr. Jones probably contracted HIV several days or weeks before developing these clinical manifestations. Other clinical manifestations of early HIV infection may include fever, sore throat, arthralgias and myalgias, headache, rash, and lymphadenopathy. Pathologic changes are also noted in the central nervous system (CNS) of many infected individuals although the mechanism of neurological dysfunction is unclear. The patient often attributes this initial manifestation of HIV infection to a common viral illness such as influenza, upper respiratory infection, or stomach virus.

4. *Which opportunistic infections are associated with AIDS?* The patient with AIDS is at risk for developing *Pneumocystis carinii* pneumonia, tuberculosis (TB), candidiasis, and *Mycobacterium avium* complex.

Case Study 2

1. *Besides latex gloves, what are some other items commonly made of latex that may have contributed to Susan's allergy to latex?* Balloons, condoms, and rubber bands. Employers should educate employees about sources of latex in their work environment.

2. *How can employers protect their employees from developing latex allergies?* Employers should select products that are latex-free whenever possible. Many latex-free products are available for healthcare workers to use. Employers should also routinely screen workers for clinical manifestations of latex allergies.

3. *Susan wants to know why powdered latex gloves are "worse" than powder-free latex gloves for people with a latex sensitivity. How should the nurse caring for Susan answer this question?* Gloves are powdered with cornstarch to aid in the donning and removal of the gloves. When the wearer removes the powdered gloves, the cornstarch particles aerosolize. The aerosolized powder contains latex and cornstarch. When a latex-sensitive person breathes in the latex particles, a respiratory and dermal exposure to the latex can result.

4. *If Susan developed a type I systemic allergic reaction as a result of a respiratory exposure, which two diagnostic tests would Susan's nurse expect to see ordered?* White blood cell count (increased eosinophil count is associated with a type I hypersensitivity); radioallergosorbent serum test (to measure the amount of IgE directed toward specific allergens).

Short Answers

The nurse is assessing the patient's immune system. Describe the findings that may accompany a patient with an infection or an immune disorder.

General appearance	Suggested answers: fatigue, weakness, appearing older than stated age, weight loss, wasting, difficulty moving, stiffness, hyperthermia
Mucous membranes in nose and mouth	Suggested answers: pale, boggy nasal mucosa; petechiae or white patches in oral mucosa
Skin	Suggested answers: pallor, jaundice, rash, lesions, petechiae, bruising, Kaposi's sarcoma, infected or unhealed wounds
Lymph nodes (cervical, axillae, and groin)	Suggested answers: swollen and tender lymph nodes
Joints	Suggested answers: reddened, swollen or tender joints; poor range of motion

NCLEX-RN® Review Questions

1. Answer: 1
   Rationale: The red blood cell count (RBC) does not provide specific information about a patient's hypersensitivity or allergic reaction. The information gained from an RBC count is used to determine the oxygen-carrying capability of blood cells. Blood type and crossmatch, Coombs' test, and complement assay testing can provide the most information about a patient's hypersensitivity or allergic reaction.
   Nursing Process: Planning
   Patient Need: Health Promotion and Maintenance

2. Answer: 3
   Rationale: Patients who have a hypersensitivity to bee venom must carry a bee sting kit with them at all times. This kit typically includes a prefilled syringe of epinephrine and an epinephrine nebulizer, which allows for prompt self-treatment. Antihistamines taken daily will not prevent a reaction if stung. The use of penicillin will not stop a hypersensitivity reaction. It is used to treat certain types of infections. The use of a steroid will not prevent a hypersensitivity reaction.
   Nursing Process: Evaluation
   Patient Need: Health Promotion and Maintenance

3. Answer: 3
   Rationale: An allograft is a graft taken from a member of the same species, such as a cadaver, and transplanted to a live patient. An autograft is a transplant using the patient's own tissue. An isograft is a graft in which the graft tissue is taken from the patient's identical twin. A xenograft is a tissue transplant from an animal to a human.
   Nursing Process: Diagnosis
   Patient Need: Physiological Integrity

4. Answer: 1
   Rationale: The CDC classification of AIDS-associated cancers currently includes Karposi's sarcoma, non-Hodgkin's lymphoma, primary lymphoma of the brain, and invasive cervical cancer.
   Nursing Process: Planning
   Patient Need: Physiological Integrity

5. Answer: 4
   Rationale: Ambulation increases circulation, decreases pressure, and helps to maintain muscle tone. The area around the blister should be massaged, but not the skin directly over the blister. Do not open and drain the blister. The blister should remain intact and dressed. Avoid the use of heat because it might further damage the patient's skin.
   Nursing Process: Implementation
   Patient Need: Physiological Integrity

Chapter 14

Terms Matching

1. C
2. E
3. H
4. A
5. O
6. L
7. R
8. B
9. T
10. P
11. K
12. G
13. I
14. D
15. Q
16. J
17. N
18. M
19. S
20. F
21. U

Focused Study

1. The person can reduce dietary intake of red meat, saturated fat, preserved meats, pickled and salty foods, high-fat foods, low-fiber foods, fried and broiled meat and fish, sodium saccharine, red food dyes, and decaffeinated and regular coffee. The person also can increase his or her dietary intake of vegetables, fiber, folate, calcium, and fruits.

2. Severe stress and cumulative stress are associated with the development of cancer. Depression, pregnancy, chronic disease, or chemotherapy treatment can weaken the patient's immune responses. Some types of losses or stressors are more commonly experienced by older adults. These losses include the death of a spouse, the death of a friend,

the loss of a position, the loss of societal status, and a decline in physical abilities. Repeated stressors are associated with immune system changes that lead to the development of cancer.

3. Benign neoplasms are localized, usually in the form of a solid mass, have a well-defined border, are encapsulated, are responsive to the body's homeostatic control mechanisms (such as contact inhibition), grow slowly, and are stable in size. They are usually harmless but can be destructive if they crowd surrounding tissue and obstruct organs from functioning appropriately. Typically, they are easy to remove and do not recur.

Malignant neoplasms grow aggressively; they do not respond to the body's homeostatic control mechanisms, are not cohesive, are irregularly shaped, cut through instead of crowding the surrounding tissue, produce bleeding, and are inflamed; necrosis of surrounding tissue occurs as the malignant neoplasm grows. They are not always easy to remove, and they can recur.

4. **a.** The goal of surgery as a primary treatment for cancer is to remove the entire tumor and any involved surrounding tissue and lymph nodes whenever feasible.

b. With chemotherapy, cytotoxic medications are administered to cure liquid or solid cancers, to decrease tumor size, or to treat or prevent suspected metastases. Chemotherapy can be given in conjunction with surgery, biotherapy, or radiation therapy. It disrupts the cell cycle during various phases, which results in interrupted cell metabolism and replication.

c. With radiation, ionizing radiations of gamma and x-rays are delivered to the patient internally or externally. External radiation involves delivering the radiation at some distance from the patient. Internal radiation involves delivering the radiation inside the body by implanting small amounts of radioactive material directly into a tumor or body cavity.

d. Biotherapy involves modifying the biologic processes that result in malignant cells, primarily through enhancing the patient's immune response mechanisms (for example, using antibodies, cytokines, or natural killer cells).

e. Photodynamic therapy is a method of treating certain kinds of superficial tumors. This type of treatment is also called phototherapy, photoradiation, and photochemotherapy. It is used to treat cancer in patients with tumors growing on the surface of the bladder, peritoneal cavity, chest wall, pleura, bronchus, or head and neck. The patient is given an intravenous dose of Photofrin® (a photosensitizing compound), which is selectively retained in higher concentrations in malignant tissue. The drug is activated by a laser treatment (three days after the drug injection and administered for three days). The drug interacts with oxygen molecules in the tissue to produce a cytotoxic oxygen molecule called singlet oxygen.

Case Study

1. *What are the American Cancer Society's guidelines for breast cancer screening?* Yearly mammograms are recommended starting at age 40. A clinical breast exam should be a part of a periodic health exam, which should take place approximately every year for a woman 40 years old and older and approximately every three years for women in their twenties and thirties. Women should promptly report any changes in their breasts to their healthcare providers. A woman with a strong family history of breast cancer or ovarian cancer or who was treated for Hodgkin's disease should receive a screening MRI.

2. *Which ethnic group experiences the highest prevalence of breast cancer?* Breast cancer is more prevalent in Caucasian women.

3. *What role does Donna's age play in her cancer?* Hormone changes that occur with the aging process are associated with cancers in postmenopausal women. Women who take estrogen supplements have an increased risk for breast and uterine cancer.

4. *During a mastectomy, the axillary lymph nodes are removed for examination. Why is this done?* The lymph nodes are removed to determine metastasis.

5. *How will the nurse assist the patient in adjusting to her new body image after the mastectomy?*
   a. Allow the patient to discuss the meaning of the loss of her breast.
   b. Observe and evaluate the interaction between the patient and her significant others.
   c. Allow denial but do not participate in it. Adopt a matter-of-fact approach and an empathetic attitude.
   d. Provide a supportive environment.
   e. Allow the patient and significant others to express feelings about her altered image.
   f. Identify new coping strategies.
   g. Enlist family and friends in reaffirming the patient's worth.
   h. Put the patient in touch with a mastectomy support group.
   i. Advise the patient to visit a mastectomy prosthetic shop.

6. *What specific tumor marker is associated with breast cancer?* CA 15-3. *Which laboratory test results may be abnormal?* All of the following tests will be elevated: acid phosphatase, alkaline phophatase, calcitonin, carcinoembryonic antigen, gamma-glutamyltransferase, haptoglobin, and estradiol serum.

7. *If the physician chose to treat Donna's breast cancer with chemotherapy, which type of chemotherapeutic drugs might the physician prescribe?* Plant alkaloids are likely to be prescribed to treat Donna's breast cancer. A common drug in this class is tamoxifen (Nolvadex®). *What side effects are associated with this medication?* Common side effects are hot flashes, nausea, and vomiting. The nurse should be prepared to administer antiemetics as ordered by the physician.

Short Answers

Cancers Associated with Different Viruses

Indicate which kind of cancer(s) are associated with each type of virus.

Virus	Cancer
Herpes simplex virus types I and II (HSV-1 and HSV-2)	**a.** Carcinoma of the lip **b.** Cervical carcinoma **c.** Kaposi's sarcoma
Human cytomegalovirus (HCMV)	**a.** Kaposi's sarcoma **b.** Prostate cancer
Epstein-Barr virus (EBV)	**a.** Burkitt's lymphoma
Human herpesvirus-6 (HHV-6)	**a.** Lymphoma
Hepatitis B virus (HBV)	**a.** Primary hepatocellular cancer
Papillomavirus	**a.** Malignant melanoma **b.** Cervical, penile, and laryngeal cancers
Human T-cell lymphotropic viruses (HTLV)	**a.** Adult T-cell leukemia and lymphoma **b.** T-cell variant of hairy cell leukemia **c.** Kaposi's sarcoma

NCLEX-RN® Review Questions

1. Answer: 2
   Rationale: The incidence of bladder cancer is four times higher in men than in women. Sun-related skin cancers are now considered to be a problem for all people. Compared to women, men are more likely to get skin cancer. Lung cancer is the leading cause of death in both men and women. The incidence of thyroid cancer is higher in women than in men
   Nursing Process: Planning
   Patient Need: Health Promotion and Maintenance

2. Answer: 3
   Rationale: Computed tomography reveals subtle differences in tissue densities and provides the greatest accuracy in tumor diagnosis. Ultrasonography is more useful in detecting masses in dense breast tissue. Magnetic resonance imaging is the tool of choice for the screening and follow-up of cranial, head, and neck tumors. Nuclear imaging can identify tumors in various body tissues and can be used to determine metastasis.
   Nursing Process: Diagnosis
   Patient Need: Health Promotion and Maintenance

3. Answer: 3
   Rationale: Chemotherapy treatment can result in the loss of taste. It is common to experience alopecia when undergoing chemotherapy. Chemotherapy depresses bone marrow, which results in an impaired ability to respond to an infection. Reproductive ability is impaired as a consequence of chemotherapy.

Nursing Process: Evaluation
Patient Need: Physiological Integrity

4. Answer: 1
   Rationale: Signs that identify anxiety include trembling, restlessness, avoidance of direct eye contact, irritability, hyperactivity, withdrawal, and a worried facial expression.
   Nursing Process: Assessment
   Patient Need: Psychosocial Integrity

5. Answer: 2
   Rationale: A patient who is willing to look at the wound and participate in wound care accepts his or her altered body image. Body image concerns are identified by the patient denying any change to his or her physical appearance, refusing visitors, and refusing to look at or care for the wound.
   Nursing Process: Evaluation
   Patient Need: Psychosocial Integrity

6. Answer: 2
   Rationale: An alcohol-based mouthwash will irritate sensitive oral mucosa and dry out an already moisture-depleted mouth. Proper oral hygiene includes using a soft-tipped toothbrush, soaking dentures in hydrogen peroxide, and using waxed dental floss.
   Nursing Process: Implementation
   Patient Need: Physiological Integrity

7. Answer: 2
   Rationale: Tumor lysis syndrome is characterized by two or more of the following metabolic abnormalities: hyperuricemia, hyperphosphatemia, hyperkalemia, and hypocalcemia.
   Nursing Process: Assessment
   Patient Need: Physiological Integrity

Chapter 15

Term Matching

1. E
2. H
3. B
4. J
5. M
6. L
7. C
8. G
9. F
10. I
11. K
12. A
13. D

Focused Study Questions

1. Pigment in an individual's skin is determined by the amount of melanin it contains. Light-skinned individuals have lesser amounts of melanin. Dark-skinned individuals have more. Exposure ot sun causes a buildup of the melanin pigment.

2. The two primary skin layers are the epidermis and the dermis. The epidermis is the outer layer. It provides protection from the environment. It also prevents water loss. Additional functions include the conversion of cholesterol to vitamin D and melanin storage.

   The dermis is the layer just beneath the epidermis. The functions of the dermis include temperature regulation and the transmission of messages to the central nervous system.

3. Hyperemeia will result in a red or bright pink skin tone. This condition may result from alcohol ingestion or increases in body or environmental temperatures. Jaundice will result in a yellow skin tone. Jaundice is the result of an excess of bilirubin. Bilirubin buildup may result from a variety of conditions. Most often jaundice is associated with liver disorders.

Case Study

1. *Is the area on the back of the patient's scalp a recurrence of her basal cell carcinoma? Why or why not?* Based on the description of the lesion, this is probably not a basal cell carcinoma; it is more likely a squamous cell carcinoma. The lesion is red, scaly, and rapid-growing with papules. There is no pearly edge or ulceration.

2. *What risk factors increase the patient's risk of developing this type of skin disorder?* Risk factors include high levels of exposure to the sun or tanning beds, fair skin and hair, immunosuppression, and previous personal or immediate family history of skin cancers.

3. *The lesion is located on the back of the patient's head, and she noticed it a week ago. The lesion is 3 mm in size now. Based on knowledge of this type of lesion, has the patient waited too long to seek treatment?* This is a rapid-growing cancer. While it is best to seek care as soon as possible for any suspected skin cancer, the key is to seek care. The location of the lesion on the back of the head makes it difficult to know how long it has been there. The fact that the lesion bleeds easily is not good.

4. *Is there a connection between the reason for the patient's admission and the lesion found on the back of her head?* No, there is probably no connection between the admission and the lesion. Bradycardia is not associated with an increased risk of basal or squamous cell carcinoma. If the nurse had not done a thorough skin assessment, the lesion may have been ignored, allowing it to grow larger and spread.

Short Answers

1.

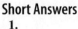

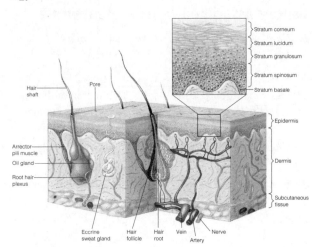

Figure 15–1 ■ Anatomy of the skin.

2.

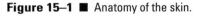

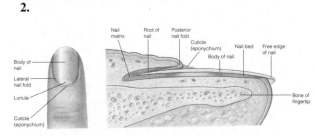

Figure 15–3 ■ Anatomy of a nail.

Crossword Puzzle

question	term answer
The outermost surface of the skin	EPIDERMIS
The second layer of skin	DERMIS
Glands responsible for producing oil	SEBACEOUS
Glands responsible for the production of sweat	SUDORIFEROUS
A yellow-to-orange pigment found in the body	CAROTENE
The total absence of melanin	ALBINISM
Retained urochrome pigments in the blood	UREMIA
Glands that regulate heat through perspiration	ECCRINE
Remnant of the sexual scent gland	APOCRINE

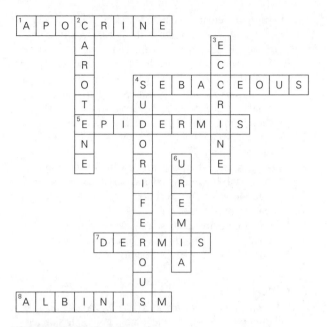

NCLEX-RN® Review Questions

1. Answer: 4

   Rationale: Exploring the background of the rash will help the nurse and the patient understand how best to approach the patient's care. Hot weather and frequent bathing can dry out the skin, but neither causes a red rash. Scratching will make it worse and may cause a secondary infection, but this statement does not help the patient understand the information. The patient never mentioned changing detergent, so assuming this is the problem will not help the patient explore the true nature of the rash.

   Nursing Process: Diagnosis

   Patient Need: Physiological Integrity

2. Answer: 3

   Rationale: Edema is best assessed by depressing the skin over the ankle or a bony prominence. A finding of 3+ edema indicates that the edema has caused the extremity to appear distorted, but the depression does not remain visible when the pressure is released. Findings of 1+ and 2+ indicate that the edema does not cause distortion. A finding of 4+ indicates that the edema caused the imprint to remain for some time after the pressure was released.

   Nursing Process: Assessment

   Patient Need: Physiological Integrity

3. Answer: 2

   Rationale: The fact that the patient has lost his natural protection, his hair, and has been exposed to the ultraviolet light of the sun for many hours a day as a construction worker significantly increases his risk of skin cancer. Smoking has a closer link to oral and lung cancer, and a high-fat diet is loosely associated with gastrointestinal cancers. There is no connection between hypothyroidism and skin cancer.

   Nursing Process: Diagnosis

   Patient Need: Health Promotion and Maintenance

4. Answer: 1

   Rationale: The tendency to burn does increase the risk of skin cancer, especially when the skin is not protected from the sun with sunscreens or the person does not avoid the harmful rays. Family history and genetics are strong indicators, but taking measures to protect skin from UVA and UVB rays can counteract that risk. Men, especially those who are older than 50, are at greater risk than women. Exposure to UVA and UVB rays, regardless of a natural tan or a tan from a tanning bed, increases the risk of skin cancers.

   Nursing Process: Diagnosis

   Patient Need: Health Promotion and Maintenance

5. Answer: 2

   Rationale: The sclera of the eye is the best place to see jaundice in a patient with a dark skin tone. Jaundice can be missed in the area under the nail or in the mucous membranes of the mouth. The forearm has too much pigment, which makes it difficult to see the yellow undertone of jaundice.

   Nursing Process: Assessment

   Patient Need: Physiological Integrity

6. Answer: 1

   Rationale: Tinea capitis, or scalp ringworm, is associated with hair loss, pustules, and scales on the scalp. Head lice may cause redness, but the nurse would see white oval-shaped nits in the hair. Seborrhea causes a greasy, flaky scalp. A boil causes a large fluid-filled area.

   Nursing Process: Assessment

   Patient Need: Physiological Integrity

7. Answer: 1 and 4

   Rationale: Both fungal infections and psoriasis can cause nails to become yellow and thicken. Trauma can cause the nail to appear dark or black-green or have red splinter hemorrhages. Pseudomonas infection will cause the nail to take on a blackish-green appearance. Thinning nails can be a sign of nutritional deficiency.

   Nursing Process: Assessment

   Patient Need: Physiological Integrity

8. Answer: 1

   Rationale: Hypothyroidism is commonly associated with coarse, dry skin because of the metabolic changes caused by the disease. Oily skin is seen in acne vulgaris. In fever, the nurse would see hot skin that could be dry, as in lacking moisture, but not dry as in flaky. Seborrhea produces a greasy, scaly appearance.

   Nursing Process: Assessment

   Patient Need: Physiological Integrity

Chapter 16

Terms Matching

1. F
2. P
3. U
4. S

5. B
6. C
7. V
8. L
9. Y
10. J
11. A
12. G
13. Z
14. AA
15. O
16. BB
17. E
18. T
19. CC
20. K
21. I
22. DD
23. D
24. M
25. N
26. W
27. X
28. Q
29. R
30. H

Focused Study

1. Therapeutic baths have a variety of uses in treating skin disorders. Depending on the agent used, therapeutic baths soothe the skin, lower the skin bacteria count, clean and hydrate the skin, loosen scales, and relieve itching.

2. When assisting a patient with a therapeutic bath, the nurse should include the following in the plan of care:
   • Ensure that the bath water is a comfortable temperature that is neither too hot nor too cool, usually 110°F–115°F (43°C–46°C).
   • Fill the tub one-third to one-half full.
   • Mix the agent well with the water.
   • Assist the patient in and out of the tub to prevent falls.
   • Dry the patient and the affected area by blotting with a towel.

3. Pressure ulcers are staged primarily by the depth and extensiveness of the wound. A stage II pressure ulcer will appear as partial thickness loss of dermis presenting as a shallow open ulcer with a red or pink wound bed. It may also present as an intact or open blister. The ulcer may be shiny or dry, without bruising or slough.

4. Retin-A®, a form of vitamin A, is often used to manage dermatological conditions. When providing education to the patient who has been prescribed Retin-A®, the nurse should include the following instructions:
   • Use the cream in a test area twice at night to test for sensitivity; if no reaction occurs, gradually increase applications to the prescribed frequency.
   • Use a pea-sized amount of the cream, which is enough to cover the entire face.

• Apply the cream to clean, dry skin.
• Do not apply the cream to the eyes, mouth, angles of the nose, or mucous membranes.
• Wash your face no more than two or three times a day using a mild soap. Do not use skin preparations (such as aftershave lotion or perfumes) that contain alcohol, menthol, spice, or lime; they may irritate your skin.
• Keep in mind that the medication may cause a temporary stinging or warm sensation but should not cause pain.
• Keep in mind that the skin on which you apply the cream will be mildly red and may peel; if you experience a more severe reaction, consult your healthcare provider.
• Because the medication may cause increased sensitivity to sunlight, use sunscreen and wear protective clothing when outdoors.

Case Study

1. *What factors place Chrissy at risk for developing malignant melanoma?* She is a naturally fair-skinned person. She is Caucasian and has a significant history of sun exposure and tanning. She is an upper middle-class professional who works indoors, and research demonstrates that these individuals have a higher-than-average incidence of developing malignant melanoma.

2. *What is Chrissy's prognosis? What factors are used to determine prognosis?* The prognosis for Chrissy will be determined by several variables, including tumor thickness, ulceration, metastasis, site, age, and gender. Younger patients and women have a somewhat better chance of survival.

3. *What treatments are available to Chrissy?* If the tumor is treatable, it can be removed by surgical excision. Malignant melanoma is also treated with chemotherapy, immunotherapy, and radiation therapy. Other successful therapies include biologic therapies with interleukin-2, interferon, and therapeutic vaccines that contain melanoma antigens.

4. *How often must Chrissy be seen for a checkup after removal of the lesion?* She should be seen every three months for the first two years, every six months for the next five years, and every year thereafter.

Short Answers

Type	Use	Examples
Creams	Moisturize the skin	Aqua Care®, Curel®, Nutraderm®
Ointments	Lubricate the skin and retard water loss	Aquaphor®, Vaseline®
Lotions	Moisturize and lubricate the skin	Alpha-Keri®, Dermassage, Lubriderm®
Anesthetics	Relieve itching	Xylocaine®

Antibiotics	Treat infection	Bacitracin, Polysporin®, gentamicin, Silvadene®
Corticosteroids	Suppress inflammation and relieve itching	Dexamethasone, clocortolone, desonide

NCLEX-RN® Review Questions

1. Answer: 2

Rationale: Nevi, more commonly called moles, are flat or raised macules or papules with rounded, well-defined borders. Cysts of the skin are benign closed sacs in or under the skin surface that are lined with epithelium and contain fluid or a semisolid material. Keloids are elevated, irregularly-shaped scars that progressively enlarge. Skin tags are soft papules on a pedicle.

Nursing Process: Assessment

Patient Need: Physiological Integrity

2. Answer: 2, 3, 4

Rationale: It is not appropriate to teach a patient with psoriasis to avoid exposure to the sun. Interventions for psoriasis include exposing the skin to sunlight but avoiding sunburn; avoiding exposure to contagious illnesses such as influenza and colds; avoiding trauma to the skin (for example, do not scrub off scales and use only an electric razor); and avoiding certain drugs [e.g., indomethacin (Indocin®), lithium, and beta-adrenergic blocking agents], which precipitate exacerbations of psoriasis. Bathing in warm water is not contraindicated for patients diagnosed with psoriasis.

Nursing Process: Implementation

Patient Need: Safe, Effective Care Environment

3. Answer: 4

Rationale: Erysipelas is an infection of the skin most often caused by group A streptococci. Cellulitis is a localized infection of the dermis and subcutaneous tissue. A carbuncle is a group of infected hair follicles. Furuncles, often called boils, are also inflammations of the hair follicle.

Nursing Process: Assessment

Patient Need: Physiological Integrity

4. Answer: 3

Rationale: The behavior that indicates the patient's understanding about caring for a vaginal *Candida albicans* infection is that the patient reports bathing more frequently. Other interventions include avoid wearing tight clothing such as jeans and pantyhose, wear cotton underwear, and ask the sexual partner to be tested to prevent the spread of infection.

Nursing Process: Evaluation

Patient Need: Health Promotion and Maintenance

5. Answer: 3

Rationale: Seborrheic dermatitis is a chronic inflammatory disorder of the skin that involves the scalp, eyebrows, eyelids, ear canals, nasolabial folds, axillae, and trunk. Contact dermatitis is a type of dermatitis that is caused by a hypersensitivity response or chemical irritation. Atopic dermatitis, also called eczema, is an inflammatory skin disorder. Exfoliative dermatitis is an inflammatory skin disorder that is characterized by excessive peeling or shedding of skin.

Nursing Process: Assessment

Patient Need: Physiological Integrity

6. Answer: 2

Rationale: Skin freezes when the temperature drops to 14°F–24.8°F (210°C–24°C).

Nursing Process: Assessment

Patient Need: Physiological Integrity

7. Answer: 4

Rationale: Laser surgery is used to treat patients with a wide variety of skin disorders, including port wine stains. Chemical destruction is the application of a specific chemical to produce destruction of skin lesions. Chemical destruction is used to treat both benign and premalignant lesions. Sclerotherapy is the removal of benign skin lesions with a sclerosing agent that causes inflammation and tissue fibrosis. Curettage is the removal of lesions with a curette, which is a semisharp cutting instrument.

Nursing Process: Planning

Patient Need: Safe, Effective Care Environment

8. Answer: 4

Rationale: A full-thickness graft contains both epidermis and dermis. These layers contain the greatest number of skin elements (sweat glands, sebaceous glands, and hair follicles) and are best able to withstand trauma. A split-thickness graft contains epidermis and only a portion of dermis of the donor site. A common donor site for a skin graft is the anterior thigh. Skin grafting is an effective way to cover wounds that have a good blood supply, that are not infected, and in which bleeding can be controlled.

Nursing Process: Planning

Patient Need: Physiological Integrity

Chapter 17

Terms Matching

1. B
2. H
3. K
4. M
5. Q
6. U
7. E
8. S
9. A
10. R
11. O
12. P
13. C
14. D
15. J
16. I

17. F
18. G
19. V
20. L
21. N
22. T

Focused Study

1. The healing process involves three phases: inflammation, proliferation, and remodeling.
   - Inflammation results immediately after the injury. Platelets come in contact with the damaged tissue aggregate. Fibrin is deposited, trapping further platelets, and a thrombus is formed. The thrombus, combined with local vasoconstriction, leads to hemostasis, which walls off the wound from the systemic circulation.
   - Proliferation begins two to three days after the burn injury. Fiberblasts occupy the wound. Granulation tissue begins to form, with complete reepithelialization. The proliferation phase lasts until complete reepithelialization occurs by epithelial cell migration, surgical intervention, or a combination of the two.
   - Remodeling may last years. Collagen fibers, which are laid down during the proliferative phase, are reorganized into more compact areas. Scars contract and fade in color.
2. Treatment is performed on an outpatient basis and generally consists of applying mild lotions, increasing liquid intake, administering mild analgesics, and maintaining warmth. If the patient is older, he or she should be observed for signs of dehydration.
3. Thermal burns result from exposure to dry or moist heat. They are the most common type of burn. They are seen most often in children and older adults. Direct exposure to the source of heat causes cellular destruction that can result in charring of vascular, bony, muscle, and nervous tissue.

   Chemical burns occur when the skin comes in direct contact with acids, alkaline agents, or organic compounds. The chemical destroys tissue protein, leading to necrosis. Burns caused by alkalis (for example, lye) are more difficult to neutralize than are burns caused by acids. They also tend to have deeper penetration with a correspondingly more severe burn than a burn from acid. Organic compound burns (caused by petroleum distillates, for example) cause cutaneous damage through fat solvent action and may cause renal and liver failure if absorbed.

   Chemical agents are further classified according to the manner by which they structurally alter proteins. Oxidizing agents such as household bleach alter protein configuration through the chemical process of reduction. Corrosives such as lye cause extensive protein denaturation.

Electrical burns result when an electrical current passes through the body. The injury is accompanied by entrance and exit wounds. Potential causes are lightning strikes. The most common cause of death for a victim of this type of burn is cardiopulmonary arrest.

Radiation burns are usually associated with sunburn or radiation treatment for cancer. These kinds of burns tend to be superficial, involving only the outermost layers of the epidermis. All functions of the skin remain intact. Symptoms are limited to mild systemic reactions: headache, chills, local discomfort, nausea, and vomiting.

4. Tissue damage following a burn is determined primarily by two factors: depth of the burn (the layers of underlying tissue affected) and the extent of the burn (the percentage of body surface area involved).

   The depth of a burn injury is determined by the elements of the skin that have been damaged or destroyed. Burns are classified as superficial, partial-thickness, or full-thickness.

Case Study

1. *What changes need to be made immediately in the patient's care?* The patient's IV fluids should be changed to lactated Ringer's solution. She should be intubated to protect her airway, especially in light of the risk of respiratory burn as evidenced by the soot on her nasal mucosa. The patient's intake and output should be carefully monitored to determine the adequacy of fluid resuscitation.
2. *To what setting will this patient likely be transferred when she is stable?* This patient will probably be transferred to a specific burn unit or to a critical care unit.
3. *Why would the patient be intubated and placed on a ventilator?* The risk of the patient's respiratory system being compromised by burn is a great risk; therefore, the airways should be protected. Intubating the patient is a safety measure. The patient's respiratory rate and oxygen saturation reading, as well as the soot around her nares, demonstrates that injury.
4. *Based on the patient's injuries, from what type of immediate surgical intervention might she benefit?* Tracheostomy

Care Plan Critical-Thinking Activity

1. Maintenance of the airway is the greatest concern for this patient.
2. The patient may have inhalation injuries. The respiratory status must be assessed. Signs and symptoms of a respiratory-related burn injury include the presence of soot, charring, edema, blisters, and ulcerations along the mucosal lining of the oropharynx and larynx. Ominous signs of hoarseness, labored breathing, or stridor indicate possible airway obstruction due to edema.

3. *Risk for Ineffective Airway Clearance* related to increasing lung congestion secondary to smoke inhalation

4. Resulting edema in the airway peaks within the first 24–48 hours of injury.

NCLEX-RN® Review Questions

1. Answer: 2

   Rationale: Lactated Ringer's (LR) is the recommended solution during the patient's fluid resuscitation. Crystalloid fluids are administered through two large-bore (14- to 16-gauge) catheters, preferably inserted through unburned skin. Warmed Ringer's lactate solution is the intravenous fluid most widely used during the first 24 hours after burn injury because it most closely approximates the body's extracellular fluid composition. Several formulas may be used to replace fluid loss. Two commonly used formulas are as follows:

   • Parkland formula, in which lactated Ringer's solution is administered 4 mL $\times$ kg $\times$ % TBSA burn

   • ABLS Consensus formula, in which lactated Ringer's solution is administered 2–4 mL $\times$ kg $\times$ % TBSA burn (Ahrns, 2004). This patient weighs 68 kg with a second-degree burn over 40% of the body, so the Parkland calculation is used: 4 mL $\times$ 68 : 40 = 10880 mL over 24 hours, with 50% to be infused over the first 8 hours and the other 50% over the remaining 16 hours.

   Nursing Process: Implementation

   Patient Need: Physiological Integrity

2. Answer: 1

   Rationale: Elevating the head of the bed to at least 30 degrees improves the patient's ability to ventilate. Oxygen should be administered at 100% via mask, not nasal cannula. Premedicating the patient and protecting the graft and skin at the burn site are extremely important, but oxygenation holds a higher priority.

   Nursing Process: Implementation

   Patient Need: Physiological Integrity

3. Answer: 3

   Rationale: A variety of tasks can be delegated to unlicensed personnel, but none should involve assessment. Encouraging the patient to use the patient-controlled analgesia and spirometer are things the patient has already been taught, so these are just reminders. Changing the dressing and documenting the change requires the nurse to assess the patient, as does checking urinary output for adequacy of fluid resuscitation. The first-time ambulating requires the nurse to assess how the patient tolerates the new activity.

   Nursing Process: Planning

   Patient Need: Physiological Integrity

4. Answer: 4

   Rationale: Wound healing and helping the body to heal are the most important and most common goals of radiation burn treatment. The other statements are true, but they are not goals of care; they are only information.

   Nursing Process: Implementation

   Patient Need: Health Promotion and Maintenance

5. Answer: 1

   Rationale: The patient's daily caloric intake dramatically increases by as much as 100% of the normal intake, possibly as high as 4000–6000 Kcal per day. Therefore, the nurse must provide 4000 Kcal per 24 hours. The Parkland formula is designed for patients with burns over more than 20% total body surface area, so it may be possible to titrate oxygen down at this point, but it should be humidified to prevent damage to the nasal mucosa. Support garments should be applied no sooner than five to seven days postgraft.

   Nursing Process: Diagnosis

   Patient Need: Physiological Integrity

6. Answer: 1

   Rationale: If the nurse does not disconnect the patient from the electrical source, the nurse will place himself or herself at risk when providing care for the patient. Electrical injuries can occur in the hospital, so the nurse cannot assume that the injury happened elsewhere. Patients with electrical burns are at greater risk of spinal injury due to the forceful contraction of the muscles during the electrical injury, but waiting to provide care until after the collar and back board are in place could cause irreversible brain injury to the patient. It is important to monitor for cardiac dysrhythmia and for fluid resuscitation requirements, but they are not the highest priority.

   Nursing Process: Diagnosis

   Patient Need: Physiological Integrity

7. Answer: 2

   Rationale: Full-thickness burns, regardless of size, require skin grafting in order to heal due to the depth of damage and location of cells needed to regenerate tissue. Partial-thickness grafting may be performed on smaller wounds, or third intention healing may be used.

   Nursing Process: Assessment

   Patient Need: Physiological Integrity

8. Answer: 3

   Rationale: The American Burn Association provides guidelines for major burns; the patient with the electrical burn meets those requirements not only because of the possible voltage, but also because of the trauma associated with the burn. Other requirements for major burns are those that involve 20% total body surface area (TBSA) in adults older than 40 years of age and 10% TBSA full-thickness burns in adults older than 40 years of age. Oxygen saturation rates may normally be below 95% for a given patient, so this is not indicative of a burn.

   Nursing Process: Assessment

   Patient Need: Physiological Integrity

9. Answer: See figure.

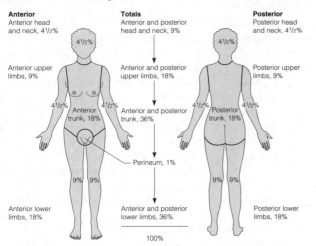

Figure 17–5 ■ The "rule of nines" is a method of quickly estimating the percentage of TBSA affected by a burn injury. Although useful in emergency care situations, the rule of nines is not accurate for estimating TBSA for adults who are short, obese, or very thin.

> Rationale: You should have shaded in the anterior trunk along with either arm or the head and neck.
> Nursing Process: Assessment
> Patient Need: Physiological Integrity

10. Answer: 2

> Rationale: Hypovolemic shock is the earliest risk and one of the greatest risks to the burn patient, in addition to sepsis. Cardiac collapse due to hypovolemia must be prevented with adequate fluid resuscitation during the first 24–36 hours. Compartment syndrome is local damage seen in the extremities that is related to circumferential burns and associated edema. Dysrhythmias are more commonly associated with electrical burns, and patients must be closely monitored. Acute renal failure is associated with hypovolemia; to avoid this complication, volume depletion must be prevented.
> Nursing Process: Diagnosis
> Patient Need: Physiological Integrity

Chapter 18

Terms Matching
1. G
2. E
3. B
4. A
5. C
6. D
7. H
8. F

Focused Study
1. Growth hormone (somatrotropin), prolactin, thyroid-stimulating hormone, adrenocorticotropic hormone, follicle-stimulating hormone, luteinizing hormone, and interstitial-cell stimulating hormone

2. The nurse should ask the patient about the onset, characteristic, severity, and course of symptoms. The nurse should ask the patient how the symptoms are precipitated and relieved. The timing and circumstances that surround the symptoms should also be determined. The nurse should explore the patient's medical history, family history, social, personal, and occupational history. The nurse should assess the patient's surgical history and list of medications.

3. Increased heart rate, increased blood pressure, increased respiratory rate, loud breath sounds, increased basal metabolic rate, increased serum glucose level, and hypoactive bowel sounds

4. The patient should be advised not to eat, smoke, or drink after midnight the day before the test. The test can take up to eight hours. The patient's weight and lying and standing blood pressures will be monitored every hour. Every hour the nurse will collect urine and serum specimens.

Case Studies

Case Study 1
1. *Which diagnostic tests might be used to correctly diagnose Ms. Aummert's health problem?*
   Magnetic resonance imaging (MRI): thyroid, pituitary gland
   Thyroid stimulating hormone (TSH)
   Thyroxine (T_4)
   Triiodothyronine (T_3)
   Thyroid antibodies (TA)
   Radioactive iodine uptake (RIA)
   Thyroid scan
   Thyroid suppression test
   Thyrotropin-releasing hormone stimulation test
   Triiodothyronine resin uptake (T_3RU)

2. *Ms. Aummert is diagnosed with hypothyroidism. What can the nurse expect to find during the physical assessment?* Skin: hypopigmentation or yellowish cast, rough, dry; nails and hair: dry, thick, brittle; thyroid gland: goiter, nodules; motor function assessment: decreased reflexes; sensory function assessment: peripheral neuropathy, paresthesias.

3. *What are some questions the nurse can ask Ms. Aummert to determine whether she's receiving adequate amounts of sleep and rest?* How many hours of sleep do you get each night? Do you ever feel nervous or unable to rest? Do you ever sweat profusely while you sleep?

4. *Ms. Aummert states that her 76-year-old mother was recently diagnosed with hypothyroidism. What are some age-related changes that occur in the endocrine system?* Her mother may have experienced age-related changes in the function of endocrine glands. Older adults are more likely to experience a lower basal metabolic rate, have an increased likelihood of being diagnosed with hypothyroidism, and have

palpable thyroid nodules. Older adults produce less glucocorticoids, 17-ketosteroids, progesterone, androgen, and estrogen. They have a higher incidence of hypertension that may be related to the effects of the sympathetic nervous system and an increased amount of circulating norepinephrine. They cannot digest fat as well as younger adults can due to a diminished production of lipase by the pancreas. They don't absorb fat-soluble vitamins well. They have difficulty metabolizing glucose.

Case Study 2

1. *What diagnostic tests may be performed to help the healthcare providers better understand the nature of Mr. Knight's health problem?* Fasting blood sugar, oral glucose tolerance test (OGTT), glycosylated hemoglobin (HbA$_1$C), and MRI of the pancreas.

2. *The nurse questions Mr. Knight regarding his family history of endocrine disorders. Mr. Knight states that his father was diagnosed with diabetes mellitus at the age of 11. Mr. Knight wants to know if other endocrine disorders can be inherited. What is the nurse's best response?* Type 1 and type 2 diabetes mellitus, Pendred syndrome, Hashimoto's disease, multiple endocrine neoplasia, and fragile X syndrome all have some genetic components.

3. *Mr. Knight is diagnosed with diabetes mellitus. What are some physical findings associated with this endocrine condition?* Skin: hypopigmentation, lesions on the lower extremities; sensory function assessment: peripheral neuropathy, paresthesias

Short Answers
Glands of the Endocrine System

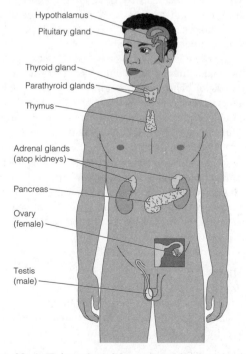

Hypothalamus

Pituitary gland

Thyroid gland

Parathyroid glands

Thymus

Adrenal glands
(atop kidneys)

Pancreas

Ovary
(female)

Testis
(male)

Figure 18–1 ■ Location of the major endocrine glands.

NCLEX-RN® Review Questions

1. Answer: 2
   Rationale: Assessment of the neck and the patient's ability to swallow may identify enlargement of the thyroid gland. While it is important to assess the abdomen for organomegaly and ascites, this is most likely not the source of the patient's health issue. Balance and gait testing may help identify weakness, but this testing is too general. Assessment of height and weight is generally important but only in comparison to a previous weight.
   Nursing Process: Assessment
   Patient Need: Physiological Integrity

2. Answer: 1
   Rationale: The pancreas produces insulin, which is responsible for making glucose available for use by the body. The pituitary is generally responsible for metabolism but not specifically insulin and carbohydrate metabolism. The thyroid increases metabolism and produces T3, T4, and calcitonin. The parathyroid secretes parathormone and controls calcium and phosphate levels.
   Nursing Process: Assessment
   Patient Need: Physiological Integrity

3. Answer: 3
   Rationale: The adrenal medulla produces epinephrine and norepinephrine. The pancreas is responsible for the production of insulin and digestive enzymes. The thyroid is responsible for the production of T$_3$, T$_4$, and calcitonin. The adrenal cortex produces corticosteroids.
   Nursing Process: Assessment
   Patient Need: Physiological Integrity

4. Answer: 3
   Rationale: The adrenal cortex secretes corticosteroids. The thyroid gland secretes thyroxine and triiodothyronine. The parathyroid secretes parathyroid hormone (PTH), or parathormone. The adrenal medulla secretes epinephrine and norepinephrine.
   Nursing Process: Assessment
   Patient Need: Physiological Integrity

5. Answer: 3
   Rationale: Follicle-stimulating hormone (FSH) stimulates the development of ovarian follicles and induces the secretion of estrogenic female sex hormones. Oxytocin causes contraction of the smooth muscles in the reproductive organs, stimulates the myometrium of the uterus to contract during labor, and induces the production of milk from the breasts. Vasopressin is responsible for decreasing urine production. Luteinizing hormone (LH) induces ovulation and the formation of the corpus luteum from an ovarian follicle.
   Nursing Process: Assessment
   Patient Need: Physiological Integrity

Chapter 19

Terms Matching

1. R
2. AA
3. I
4. N
5. U
6. J
7. A
8. Y
9. C
10. E
11. L
12. G
13. P
14. B
15. T
16. Q
17. H
18. M
19. Z
20. K
21. X
22. V
23. O
24. W
25. D
26. F
27. S

Focused Study

1. **a.** Manifestations
   - Increased appetite
   - Changes in weight, usually weight loss
   - Increased peristalsis, diarrhea
   - Hypermetabolism: heat intolerance, insomnia, palpitations, increased sweating
   - Smooth, warm skin
   - Fine hair; hair loss in the scalp, eyebrow, axilla, or pubic area
   - Emotional lability

   b. Treatment

   Hyperthyroidism is treated with antithyroid medications that reduce TH production. Examples include methimazole (Tapazole®), carbimazole, and propylthiouracil (PTU, Propyl-Thyracil®). Beta blockers such as propanolol (Inderal®) and esmolol are prescribed to decrease the cardiovascular manifestations associated with hyperthyroidism.

2. Goiter and hoarseness
   - Fluid retention and edema
   - Decreased appetite and weight gain
   - Constipation
   - Dry skin and pallor
   - Muscle stiffness
   - Decreased sense of taste and smell
   - Menstrual disorders
   - Anemias
   - Cardiac enlargement
   - Bradycardia
   - Elevated serum cholesterol and triglyceride levels
   - Hyponatremia
   - Sleep apnea

3. Cushing's syndrome that results from a pituitary tumor is treated with medications and surgery or radiation. Medications are prescribed for patients with inoperable pituitary or adrenal malignancies. The following medications may be used:
   - Mitotane suppresses adrenal cortex activity and decreases corticosteroid metabolism.
   - Aminoglutethimide and ketoconazole inhibit cortisol synthesis.
   - Somatostatin analog (octreotide) suppresses ACTH secretion in some patients.

   An adrenalectomy may be performed to remove an adrenal cortex tumor.

4. Gigantism is a result of GH hypersecretion. It begins before puberty and the closure of the epiphyseal plates. The person becomes abnormally tall, often exceeding 7 feet in height. However, the person's body proportions are relatively normal. It is most often the result of a tumor.

   Acromegaly also is the result of GH hypersecretion. However, the affected person is already an adult. It is most commonly a result of pituitary tumors. The person's hands and feet, connective tissue, membraneous bones of the skull, and soft tissues continue to grow. The forehead enlarges, the maxilla lengthens, the tongue enlarges, and the voice deepens. Peripheral nerve damage can occur from entrapment of nerves. The person may develop problems such as headaches, arthralgias, hypertension, congestive heart failure, skin thickening and copious sweating, seizures, and visual disturbances. The person may develop impaired glucose tolerance and diabetes.

5. Diabetes insipidus, a deficit of ADH, causes polyuria. The patient has extreme thirst and demonstrates polydipsia. The patient becomes dehydrated and hypernatremic if unable to replace lost fluids. Even though serum hyperosmolality is present, the urine is dilute and has a low specific gravity.

   SIADH is usually nonspecific but is related to hyponatremia and water intoxication. The patient retains fluids and is thirsty. Brain cells may swell, causing neurological manifestations, including headache, changes in mental status or personality, lethargy, and irritability. The patient gains weight due to fluid retention.

Case Study

1. *How should the nurse explain Addison's disease to Ms. Moss?* The nurse should explain that Addison's disease is a condition resulting from destruction or dysfunction of the adrenal cortex.

2. *What manifestations should the nurse look for during the assessment of Ms. Moss?* The nurse should look for any of the following symptoms: confusion, lethargy, tremors, emotional lability, postural hypotension, tachycardia, cardiac arrhythmias, lethargy, weakness, muscle wasting, joint pain, muscle pain, anorexia, nausea, vomiting, and diarrhea.

3. *What skin changes should the nurse expect Ms. Moss to experience?* Ms. Moss's skin may appear deeply tanned or bronzed due to hyperpigmentation. The patient may experience delayed wound healing.

4. *What diagnostic testing procedures may have been used to diagnose Ms. Moss's condition?* The following diagnostic studies are used to diagnose Addison's disease: serum cortisol, blood glucose, serum sodium, serum potassium, blood urea nitrogen (BUN), urinary 17-hydroxycorticoids and 17-ketosteroids, plasma ACTH, (a cortisol) ACTH stimulation test, and a computed tomography (CT) scan.

5. *What medications can be used to treat Ms. Moss?* Cortisone (Cortone, Cortogen); hydrocortisone (Cortisol, Hydrocortone®, Cortef®); fludrocortisone acetate (Florinef®, F-Cortef®); dexamethasone (Decadron®, Hexadrol®, Dexasone®); prednisone (Meticorten®, Deltasone®, Orasone®); prednisolone (Meticortelone®)

6. *What should the nurse include when educating Ms. Moss about self-care techniques?* The medications used to replace cortisol should be taken with food or milk. The patient should report any gastric distress or dark stools. Most people take these medications for the remainder of their lives. The patient's diet should be low in potassium and high in sodium and protein. The patient should weigh herself at the same time each day and report any weight gain. The patient should use safety measures to prevent injuries and falls. Corticosteroids may reduce the effectiveness of oral contraceptives. The patient should take the medication as ordered on a regular schedule. Ms. Moss should wear a medical alert bracelet. The patient should monitor herself for increased stressors and increase the dose as indicated by the physician. Anticoagulant medication may decrease the effectiveness of corticosteroids. Ms. Moss should report to her physician dizziness upon sitting or standing, nausea and vomiting, pain, thirst, feelings of anxiety, malaise, or infection.

Short Answers

Fill in the missing pieces regarding the pathophysiology of Cushing's syndrome.

Manifestations	Pathophysiology
Fat deposits in the abdominal region, fat pads under the clavicles, a "buffalo hump" over the upper back, and a round "moon" face	Excess glucocorticoids affect normal carbohydrate metabolism, resulting in a redistribution of body fat and a breakdown of fats to fatty acids.
Muscle weakness and wasting, especially in the extremities	Excess cortisol results in changes in protein metabolism and changes in protein catabolism from mobilization of amino acids for gluconeogenesis.
Thinning of skin, abdominal striae, easy bruising, poor wound healing, and frequent skin infections	Inhibition of fibroplasts by excess glucocorticoids with loss of collagen and connective tissue. Excess glucocorticoids depress the inflammatory response and inhibit immune system effectiveness.
Osteoporosis, compression fractures of the vertebrae, and rib fractures	Excessive mineralocorticoids result in changes in absorption of calcium.
Hypokalemia	Loss of potassium
Hypertension and hypernatremia	Excess aldosterone alters the absorption of sodium by the distal tubules of the kidneys (via the rennin–angiotensin–aldosterone system), and sodium is retained. As potassium is lost, sodium is retained.
Hyperglycemia, polyuria, and polydipsia	Altered glucose metabolism
Increased risk of gastric ulcers	Increased gastric acid secretion
Hirsutism, acne, and menstrual irregularities	Increased androgen levels
Emotional instability	Decreased response to stress

NCLEX-RN® Review Questions

1. Answer: 4
   Rationale: The patient with hyperthyroidism will experience diarrhea, not constipation. The patient with hyperthyroidism will have the following manifestations: increased appetite, increased peristalsis, heat intolerance, insomnia, palpitations, increased sweating, and emotional lability.
   Nursing Process: Assessment
   Patient Need: Physiological Integrity

2. Answer: 2
   Rationale: Reducing the patient's temperature with aspirin will increase the free thyroid hormone in the body and worsen the crisis. The patient's body temperature should be reduced with aspirin-free medication. The patient's fluids and electrolytes should be replaced, and oxygen should be administered due to increased oxygen needs.
   Nursing Process: Implementation
   Patient Need: Safe, Effective Care Environment

3. Answer: 2

Rationale: Patients with hyperthyroidism must learn to keep the environment as distraction-free as possible. Decreasing stress lowers the cardiac output and circulating catecholamines. Patients must learn to balance periods of activity with periods of rest. Patients must monitor their weight closely and weigh themselves at the same time every day. They must add carbohydrates and proteins to their diet.

Nursing Process: Evaluation

Patient Need: Health Promotion and Maintenance

4. Answer: 2

Rationale: Estrogen increases thyroid function. Other medications that increase thyroid function include clofibrate, methadone, amiodarone, and birth control pills. Anabolic steroids, lithium, and propanolol may decrease thyroid function.

Nursing Process: Assessment

Patient Need: Physiological Integrity

5. Answer: 1

Rationale: Hashimoto's thyroiditis is more common in women than men. It is an autoimmune disease that causes a goiter. It does have a familial link.

Nursing Process: Diagnosis

Patient Need: Health Promotion and Maintenance

6. Answer: 2

Rationale: Cushing's syndrome is a chronic disorder in which hyperfunction of the adrenal cortex produces excessive amounts of circulating cortisol or ACTH. Cushing's syndrome is more common in women, with the average age of onset between 30 and 50 years, and in patients undergoing long-term steroid treatment and chemotherapy.

Nursing Process: Assessment

Patient Need: Health Promotion and Maintenance

7. Answer: 3

Rationale: The behavior that demonstrates the patient's understanding of treatment for Cushing's syndrome includes restricting fluid intake. Patients who understand health teaching will discuss their altered body image, increase their dietary intake of vitamins A and C, and use bright lighting in their rooms to avoid falls and injury.

Nursing Process: Evaluation

Patient Need: Health Promotion and Maintenance

8. Answer: 4

Rationale: The onset of Addison's is slow, and symptoms appear after 90% of the gland function is lost. Symptoms may not appear in patients with less than a 90% loss of gland function.

Nursing Process: Assessment

Patient Need: Physiological Integrity

Chapter 20

Terms Matching

1. K
2. P
3. B
4. J
5. A
6. G
7. C
8. I
9. L
10. M
11. H
12. D
13. F
14. E
15. N
16. O

Focused Study

1. Type 1 DM is the result of pancreatic islet cell destruction and a total deficit of circulating insulin. Type 2 DM results from insulin resistance with a defect in compensatory insulin secretion.

   Type 1 DM most often occurs in childhood and adolescence, but it may occur at any age, even in the eighties and nineties. Type 1 DM is the result of destruction of the beta cells of the islets of Langerhans in the pancreas, the only cells in the body that make insulin. Patients with Type 1 DM make no insulin and must be managed with injected insulin.

   Type 2 DM is a condition of fasting hyperglycemia that occurs despite the availability of endogenous insulin. Type 2 DM can occur at any age, but it is usually seen in middle age. Level of insulin produced varies in Type 2 DM. Patients with Type 2 DM are managed with diet and oral and/or injected insulin.

2. The following diagnostic tests are used to manage diabetes:
   • Fasting blood glucose (FBS)
   • Glycosylated hemoglobin (A1C)
   • Urine glucose and ketone
   • Self-monitoring of blood glucose (SMBG)

3. Preparations of insulin are derived from animal (pork pancreas) or synthesized in the laboratory from an alteration of pork insulin or from recombinant DNA technology. Insulins are available in rapid-acting, short-acting, intermediate-acting, and long-acting preparations.

4. Diabetic ketoacidosis (DKA) develops when there is an absolute deficiency of insulin and an increase in the insulin counterregulatory hormones (for example, cortisol). The processes of DKA result in a series of metabolic problems including hyperosmolarity from hyperglycemia and dehydration, metabolic acidosis from an accumulation of ketoacids, extracellular volume depletion from osmotic diuresis, and electrolyte imbalances (such as loss of potassium and sodium) from osmotic diuresis.

   The management of manifestations of DKA includes the following:
   • The administration of fluids to correct the dehydration. An infusion of 0.9% saline solution is

used initially. After a few hours, the solution is changed to 0.45% saline. When the glucose level are reduced to 250 mg/dL, dextrose is added to the IV infusion.
- Regular insulin may be administered intravenously.
- Electrolyte levels are assessed.
- Electrolyte replacement is initiated.

5. The following treatments are used to manage hyperosmolar hyperglycemic state:
- Establishing and maintaining adequate ventilation
- Correcting shock with adequate intravenous fluids
- Instituting nasogastric suction to prevent aspiration if the patient is comatose
- Maintaining fluid volume with intravenous isotonic or colloid solutions
- Administering potassium intravenously to replace losses
- Administering insulin to reduce blood glucose

Case Study

1. *With what type of diabetes would Mr. Brown be diagnosed? Why?* Mr. Brown would be diagnosed with type 2 diabetes. He is being discharged with prescriptions for an oral hypoglycemic. Type 2 diabetes can occur at any age, but it is usually seen in middle-age and older people. Mr. Brown is middle-aged at age 56.
2. *How do oral hypoglycemics regulate blood sugar?* Hypoglycemic agents lower blood sugar by stimulating or increasing insulin secretion, preventing breakdown of glycogen to glucose by the liver, and increasing peripheral uptake of glucose by making cells less resistant to insulin. Some hypoglycemics keep blood sugar low by blocking absorption of carbohydrates in the intestines.
3. *What modifications will Mr. Brown need to make to his diet?* There are no specific dietary guidelines for type 2 diabetes mellitus (DM). The general dietary guidelines are to decrease kilocalories and to consume three meals of equal size that are evenly spaced approximately four to five hours apart, with one or two snacks. The person with type 2 DM should also decrease fat intake.
4. *How should Mr. Brown be taught to manage an episode of hypoglycemia?* When mild hypoglycemia occurs, immediate treatment is necessary. Mr. Brown should take about 15 grams of a rapid-acting sugar. This amount of sugar is found, for example, in three glucose tablets, ½ cup of fruit juice or regular soda, 8 ounces of skim milk, five Life Savers® candies, three large marshmallows, or 3 teaspoons of sugar or honey. If Mr. Brown continues to experience symptoms of hypoglycemia, he should follow the 15/15 rule: wait 15 minutes; monitor blood glucose; and if it is low, eat another 15 grams of carbohydrate. This procedure can be repeated until the blood glucose levels return to normal. If the symptoms are not relieved or if they get worse, he should call his healthcare provider immediately or go to the nearest emergency room.

5. *Mr. Brown asks about the types of complications that may accompany his condition. What disorders are linked to diabetes mellitus?* Patients with diabetes are at an increased risk for the development of vascular complications. Atherosclerosis, myocardial infarction, and hypertension are increased in those with diabetes. Other complications include diabetic nephropathy and retinopathy. Diabetic patients also have an increased susceptibility to infection.

Short Answers
Fill in the table.

Drug Name	Classification	Onset (hrs)	Peak (hrs)	Duration (hrs)
Lispro	Rapid-acting	0.25	1.0–1.5	3–4
Regular	Short-acting	0.5–1.0 minute	2–3	4–6
Humulin R®	Intermediate-acting	2	6–8	12–16
NPH	Intermediate-acting	2	6–8	12–16
Lantus®	Long-acting	Not defined	Not defined	24

NCLEX-RN® Review Questions

1. Answer: 2
Rationale: Type 2 diabetes mellitus (DM) is a nonketonic form of diabetes. Type 1 DM begins most often in childhood, is a ketonic form of diabetes, can be triggered by a virus, and requires an exogenous form of insulin. Type 2 DM can occur at any age, but it is usually seen in middle-age and older people. Type 2 DM requires a diet change, increased exercise, and weight loss. Oral hypoglycemics may be ordered to assist in lowering patients' blood sugar.
Nursing Process: Assessment
Patient Need: Health Promotion and Maintenance
2. Answer: 3
Rationale: Manifestations of type 2 diabetes mellitus (DM) include blurred vision, fatigue, paresthesias, and skin infections. Type 2 symptoms do not include polydipsia, polyuria, or polyphagia.
Nursing Process: Assessment
Patient Need: Physiological Integrity
3. Answer: 3
Rationale: Normal fasting blood glucose is 100mg/dL. A fasting blood glucose of < 100 mg/dL is abnormal. A fasting blood glucose of 200 mg/dL and over is also abnormal.
Nursing Process: Assessment
Patient Need: Physiological Integrity
4. Answer: 4
Rationale: Syringes for administering U-100 insulin can be purchased in 0.3 mL (30 U), 0.5 mL (50 U), and 1.0 mL (100 U) sizes.

Nursing Process: Implementation

Patient Need: Safe, Effective Care Environment

5. Answer: 2

Rationale: Do not massage the site after administering the insulin injection because this may interfere with absorption. Correct insulin administration includes injecting the needle at 90 degrees, rotating the sites of injection, and not injecting insulin into an area that will be exercised.

Nursing Process: Implementation

Patient Need: Safe, Effective Care Environment

6. Answer: 3

Rationale: The dawn phenomenon is a rise in blood glucose between 4 AM and 8 AM and is not a response to hypoglycemia. This condition occurs in people with both type 1 and type 2 diabetes mellitus (DM). The exact cause is unknown but is believed to be related to nocturnal increases in growth hormone, which decreases peripheral uptake of glucose.

Nursing Process: Planning

Patient Need: Physiological Integrity

7. Answer: 4

Rationale: The patient should carefully pat the feet dry and ensure that the areas between the toes are thoroughly dry after bathing. Patting the feet dry and ensuring that the areas between the toes are dry can help the patient prevent the development of skin integrity issues that often accompany diabetes. The patient must inspect the feet each day, not each month. Tight-fitting shoes can contribute to skin integrity issues because they can impair circulation within the feet. The patient should elevate the lower extremities to prevent edema. Edema can contribute to poor circulation and contribute to the development of skin integrity issues.

Nursing Process: Assessment

Patient Need: Physiological Integrity

Chapter 21

Terms Matching

1. Q
2. E
3. M
4. A
5. O
6. I
7. B
8. J
9. L
10. R
11. C
12. G
13. D
14. N
15. K
16. H
17. P
18. F

Focused Study

1.

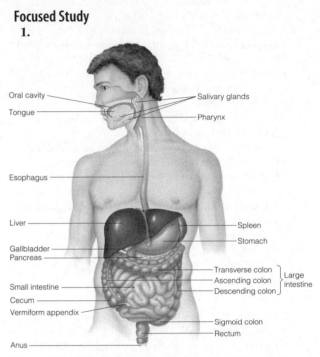

Figure 21–1 ■ Organs of the gastrointestinal system and accessory digestive organs.

2. **a.** The primary sources of carbohydrates are from plants. Monosaccharides and disaccharides come from milk, sugar cane, sugar beets, honey, and fruits. Polysaccharide starch is found in grains, legumes, and root vegetables. Carbohydrates are converted primarily to glucose and are used to make adenosine triphosphate (ATP).

   b. Proteins are either complete or incomplete. Complete proteins are found in animal products such as eggs, milk, milk products, and meat. Complete proteins contain the greatest amount of amino acids and meet the body's requirements for tissue growth and maintenance. Incomplete proteins are found in legumes, nuts, grains, cereals, and vegetables. These sources lack one or more of the amino acids essential for building complete proteins. Protein is used to build the skin's keratin, the connective tissue's elastin, and muscles. Proteins are used to make enzymes, hemoglobin, plasma proteins, and some hormones.

   c. Fats, also known as lipids, include phospholipids, steroids, and neutral fats. Neutral fats are the most abundant fats in the diet. They may be either saturated or unsaturated. Saturated fats are found in animal products and in some plant products. Unsaturated fats are found in seeds, nuts, and most vegetable oils. Sources of cholesterol include meats, milk products, and egg yolks. Fats are a necessary part of the structure and function of the body. Phospholipids can be found in cell membranes. Triglycerides are a major energy source for cells in the liver and skeletal muscles. Dietary fats assist the body in absorbing fat-soluble vitamins. Linoleic acid is an essential fatty acid that helps form prostaglandins, regulatory molecules that assist in smooth muscle contraction, maintenance of blood pressure, and control of inflammatory responses. Cholesterol is the essential component of bile salts, steroid hormones, and vitamin D. Adipose tissue serves as protection around body organs, as a layer of insulation under the skin, and as a concentrated source of fuel for cellular energy.

3. Stimulation of the parasympathetic vagus nerve increases gastric secretory activity. Stimulation of sympathetic nerves decreases secretory activity.

4. The following two formulas can be used:
   Weight (kilograms) ÷ height (meters) squared = BMI
   Weight (pounds) × 705 divided by height (inches) = BMI

Case Studies

Case Study 1

1. *What questions should the nurse ask this patient?* Ask the patient to describe any heartburn, indigestion, abdominal discomfort, or pain. Explore where the pain is located, what type of pain it is, when it occurs, what foods aggravate and relieve it, and how it is relieved. Abdominal pain is often referred to other sites. Ask the patient whether the pain more intense before or after he eats. Ask whether the pain is associated with positioning. Ask what makes the pain better or worse. Ask what the patient did to relieve the pain and whether those methods worked.

2. *Epigastric pain can be associated with what disorders?* A patient with a liver disorder may experience pain over the right shoulder (Kehr's sign). Epigastric (middle upper abdominal) pain may be a sign of acute gastritis, obstruction of the small intestine, or acute pancreatitis. Pain in the right upper quadrant is associated with cholecystitis. Pain in the left upper quadrant may be related to a gastric ulcer.

3. *The patient has been scheduled for an esophagogastroduodenoscopy. What are the nurse's responsibilities regarding caring for this patient?* The patient's dentures and eyeglasses should be removed. The patient should be not allowed to eat food or drink fluids for six to eight hours prior to the procedure. The patient should be informed that the procedure takes 20–30 minutes and that a local anesthetic will be administered to his throat to help prevent discomfort. After the procedure, the patient is allowed to eat and drink as soon as he can safely swallow. The patient may experience mild bloating, belching, or flatulence after the procedure. The patient should be instructed to contact the physician post-examination for difficulty swallowing; epigastric, substernal or shoulder pain; fever; or black tarry stools or if he is vomiting blood.

Case Study 2

1. *Mr. Parsons states, "It seems as though my problems with constipation have gotten worse as I have gotten older." How should the nurse respond?* The patient

should be educated about how aging affects the gastrointestinal system. The large intestine produces less mucus. The elasticity of the wall of the rectum decreases. There is a loss of tone in the internal sphincter with decreased awareness of need to defecate. All of these factors increase the patient's risk for developing constipation.

2. *What could result from frequent bouts of constipation?* External hemorrhoids may develop.

3. *What radiographic study may be performed to assess Mr. Parsons' rectum and colon?* Barium enema

Short Answers

The nurse is assessing a patient who is experiencing malnutrition. Complete the table by identifying the expected assessment findings.

Body System	Assessment Findings
Nails	Soft and spoon-shaped with iron deficiency. Splinter hemorrhages with vitamin C deficiency.
Hair	Dry, dull, and scarce in zinc, protein, and linoleic acid deficiencies.
Skin	Flaky and dry in vitamin A, vitamin B, and/or linoleic acid deficiency. Cracks and/or hyperpigmentation in niacin deficiency. Bruising in vitamin C or vitamin K deficiency.
Eyes	Dry and soft with decrease in vitamin A. Pale conjunctiva with a decrease in iron; red conjuctiva with a decrease in riboflavin.
Nervous system	Decreased reflexes and possible peripheral neuropathies with thiamine deficiency. Possible irritability and/or disorientation with thiamine deficiency.
Musculoskeletal system	Muscle wasting with deficits in protein, carbohydrate, and fat metabolism. Calf pain with thiamine deficiency; possible joint pain with vitamin C deficiency.
Cardiovascular system	Possible increase in heart size and rate with thiamine deficiency. Possible increase in diastolic blood pressure with a high intake of fat. Possible lowered cardiac output and decreased blood pressure with caloric deficiencies over a long time period.
GI system	Cheilosis (sores at corner of the mouth) in vitamin B-complex deficiencies, especially riboflavin. Possible stomatitis and spongy, bleeding gums in malnutrition.

NCLEX-RN® Review Questions

1. Answer: 1
   Rationale: Nutrients from food begin absorption in the duodenum, and absorption continues through the

small bowel. While the patient will absorb nutrients through the remaining small bowel, the amount of loss will determine the body's ability to compensate. Water is absorbed in both the large and small bowel. Vitamin D is produced in the skin with exposure to sunlight. Bile is produced in the liver, stored in the gallbladder, and delivered to the small bowel. Depending on the extent of the injury, it may be important to decrease fat intake.
Nursing Process: Assessment
Patient Need: Health Promotion and Maintenance

2. Answer: 3
Rationale: The patient's body mass index should be 20–25. A BMI of 18 is too low and indicates that the patient is malnourished. The patient's triceps skinfold thickness should be greater than 125 mm. The patient's midarm muscle circumference should be greater than 253 mm. The patient's midarm circumference should be greater than 293 mm.
Nursing Process: Assessment
Patient Need: Physiological Integrity

3. Answer: 3
Rationale: This is a normal assessment finding. The liver may be enlarged and can be percussed in an area lower than the costal margin in patients with hepatitis, cirrhosis, or venous congestion of the liver.
Nursing Process: Assessment
Patient Need: Physiological Integrity

4. Answer: 2
Rationale: To determine that a patient's bowel sounds are absent, the nurse must listen for five minutes in each quadrant. It could take up to 20 minutes to completely assess all quadrants for bowel sounds. Bowel sounds are most active in the lower right quadrant, and the activity may vary from one quadrant to another. The bowel sounds can normally be heard after 5–15 seconds of auscultation. High-pitched, tinkling, or rushing bowel sounds are associated with diarrhea or at the onset of a bowel obstruction.
Nursing Process: Assessment
Patient Need: Physiological Integrity

5. Answer: 2
Rationale: When the patient becomes dehydrated, the patient may develop vertical fissures on the tongue. Cheliosis are painful lesions that occur at the corners of the mouth and can be associated with a riboflavin or niacin deficiency. Atrophic smooth glossitis is characterized by a bright red tongue. It is seen in B_{12}, folic acid, and iron deficiencies. Black, hairy tongues can be found in patients who have recently taken antibiotics.
Nursing Process: Assessment
Patient Need: Physiological Integrity

6. Answer: 2
Rationale: The nurse should inspect the abdomen as the first step of the assessment. The second step is to auscultate the abdomen. The abdomen should then be percussed. The abdomen is palpated last.

Nursing Process: Assessment
Patient Need: Physiological Integrity

7. Answer: 2
Rationale: The advanced practice nurse will insert a gloved and lubricated finger slowly into the patient's anus. The nurse should point the finger toward the patient's umbilicus to assess the patient' rectum. The nurse should not point the finger toward the descending colon, the right lung, or the liver because these actions may result in pain or discomfort.
Nursing Process: Assessment
Patient Need: Safe, Effective Care Environment

Chapter 22

Terms Matching
1. G
2. L
3. P
4. R
5. A
6. M
7. Q
8. J
9. B
10. K
11. O
12. D
13. E
14. N
15. H
16. C
17. I
18. F

Focused Study
1. Obesity, an excess of adipose tissue, is one of the most prevalent, preventable health problems in the United States. Obesity occurs when excess calories are stored as fat. It can result from excess energy intake, decreased energy expenditure, or a combination of both. However, the etiology of obesity is not as simple as excess kilocalorie intake in relation to energy expenditure. The systems that regulate food intake, energy storage, and energy expenditure are complex and not fully understood. Obesity has serious physiological and psychologic consequences and is associated with increased morbidity and mortality. It contributes to poor health-related quality of life to a greater extent than do smoking, excess alcohol use, or poverty. The obesity epidemic has prompted rapid growth in bariatrics, the healthcare science that focuses on patients who are extremely obese.

   Obesity is a major health risk factor, increasing the risk of mortality from all causes over that of normal-weight people. As obesity increases, so does the risk of dying.

Cardiovascular Disease. Obesity is a significant risk factor, for hypertension, coronary heart disease (CHD), and heart failure. The prevalence of hypertension in obese men and women is approximately twice that in people with a BMI of less than 25 (NHLBI, 1998). Several factors contribute to hypertension in obese individuals, including sodium retention with associated increased vascular resistance, blood volume, and cardiac output. The increases in blood pressure seen with obesity increase the risk for CHD and stroke.

Patients who are obese, particularly those who have abdominal obesity, often have a lipid profile that promotes atherosclerosis. Levels of low-density lipoprotein (LDL) and very low-density lipoprotein (VLDL) cholesterol and triglycerides are increased, and levels of high-density lipoprotein (HDL or desirable) cholesterol are reduced. Furthermore, adipose tissue secretes cytokines that stimulate the liver to produce C-reactive protein (CRP), now recognized as a risk factor for CHD.

These factors account for the fact that many obese individuals have *metabolic syndrome,* a constellation of cardiovascular risk factors, including increased waist circumference, hypertension, elevated blood triglycerides and fasting blood glucose, and low HDL cholesterol. The metabolic syndrome is an identified risk factor for atherosclerosis and CHD.

Obesity also increases the risk for heart failure. Left ventricular muscle mass increases, and the ventricle dilates in obese individuals, possibly related to increased blood volume and cardiac output.

Respiratory Disorders. Being overweight and obese increase the risk for developing asthma in both adults and children. The relationship between obesity and asthma is not clear but may be related to genetic factors and the connection between obesity and inflammation. Obesity is the major risk factor for obstructive sleep apnea, intermittent airflow obstruction due to upper airway collapse during sleep. As obesity is a risk factor for sleep apnea, the reverse also may be true: Sleep apnea may predispose patients for weight gain (NHLBI, 2004).

Diabetes Mellitus. Obesity increases the risk of insulin resistance and type 2 diabetes. While not all obese people develop diabetes, up to 80% of people with type 2 diabetes are obese. Weight gain in adulthood and abdominal (central) obesity are positively correlated with the risk of developing type 2 diabetes (Fauci et al., 2008).

Other Disorders. Obesity affects reproductive function in both men and women. Androgen (male sex hormone) levels are reduced in obese men; menstrual irregularities and polycystic ovarian syndrome (PCOS) are more common in obese women. PCOS is an additional risk factor for hyperinsulinemia and insulin resistance. Increased weight also increases the risk for gallstones in men

and women. The risk for developing several types of cancer, including colon, breast, and endometrial, increases in obesity. Increased weight places abnormal stress on joints, increasing the prevalence of joint pain and osteoarthritis, particularly in weight-bearing joints (especially the knee joints).

2. The most common bariatric surgical procedures are adjustable gastric band, gastric bypass, gastric sleeve, and biliopancreatic bypass with duodenal switch. These procedures restrict stomach capacity, limiting food intake, and in most cases bypass a portion of the small intestine to restrict absorption of calories and nutrients. In many cases, they can be performed laparoscopically.

In the Roux-en-Y gastric bypass (RGB), a small stomach pouch is created to restrict food intake. A Y-shaped section of the jejunum is then attached to the pouch to allow food to bypass the lower stomach and duodenum. As a result, calorie and nutrient absorption is limited. The biliopancreatic diversion (BPD) is a more complex procedure that carries a higher risk of nutritional deficiencies. This surgery may be performed in two stages, with the majority of the stomach removed and a gastric sleeve created during the first stage. In BPD, the duodenum and jejunum are bypassed by connecting the ileum directly to the stomach pouch or just distal to the pyloric valve.

Surgeries that restrict nutrient intake and absorption produce rapid weight loss that is maintained over time. Many patients maintain a significant weight loss for 10 years or more, with improvement in obesity-associated health problems such as type 2 diabetes, hypertension, and sleep apnea. Because these procedures allow food to bypass the duodenum and jejunum, nutrient deficiencies are common, particularly deficiencies of iron, calcium, vitamin B_{12}, and possibly the fat-soluble vitamins.

Restrictive procedures such as adjustable gastric banding (AGB) are safer but generally less effective in the long term. In AGB, a hollow band of silicone rubber is placed around the upper (proximal) portion of the stomach. The band is inflated with saline solution to create a small stomach pouch with a narrow passage through to the rest of the stomach. The amount of band inflation can be adjusted using a port implanted under the skin. Few nutritional deficiencies are associated with restrictive bariatric procedures. Vomiting is a common postoperative risk with restrictive procedures. The band may slip or break, necessitating a return to surgery. While patients typically lose about 50% of their excess body weight within the first year after these procedures, fewer maintain that weight loss over a 10-year period than those who undergo gastric bypass.

3. The manifestations of malnutrition may vary among patients. Weight loss is the most apparent manifestation: The malnourished patient may have a body weight of less than 90% of ideal. Body mass also is reduced, as is skinfold thickness. Other manifestations include a wasted appearance, dry and

brittle hair, and pale mucous membranes. Peripheral or abdominal edema may be present. Older adults may show general symptoms of frailty, including weakness, slow walking speed, low physical activity level, unintentional weight loss, and exhaustion.

4. Anorexia nervosa typically begins during middle to late adolescence. Patients with anorexia nervosa have a distorted body image and irrational fear of gaining weight. Refusal to maintain body weight at or above a minimally normal level for height and body type is a common manifestation of anorexia nervosa. Patients maintain weight loss through restricted calorie intake, often accompanied by excessive exercise. Some may exhibit binge–purge behavior.

Bulimia nervosa develops in late adolescence or early adulthood. Unlike patients with anorexia nervosa, the weight of patients with bulimia is within or above the normal range. Like anorexia nervosa, however, the likely cause is multifactorial, including cultural, psychosocial, and biologic factors. The patient with bulimia often restricts caloric intake, leading to increased hunger and overeating. Foods consumed during a binge often are high-calorie, high-fat, and sweet. After binge eating, the patient induces vomiting (usually by stimulating the gag reflex) or may take excessive quantities of laxatives or diuretics. Fluid and electrolyte balance may be severely disrupted by loss of fluid and gastrointestinal secretions.

Case Study

1. *What psychosocial factors may have contributed to Ms. Spencer's eating disorder?* Depression, anxiety, or a personality disorder
2. *What diagnostic studies may be ordered to assess Ms. Spencer's nutritional status?* There is no specific diagnostic test for binge-eating disorder (BED). In patients with BED, the blood glucose and lipid levels may be elevated. The BMI usually is above the normal range and may identify the patient as obese or morbidly obese. A mental health evaluation is indicated for patients with eating disorders to identify contributing factors and to help direct treatment.
3. *What treatments are instituted for patients with a binge-eating disorder?* Treatment for patients with binge-eating disorder focuses on establishment of healthy eating patterns, psychosocial therapy (including cognitive-behavioral therapy and group counseling) to address underlying issues, and management of obesity and its complications. Patients with BED also may benefit from an SSRI or another antidepressant drug.
4. *What role can Ms. Spencer's family play in assisting her to be successful with her treatment regimen?* Involvement of the family and social support people is vital to success. Encourage family members to participate in teaching and nutritional counseling sessions. Discuss the value of family therapy to address issues that have contributed to the disorder.

Emphasize the need to provide consistent messages of support for healthy eating habits. Discuss using rewards for food and calorie intake rather than weight gain. Provide referrals to a dietitian, a nutritional support team, counseling, and support groups for people with eating disorders.

Short Answers

Fill in the table regarding nutritional deficiencies. Identify assessment data related to each nutritional deficiency listed.

Deficiency	Assessment Data
Calorie	Weight loss
	Weakness, listlessness
	Loss of subcutaneous fat
	Muscle wasting
Protein	Thin or sparse hair
	Flaking skin
	Hepatomegaly
Vitamin A	Night blindness
	Altered taste and smell
	Dry, scaling, rough skin
Thiamine	Confusion, apathy
	Cardiomegaly, dyspnea
	Muscle cramping and wasting
	Paresthesias, neuropathy
	Ataxia
Riboflavin	Cheilosis, stomatitis
	Neuropathy, glossitis
Vitamin C	Swollen, bleeding gums
	Delayed wound healing
	Weakness, depression
	Easy bruising
Iron	Smooth tongue
	Listlessness, fatigue
	Dyspnea

NCLEX-RN® Review Questions

1. Answer: 4
   Rationale: Obesity is defined as excess adipose tissue and a BMI greater than 30 kg/m^2.
   Nursing Process: Assessment
   Patient Need: Physiological Integrity
2. Answer: 1
   Rationale: Physical inactivity is probably the most important factor contributing to obesity.
   Nursing Process: Assessment
   Patient Need: Health Promotion and Maintenance

3. Answer: 2

Rationale: A low HDL cholesterol is not a manifestation of metabolic syndrome. The following are manifestations of metablic syndrome: increased waist circumference, hypertension, elevated blood triglycerides and fasting blood glucose, and low HDL cholesterol.

Nursing Process: Assessment

Patient Need: Physiological Integrity

4. Answer: 4

Rationale: The adverse effects of Xenical® (orlistat) relate to its inhibition of fat absorption: oily stools, flatulence, and fecal urgency.

Nursing Process: Implementation

Patient Need: Safe, Effective Care Environment

5. Answer: 2

Rationale: In the Roux-en-Y gastric bypass (RGB), a small stomach pouch is created to restrict food intake. A Y-shaped section of the jejunum is then attached to the pouch to allow food to bypass the lower stomach and duodenum. As a result, calorie and nutrient absorption is limited.

Nursing Process: Assessment

Patient Need: Physiological Integrity

6. Answer: 2

Rationale: A gradual, slow weight loss of no more than 1–2 pounds per week is recommended. Researchers have found that most overweight people are stimulated to eat by external cues, such as the proximity to food and the time of day. In contrast, hunger and satiety are the cues that regulate eating in adults of normal weight. Strategies to control food cues include keeping food out of view, eliminating snack foods, and eating only in designated areas. A well-balanced food menu is appropriate in a weight reduction plan. Laboratory values should be monitored for nutritional deficiencies.

Nursing Process: Implementation

Patient Need: Safe, Effective Care Environment

7. Answer: 2

Rationale: The manifestations of malnutrition may vary among patients. Weight loss is the most apparent manifestation: The malnourished patient may have a body weight of less than 90% of ideal. Body mass also is reduced (see Box 22–1), as is skinfold thickness. Other manifestations include a wasted appearance, dry and brittle hair, and pale mucous membranes. Peripheral or abdominal edema may be present. Older adults may show general symptoms of frailty, including weakness, slow walking speed, low physical activity level, unintentional weight loss, and exhaustion.

Nursing Process: Assessment

Patient Need: Physiological Integrity

8. Answer: 2

Rationale: When given separately, fat emulsions may be administered through a peripheral vein or via the same intravenous catheter as parenteral nutrition (PN).

PN solutions are always administered with an infusion pump to ensure the correct rate of infusion.

Nursing Process: Implementation

Patient Need: Safe, Effective Care Environment

9. Answer: 3

Rationale: Dumping syndrome, which can be precipitated by a meal high in simple carbohydrates, may develop following gastric bypass surgeries. In dumping syndrome, stomach contents move rapidly through the small intestine, drawing fluid into the intestine by osmosis. The patient experiences nausea, bloating, abdominal pain, weakness, sweating, and possibly syncope.

Nursing Process: Assessment

Patient Need: Physiological Integrity

Chapter 23

Terms Matching

1. D
2. I
3. JJ
4. A
5. X
6. U
7. N
8. LL
9. L
10. Q
11. V
12. T
13. BB
14. F
15. P
16. Z
17. HH
18. H
19. S
20. J
21. FF
22. DD
23. MM
24. K
25. II
26. G
27. M
28. W
29. Y
30. AA
31. EE
32. E
33. C
34. GG
35. KK
36. O
37. CC
38. B
39. R

Focused Study

1. Patients who are 65 years old and older; are immunocompromised; have been diagnosed with heart failure or chronic renal failure; have had chemotherapy, radiation therapy, or a stem cell transplant; receive oxygen; breathe frequently through the mouth; receive certain medications (antibiotics, phenytoin, anticholinergics, corticosteroids); have poor oral hygiene or ill-fitting dentures; use alcohol or tobacco

2. The patient may develop the following problems in the oral cavity: leukoplakia; erythroplakia; ulcers; masses; brown or black pigmented areas; fissures; or asymmetry of the head, face, jaw, or neck.

3. Patients with peptic ulcer disease may experience nighttime ulcer pain, which typically occurs between 1 AM and 3 AM. This can disrupt the patient's sleep cycle and result in inadequate rest. Anticipation of pain may lead to insomnia or other sleep disruptions. The patient should be educated about the importance of taking medications as ordered. The patient may be prescribed a proton pump inhibitor or H_2-receptor blocker that can be used to minimize the production of hydrochloric acid at night. The patient should be educated about the importance of limiting food intake following the evening meal because eating before bed can stimulate the production of gastric acid and pepsin, increasing the likelihood of nighttime pain. The patient should be encouraged to use relaxation techniques and comfort measures to promote sleep. Once the pain associated with PUD has been controlled, these measures help reduce anxiety and reestablish a normal sleep pattern.

4. Patients with acute and chronic gastritis are typically managed in community settings. The patient requires acute care only when nausea and vomiting are severe enough to interfere with normal fluid and electrolyte balance and nutritional status. If a hemorrhage occurs, surgical intervention may be required. Acute gastritis is usually diagnosed in the history and clinical presentation. The vague symptoms of chronic gastritis may require more extensive diagnostic testing.

Case Study

1. *What role does Mr. Hess's age, smoking history, and ibuprofen use play in his peptic ulcer disease?* Duodenal ulcers are the most common type of peptic ulcer disease. They usually develop in patients who are between the ages of 30 and 55. Duodenal ulcers are more commonly found in men than in women. Ulcers are also more common in people who smoke and who are chronic users of NSAIDs.

2. *Why might Mr. Hess be screened for* H. pylori *infection?* H. pylori infection is found in about 50% of people who have peptic ulcer disease. *H. pylori* contributes to gastric epithelial cell damage without producing immunity to the infection. This may be related to the increased gastric acid production that is associated with *H. pylori* infection.

3. *As the nurse assesses Mr. Hess, what are some expected findings regarding his description of symptoms?* The nurse would expect to learn that Mr. Hess describes his pain as gnawing, burning, aching, or hungerlike and that it occurs in the epigastric region, sometimes radiating to the back. Mr. Hess may report heartburn or regurgitation and may vomit. The nurse would monitor the patient for clinical manifestations associated with bleeding, such as weakness, fatigue, dizziness, and orthostatic hypotension.

4. *Describe the clinical manifestations Mr. Hess may experience if he develops the most lethal complication of peptic ulcer disease.* The most lethal complication of peptic ulcer disease is perforation of the ulcer through the mucosal wall. When an ulcer perforates, the patient has immediate, severe upper abdominal pain that radiates throughout the abdomen and possibly to the shoulder. The abdomen becomes rigid and boardlike, with absent bowel sounds. Signs of shock may be present, including diaphoresis, tachycardia, and rapid and shallow respirations.

5. *Mr. Hess's physician has prescribed lansoprazole (Prevacid®). How should the nurse educate Mr. Hess regarding how he should take this medication?* He should take the drug as ordered for the full course of therapy even if symptoms are relieved. He should not crush, break, or chew tablets. He should increase his calcium intake or take a calcium supplement while using this drug because it can interfere with calcium absorption. He should avoid cigarette smoking, alcohol, aspirin, and NSAIDs while taking this drug because they may interfere with healing. He should report to his physician any episodes of black, tarry stools; diarrhea; or abdominal pain.

6. *During the nurse's assessment of Mr. Hess, he begins to hemorrhage. What are some clinical manifestations the nurse may discover with this?* Mr. Hess states that he has blood in his stool, or the nurse is able to find occult blood in his stool. He may begin to vomit blood or become fatigued, weak, or dizzy. He develops orthostatic hypotension and eventually hypovolemic shock.

7. *What are several nursing diagnoses the nurse may use when developing Mr. Hess's plan of care?* Deficient Fluid Volume related to acutely bleeding duodenal ulcer; *Risk for Injury* related to acute blood loss; *Fear* related to threat to well-being; *Ineffective Self-Health Management* related to lack of knowledge regarding pud and its treatment

Care Plan Critical-Thinking Activity

1. The nurse should educate Mr. Chavez about the dangers of smoking cigarettes. Smoking cigarettes is a primary risk factor for developing oral cancer. The first component of treatment is eliminating any causative factors. The nurse should refer Mr. Chavez to a smoking cessation clinic or program.

2. Oral surgery can interfere with communication. Effective communication is vital to postoperative

recovery and prevention of complications. Before surgery, the nurse should establish and practice a communication plan such as using a magic slate or flash cards. The nurse should provide ample time for communication efforts and should not answer for the patient. The nurse should watch for nonverbal communication. The nurse should use yes/no questions and simple phrases. The nurse may need to refer Mr. Chavez to or consult with a speech therapist.

3. The patient denies any complaints of heart palpitations, muscle weakness and tension, nausea, chest pain, or dyspnea. The patient is not demonstrating any diaphoresis, pallor, dilated pupils, or trembling.

Short Answers

Fill in the table. Identify the pathophysiology associated with each clinical manifestations of GERD.

Manifestation	Pathophysiology *Suggested answers are provided.*
Heartburn *Chest pain* *Regurgitation* *Belching*	Reflux of gastric juices through the lower esophageal sphincter into the lower esophagus exposes esophageal mucosa to corrosive pepsin, acid, and bile. Gastric juices normally are cleared by esophageal peristalsis or are neutralized by saliva; when these mechanisms are impaired, esophageal mucosa becomes inflamed and may eventually ulcerate. Further exposure of the inflamed and ulcerated mucosa to corrosive gastric juices leads to heartburn or angina-like or atypical chest pain.
Dysphagia	Untreated esophagitis leads to inflammatory cell infiltrates, fibrosis, and scarring of esophageal tissue, constricting its lumen and causing difficult, painful swallowing.
Pain after eating	Increased gastric volume increases pressure in the stomach relative to the ability of the lower esophageal sphincter to prevent reflux into the esophagus. Reflux irritates already inflamed tissue, causing pain.
Chronic cough *Hoarseness* *Laryngitis,* *pharyngits*	Reflux of gastric contents into the pharynx and mouth allows aspiration of gastric contents into the tracheobronchial tree. This usually occurs during sleep, when a recumbent position increases gastroesophageal reflux and relaxation of tissues and muscles in the oropharynx increases the risk of aspiration.

NCLEX-RN® Review Questions

1. **Answer: 2**
   Rationale: The upper lip is not a common site for oral cancers to develop. The most common sites are the tongue, lower lip, and floor of the mouth.
   Nursing Process: Diagnosis
   Patient Need: Health Promotion and Maintenance

2. **Answer: 3**
   Rationale: If the patient will not be able to verbally communicate with the staff after surgery, have a writing tablet with pens or a picture menu ready at the bedside for the patient to use for communication. Recording questions preoperatively does not allow for all of the situations and questions that may arise after surgery. Having a spokesperson available for the patient at all times is not feasible, and the spokesperson may not be able to interpret the patient's needs anyway. Providing cell phone numbers of staff will not aid a patient who cannot speak.
   Nursing Process: Planning
   Patient Need: Safe, Effective Care Environment

3. **Answer: 1**
   Rationale: A barium enema is performed to diagnose diseases of the colon. Diagnostic studies that may be performed for gastroesophageal reflux disease (GERD) include a 24-hour ambulatory pH monitoring, a barium swallow, and an upper gastrointestinal endoscopy.
   Nursing Process: Planning
   Patient Need: Health Promotion and Maintenance

4. **Answer: 1**
   Rationale: There are two types of esophageal tumors, adenocarcinoma and squamous cell carcinoma. Over the past two decades, the incidence of squamous cell tumors of the esophagus has been decreasing. Basal cell, epithelial cell, and stratus cell are not causes of esophageal cancer.
   Nursing Process: Assessment
   Patient Need: Health Promotion and Maintenance

5. **Answer: 1**
   Rationale: Hyperkalemia is not a complication of vomiting. Potential complications of vomiting include dehydration, hypokalemia, metabolic alkalosis (from loss of hydrochloric acid from the stomach), aspiration with resulting pneumonia, and rupture or tears of the esophagus.
   Nursing Process: Planning
   Patient Need: Health Promotion and Maintenance

6. **Answer: 4**
   Rationale: Ginger, an aromatic root that is frequently used in cooking, may be helpful in relieving nausea and vomiting, particularly when they are due to motion sickness. Anise, catmint, and sage are not known to relieve nausea and vomiting due to motion sickness.
   Nursing Process: Implementation
   Patient Need: Health Promotion and Maintenance

7. Answer: 2

Rationale: To prevent dumping syndrome, liquids and solids should not be mixed at meal time, but consumed separately. The patient must eat smaller, more frequent meals throughout the day. Protein must be increased in the diet, while sugars should be decreased.

Nursing Process: Evaluation

Patient Need: Health Promotion and Maintenance

Chapter 24

Terms Matching

1. D
2. F
3. V
4. J
5. T
6. N
7. L
8. Q
9. X
10. G
11. R
12. O
13. B
14. C
15. H
16. A
17. K
18. U
19. P
20. S
21. M
22. W
23. I
24. E

Focused Study

1. Lack of exercise; bedrest; low-fiber foods; highly refined foods; inadequate fluid intake; antacids that contain aluminum or calcium salts; narcotic analgesics; anticholinergics; many antidepressants, tranquilizers, and sedatives; many antihypertensives; iron salts; diverticular disease; inflammatory diseases; tumor; obstruction; changes in rectal or anal structure or function; voluntary suppression of urge to have bowel movement; perceived need to defecate on schedule; depression; advanced age; pregnancy; trauma; multiple sclerosis; cerebrovascular accident; Parkinsonism; hypothyroidism; hypercalcemia; uremia; porphyria

2. Peritonitis: diffuse or localized pain, rebound tenderness, abdomen that becomes rigid and boardlike, diminished or absent bowel sounds, distended abdomen, anorexia, nausea, vomiting

   Systemic infection due to peritonitis: fever, malaise, tachycardia, tachypnea, confused, disoriented, oliguria

3. Medications: antibiotics (oral or intravenous), stool softeners. Nutrition: high-fiber diet, bulk-forming products, avoidance of seeds, bowel rest during an acute episode. Surgery: treatment of peritonitis or abscess that hasn't responded to medical treatment, control of hemorrhage, bowel resection, two-stage Hartmann's procedure

4. Adenomatous polyps, tubular adenomas (pedunculated polyps), villous adenomas (sessile polyps)

   Most of the time, polyps are asymptomatic. They are often found coincidentally during a routine examination or during diagnostic testing. The most common presenting complaint is intermittent painless rectal bleeding that is bright or dark red. A large polyp may cause abdominal cramping, pain, or manifestations of obstruction. Diarrhea and mucus discharge may be associated with a large villous adenoma.

Case Study

1. *Where is McBurney's point located?* McBurney's point is located midway between the umbilicus and the anterior iliac crest in the right lower quadrant.

2. *What are possible complications of untreated appendicitis?* Potential complications of untreated appendicitis include local peritonitis, abscess, and generalized peritonitis.

3. *What diagnostic studies may be used to diagnose appendicitis?* The following diagnostic studies will likely be performed: CBC, chemistry profile, urinalysis, abdominal ultrasound, abdominal x-rays, WBC with differential, intravenous pyelogram, urinalysis, and pelvic examination.

4. *Prior to an appendectomy, what medications may be ordered for Ms. Bowman?* Intravenous fluids restore or maintain vascular volume and prevent electrolyte imbalance. Antibiotics such as third-generation cephalosporin are used to kill gram-negative bacteria. Examples include cefoperazone (Cefobid®), cefotaxime (Claforan®), ceftazidime (Fortaz®), and ceftriaxone (Rocephin®). Pain medications are administered as prescribed.

5. *Ms. Bowman undergoes an appendectomy. What should the nurse's postoperative teaching include?* Teaching topics should include wound care instructions, symptoms of infection that need to be reported to the healthcare provider, activity limitations, abdominal splinting technique, and at what point the patient may return to work.

6. *What two nursing diagnoses might the nurse use in Ms. Bowman's plan of care following surgery?* Suggested answers: *Impaired Skin Integrity* related to surgical incision, *Acute Pain* related to surgical intervention, *Anxiety* related to situational crisis

Short Answers

Fill in the table. Note whether the laboratory value will be "increased," "decreased," or "within normal limits" when the patient has been experiencing severe diarrhea.

Test

Normal Value	Change with Severe Diarrhea
Serum osmolality	
280–300 mOsm/kg	Increased
Serum potassium	
3.5–5.3 mEq/L	Decreased
Serum sodium	
135–145 mEq/L	Decreased
Serum chloride	
95–105 mEq/L	Increased when sodium loss is greater than chloride loss; decreased with severe diarrhea and vomiting
Blood gases	
pH	
Arterial: 7.35–7.45	Decreased (metabolic acidosis)
PCO_2	
Arterial: 35–45 mmHg	Decreased (metabolic acidosis)
Bicarbonate	
24–28 mEq/L	Decreased (metabolic acidosis)
Hematocrit	
Males: 40%–54%	Increased
Females: 36%–46%	Increased
Urine specific gravity 1.005–1.030	Increased

NCLEX-RN® Review Questions

1. Answer: 2
   Rationale: Managing diarrhea involves teaching the patient to eat small, frequent meals; drink electrolyte solutions such as Gatorade®; limit food intake during acute episodes; and avoid foods high in fiber, milk products, and caffeine.
   Nursing Process: Implementation
   Patient Need: Health Promotion and Maintenance

2. Answer: 3
   Rationale: The patient would demonstrate understanding of teaching about managing constipation by following a diet high in fiber including prunes. The patient should add more fluids to his or her diet and exercise daily. Drinking a glass of warm water before breakfast helps stimulate peristalsis.
   Nursing Process: Evaluation
   Patient Need: Health Promotion and Maintenance

3. Answer: 1
   Rationale: An abdominal ultrasound is the most effective diagnostic study for diagnosing acute appendicitis. An abdominal x-ray, an intravenous pyelogram, and a urinalysis can be used to diagnose acute appendicitis, but none of them provide as much information as an abdominal ultrasound.

Nursing Process: Assessment
Patient Need: Safe, Effective Care Environment

4. Answer: 1
   Rationale: Urine output of less than 30 mL/hr may indicate hypovolemia, decreased cardiac output, and impaired tissue perfusion.
   Nursing Process: Assessment
   Patient Need: Physiological Integrity

5. Answer: 4
   Rationale: *Salmonellosis* is a food poisoning caused by ingesting raw or improperly cooked meat, eggs, and dairy products. Manifestations of *salmonellosis* develop 8–48 hours after ingestion. *Shigellosis* is caused by the *shigella* organism and is transferred via the fecal–oral route through contaminated food. Its incubation period is 1–4 days. Travelers' diarrhea develops when traveling to another country and is caused by a difference in climate, sanitation standards, food, or drink. Cholera is diarrhea caused by *Vibrio cholerae* found in contaminated food and water.
   Nursing Process: Assessment
   Patient Need: Health Promotion and Maintenance

6. Answer: 3
   Rationale: Amebiasis is an infection that affects the cecum, appendix, ascending colon, sigmoid colon, and rectum. Giardiasis is a protozoal infection of the proximal small intestine. Helminths are parasitic worms capable of causing bowel infections. Coccidiosis secretes an enterotoxin that causes watery diarrhea.
   Nursing Process: Assessment
   Patient Need: Health Promotion and Maintenance

7. Answer: 2
   Rationale: The patient with IBD must increase fluid intake to 2–3 quarts of liquids per day. The patient should add nutritional supplements such as Ensure® and vitamins to his diet. The patient must adhere to the prescribed medication regimen as ordered by the physician. Participation in smoking cessation classes can help the patient manage IBD.
   Nursing Process: Evaluation
   Patient Need: Health Promotion and Maintenance

8. Answer: 4
   Rationale: Patients with celiac disease are placed on gluten-free diets. The patient must add calories and protein to his or her diet to correct nutritional deficits. The patient must avoid fats and lactose.
   Nursing Process: Implementation
   Patient Need: Health Promotion and Maintenance

Chapter 25

Terms Matching
1. C
2. F
3. H
4. L
5. J
6. W

7. Q
8. N
9. S
10. U
11. D
12. E
13. P
14. A
15. O
16. G
17. M
18. R
19. T
20. V
21. B
22. K
23. I

Focused Study

1. Increased age, family history of gallstones, Native American, Northern European heritage, obesity, hyperlipidemia, rapid weight loss, female, use of oral contraceptives, pregnancy, fasting, prolonged parenteral nutrition, diabetes mellitus, cirrhosis, ileal disease or resection, and sickle cell anemia

2. Normally, when red blood cells are destroyed, hemoglobin is released. The hemoglobin molecule breaks up into globin, a protein, and heme, the iron-containing portion of the molecule. In this process, biliverdin, later converted to fat-soluble bilirubin, is released. The bilirubin binds with albumin to be transported to the liver. In the liver, it is converted to a water-soluble form that can be excreted by the body. When the process of metabolizing and excreting bilirubin is disrupted, bilirubin accumulates in the patient's tissues, which leads to jaundice. There are three types of jaundice: hemolytic, hepatic, and obstructive.

3. Chronic pancreatitis: recurrent epigastric and left upper quadrant (LUQ) pain, which radiates to back; anorexia; nausea and vomiting; weight loss; flatulence; constipation; steatorrhea. Acute pancreatitis: abrupt onset of severe epigastric and LUQ pain, which may radiate to back; nausea; vomiting; fever; decreased bowel sounds; abdominal distention and rigidity; tachycardia; hypotension; cold, clammy skin; possible jaundice; positive Turner's sign or Cullen's sign

4.
   • Educate the patient about the relationship between fat intake and the pain. Teach the patient ways to reduce fat intake. Rationale: Fat entering the duodenum initiates gallbladder contractions, causing pain when gallstones are present in the ducts.
   • Withhold oral food and fluids during episodes of acute pain. Insert nasogastric tube and connect to low suction if ordered. Rationale: Emptying the stomach reduces the amount of chyme entering the duodenum and the stimulus for gallbladder contractions, thus reducing pain.

   • Administer morphine, meperidine, or other narcotic analgesia as ordered for severe pain. Rationale: Recent research indicates that morphine is no more likely than meperidine to cause spasms of the sphincter of Oddi.
   • Place patient in Fowler's position. Rationale: Fowler's position decreases pressure on the inflamed gallbladder.

Case Study

1. *What role does Mr. Wales's past medical history play in his current episode of acute pancreatitis?* Alcoholism and gallstones are the primary risk factors for the development of acute pancreatitis. Gallstones may obstruct the pancreatic duct or cause bile reflux, activating pancreatic enzymes in the pancreatic duct system. Alcohol causes duodenal edema and may increase pressure and spasm in the sphincter of Oddi, obstructing pancreatic outflow. It also stimulates pancreatic enzyme production, thus increasing pressure in the pancreas.

2. *What clinical manifestations are associated with acute pancreatitis?* Mr. Wales will likely present with the following manifestations: acute onset of severe epigastric and left upper abdominal pain that may radiate to his back, nausea, vomiting, abdominal distention, abdominal rigidity, decreased bowel sounds, increased heart rate, hypotension, fever, cold and clammy skin, mild jaundice, retroperitoneal bleeding, Turner's sign, or Cullen's sign.

3. *The nurse is monitoring Mr. Wales for the development of complications related to acute pancreatitis. What are some complications of acute pancreatitis?* Systemic complications of acute pancreatitis include intravascular volume depletion with shock, acute tubular necrosis and renal failure, and acute respiratory distress syndrome (ARDS). Localized complications include pancreatic necrosis, abscess, pseudocysts, and pancreatic ascites.

4. *What is one common nursing diagnosis that is associated with acute pancreatitis?* Fatigue and Imbalanced Nutrition: Less Than Body Requirements.

5. *The nurse reviews Mr. Wales's laboratory results. Which laboratory results does the nurse expect to be abnormal?* Serum amylase (may be elevated), serum lipase (may be elevated), urine amylase (may be elevated), serum glucose (may be elevated), serum bilirubin (may be elevated), serum alkaline phosphatase (may be elevated), serum calcium (may be decreased), and white blood cells (may be elevated).

6. *Describe discharge teaching the nurse should provide for Mr. Wales.*
   • Alcohol can cause stones to form, blocking pancreatic ducts and the outflow of pancreatic juice. Continued alcohol intake is likely to cause further inflammation and destruction of the pancreas. Mr. Wales should avoid alcohol entirely.
   • Smoking and stress stimulate the pancreas and should be avoided.

- If pancreatic function has been severely impaired, discuss appropriate use of pancreatic enzymes, including timing, dose, potential side effects, and monitoring of effectiveness.
- A low-fat diet is recommended for Mr. Wales. Provide a list of high-fat foods to avoid. Crash dieting and binge eating also should be avoided as they may precipitate attacks. Spicy foods, coffee, tea, colas, and gas-forming foods stimulate gastric and pancreatic secretions and may precipitate pain.
- Mr. Wales should report any signs or symptoms of infection (fever of 102°F or more, pain, rapid pulse, malaise) because a pancreatic abscess can develop after initial recovery.

Care Plan Critical-Thinking Activity

1. Native Americans have a higher incidence of gallstones than do Caucasians. This is thought to result from the Native Americans' genetic makeup that has been responsible for promoting efficient calorie and fat storage.
2. Mrs. Red Wing should be educated about the importance of reducing her dietary intake of high-fat foods and eating a low-carbohydrate, low-fat, higher-protein diet. She can be referred to a dietician or nutritionist to promote healthy weight loss and reduce episodes of pain. It is important to assess her nutritional status, diet history, height and weight, and skin fold measurement. Patients with cholelithiasis often have imbalanced diets and vitamin deficiencies. The nurse should evaluate Mrs. Red Wing's laboratory results (serum bilirubin, albumin, glucose, and cholesterol levels). She should take vitamin supplements as ordered. She likely has difficulty absorbing fat-soluble vitamins.

Short Answers

Fill in the blanks regarding the various types of viral hepatitis.

NCLEX-RN® Review Questions

1. Answer: 1
   Rationale: Most gallstones (80%) consist primarily of cholesterol. The rest contain a mixture of bile components.
   Nursing Process: Planning
   Patient Need: Health Promotion and Maintenance
2. Answer: 4
   Rationale: Diarrhea is not a clinical manifestation typically associated with acute cholecystitis. Manifestations of acute cholecystitis include anorexia, nausea, vomiting, fever, and right upper quadrant pain.
   Nursing Process: Assessment
   Patient Need: Physiological Integrity
3. Answer: 1
   Rationale: Patients with abnormal liver function studies and impaired consciousness with mental status changes are experiencing portal systemic encephalopathy. Portal systemic encephalopathy is the accumulation of toxic waste products in the blood as blood bypasses the congested liver and is not filtered. Ascites is the accumulation of fluid in the peritoneal cavity. Hepatorenal syndrome is acute renal failure caused by the disruption of blood flow to the kidneys. Splenomegaly is the enlargement of the spleen.
   Nursing Process: Diagnosis
   Patient Need: Physiological Integrity
4. Answer: 1
   Rationale: Hepatitis A and B are preventable because vaccines are available. No vaccine is available for hepatitis D, C, and E.
   Nursing Process: Planning
   Patient Need: Health Promotion and Maintenance
5. Answer: 4
   Rationale: *Altered Body Image* related to bruising would be an unexpected nursing diagnosis for the patient with liver trauma. Nursing diagnoses for

Virus	Hepatitis A (HAV)	Hepatitis B (HBV)	Hepatitis C (HCV)	Hepatitis D (HDV)	Hepatitis E (HEV)
Mode of transmission	Fecal–oral	Blood and body fluids; perinatal	Blood and body fluids	Blood and body fluids; perinatal	Fecal–oral
Incubation (in weeks)	2–6	6–25	5–12	3–13	3–6
Onset	Abrupt	Slow	Slow	Abrupt	Abrupt
Carrier state	No	Yes	Yes	Yes	Yes
Possible complications	Rare	Chronic hepatitis	Chronic hepatitis	Chronic hepatitis	May be severe in pregnant women
		Cirrhosis	Cirrhosis	Cirrhosis	
		Liver cancer	Liver cancer	Fulminant hepatitis	
Laboratory findings	Anti-HAV antibodies present	Positive HBsAg (HBV surface antigen); anti-HBV antibodies present	Anti-HCV antibodies present	Positive HDVAg (delta antigen) early; anti-HDV antibodies later	Anti-HEV antibodies present

patients with liver trauma include the following: *Deficient Fluid Volume* related to hemorrhage, *Risk for Infection* related to wound or abdominal contamination, and *Risk for Bleeding* related to impaired coagulation.

Nursing Process: Diagnosis

Patient Need: Physiological Integrity

6. Answer: 2

Rationale: Following a low-fat diet is not a known risk factor for developing pancreatic cancer. Some risk factors for developing pancreatic cancer include consuming a high-fat diet, being exposed to industrial chemicals or environmental toxins, having chronic pancreatitis or diabetes mellitus, and smoking.

Nursing Process: Assessment

Patient Need: Health Promotion and Maintenance

Chapter 26

Terms Matching

1. E
2. H
3. I
4. F
5. D
6. A
7. J
8. G
9. C
10. B

Focused Study

1. The organs of the renal system are the paired kidneys, the paired ureters, the urinary bladder, and the urethra.

Kidneys
- The kidneys are located outside the peritoneal cavity on either side of the vertebral column at the levels of T_{12} through L_3.
- These highly vascular bean-shaped organs are approximately 4.5 inches (11.4 cm) long and 2.5 inches (6.4 cm) wide.
- Each kidney contains approximately 1 million nephrons, which process the blood to make urine.

Ureters
- These bilateral tubes are approximately 10–12 inches (26–30 cm) long.
- They transport urine from the kidney to the bladder through peristaltic waves originating in the renal pelvis.

Urinary bladder
- The bladder is posterior to the symphysis pubis and serves as a storage site for urine.
- In males, the bladder lies immediately in front of the rectum; in females, the bladder lies in front of the vagina and the uterus.

Urethra
- This thin-walled muscular tube channels urine outside the body.

- In females, the urethra is approximately 1.5 inches (3–5 cm) long and the urinary meatus is anterior to the vaginal orifice. In males, the urethra is approximately 8 inches (20 cm) long and serves as a channel for semen as well as urine.

2.

- A urinalysis (UA) is an examination of the constituents of a sample of urine to establish a baseline, to provide data for diagnosis, or to monitor results of treatment through normal findings and abnormal findings.
- Blood urea nitrogen measures urea, the end product of protein metabolism. Increased levels may result from dehydration, vomiting, diarrhea, digested blood, or prerenal/renal failure.
- Creatinine (serum) is used to diagnose kidney dysfunction. Creatinine is a by-product of the breakdown of muscle and is excreted by the kidneys. When 50% or more nephrons are destroyed, serum creatinine levels rise.
- A creatinine clearance test is a 24-hour urine test used to identify renal dysfunction and to monitor renal function.
- Cystatin C is a blood test that may be used as an alternative to creatinine and creatinine clearance to screen for and monitor kidney dysfunction in people suspected of having kidney diseases. Cystatin C is a cysteine proteinase inhibitor that is filtered by the kidneys; increased concentrations in the blood indicate kidney dysfunction.
- A CT scan of the kidneys is a radiological scan that allows for evaluation of kidney size, tumors, abscesses, suprarenal masses, and obstructions. A contrast dye may be administered orally or injected intravenously, allowing increased visualization of the density of renal tissue and masses in comparison to an ultrasound.
- A cystometrogram (CMG) (voiding cystogram) evaluates bladder capacity and neuromuscular functions of the bladder, urethral pressures, and causes of bladder dysfunction. A measured quantity of fluid is instilled into the bladder, and the filling capacity and voiding pressures are measured.
- A cystoscopy (cystogram) and cystography provide direct visualization of the bladder wall and urethra through use of a cystoscope. During the procedure, small renal calculi can be removed from the ureter, bladder, or urethra and tissue biopsy can be done. It also permits determination of the cause of hematuria or UTI.
- Measured GFR is considered the most accurate means of detecting changes in kidney function. Because the GFR is a complicated measurement to obtain, an estimated GFR (eGFR) can be used. The eGFR is calculated based on the serum creatinine, age, gender, and (in some instances) racial origin.
- An intravenous pyelogram (IVP) is a radiological examination done to visualize the entire renal tract to identify abnormal size, shape, and function of the kidneys or to detect renal calculi (stones), tumors,

or cysts. A radiopaque substance is injected intravenously, and a series of x-rays are taken.

- An MRI of the kidneys is used to visualize the kidneys by assessing computer-generated films of radiofrequency waves and changes in magnetic fields.
  - A portable ultrasonic bladder scan is used to obtain information about residual urine. Warmed ultrasound gel is applied over the lower abdomen, and the ultrasound probe is placed just above the pubic bone. The scanner shows an outline of the bladder and displays the amount of urine in the bladder in milliliters.
  - A renal arteriogram or angiogram is a radiological test used to visualize renal blood vessels to detect renal artery stenosis; renal thrombosis; or an embolism, tumors, cysts, or an aneurysm. It also is used to determine the causative factor for hypertension and to evaluate renal circulation.
  - A renal biopsy is performed to determine the cause of renal disease, to rule out cancer metastasis to the kidney, or to determine whether rejection is occurring with a kidney transplant. It is performed with a cystoscope, excising a wedge of kidney tissue, or through the skin with a biopsy needle (percutaneous route).
  - A renal scan evaluates kidney blood flow, location, size, and shape and assesses kidney perfusion and urine production.
  - A renal ultrasound is a noninvasive test conducted to detect masses, identify obstructions, and diagnose renal cysts. It is done by applying a conductive gel to the skin and placing a small external ultrasound probe on the patient's skin.
  - Residual urine (postvoiding residual urine) is a test that measures the amount of urine left in the bladder after voiding.
3. Each kidney contains approximately 1 million nephrons, which process the blood to make urine. The kidneys process about 180 L (47 gal) of blood-derived fluid each day. Of this amount, only 1% is excreted as urine; the rest is returned to circulation. Urine formation is accomplished entirely by the nephron through three processes: glomerular filtration, tubular reabsorption, and tubular secretion.
   - Glomerular filtration is a passive process in which forces push fluid and solutes through a membrane. The rate of filtration is controlled by hydrostatic pressure and osmotic pressure.
   - Tubular reabsorption is a process that begins as filtrate enters the proximal tubules. These tubules regulate the rate and degree of water and ion reabsorption in response to hormonal signals.
   - Tubular secretion is the final process in urine formation. Substances move from the blood into the tubules as filtrates. Tubular secretion is important for disposing of substances not already in the filtrate, such as medications. This process eliminates undesirable substances that have been reabsorbed by passive processes and rids the body of excessive potassium ions. It is also a vital force in the regulation of blood pH.

Case Study

1. *Explain the functions of the kidney.* The functions of the kidney are to form urine; balance solute and water transport; excrete metabolic waste products; conserve nutrients; regulate acid–base balance; and secrete hormones to help regulate blood pressure, erythrocyte production, and calcium metabolism.
2. *What could tenderness and pain on percussion of the costovertebral angle suggest?* Tenderness and pain on percussion of the costovertebral angle could suggest glomerulonephritis or glomerulonephrosis.
3. *What could pallor of the skin and mucous membranes indicate?* Pallor of the skin and mucous membranes may indicate kidney disease with resulting anemia.

Crossword Puzzle

question	term answer
The functional unit of the kidney	NEPHRON
Channels urine from the kidney to the bladder	URETER
Acts on a plasma globulin, angiotensinogen, to release angiotensin I, which in turn is converted to angiotensin II	RENIN
The substance necessary for the absorption of calcium	VITAMIND
The color of normal urine	STRAW
Milky urine is the result of this	PYURIA
The by-product of muscle breakdown that is excreted by the kidney	CREATININE
The test used to directly visualize the bladder wall	CYSTOSCOPY
Urine remaining in the bladder after voiding	RESIDUAL

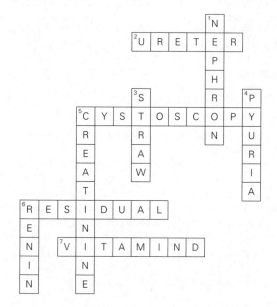

NCLEX-RN® Review Questions

1. Answer: 4

   Rationale: Urine may be discolored as a result of medication therapies. Medications that may be associated with orange urine include phenazopyridine (Pyridium®), amidopyrine, nitrofurantoin, sulfonamides and on rarer occasions due to iron supplements. Sexual activity is not linked to orange urine. Dietary factors may be noted with orange-colored urine. Saturated fats are not associated with orange-colored urine. Dietary intake high in carrots, beets, or food colorings are associated with this color change.

   Nursing Process: Implementation

   Patient Need: Physiological Integrity

2. Answer: 1

   Rationale: The functions of the kidney are to form urine; balance solute and water transport; excrete metabolic waste products; conserve nutrients; regulate acid–base balance; and secrete hormones to help regulate blood pressure, erythrocyte production, and calcium metabolism.

   Nursing Process: Assessment

   Patient Need: Physiological Integrity

3. Answer: 1

   Rationale: Glomerular filtration is a passive, nonselective process in which hydrostatic pressure forces fluid and solutes through a membrane. The amount of fluid filtered from the blood into the capsule per minute is called the glomerular filtration rate (GFR). Three factors influence this rate: the total surface area available for filtration, the permeability of the filtration membrane, and the net filtration pressure. The glomerulus is a far more efficient filter than most capillary beds because the filtration membrane of the glomerulus is more permeable to water and solutes than are other capillary membranes.

   Nursing Process: Assessment

   Patient Need: Physiological Integrity

4. Answer: 1

   Rationale: Urine is composed, by volume, of about 95% water and 5% solutes. The largest component of urine by weight is urea. Other solutes normally excreted in urine include sodium, potassium, phosphate, sulfate, creatinine, uric acid, calcium, magnesium, and bicarbonate.

   Nursing Process: Assessment

   Patient Need: Physiological Integrity

5. Answer: 2

   Rationale: Vitamin D is necessary for the absorption of calcium and phosphate by the small intestine. The stimulus for the production of erythropoietin by the kidneys is decreased oxygen delivery to kidney cells. Erythropoietin stimulates the bone marrow to produce red blood cells in response to tissue hypoxia. Hormones that are activated or synthesized by the kidneys include the active form of vitamin D, erythropoietin, and natriuretic hormone.

   Nursing Process: Assessment

   Patient Need: Physiological Integrity

6. Answer: 1

   Rationale: The layers of the bladder wall (from internal to external) are the epithelial mucosa lining the inside, the connective tissue submucosa, the smooth muscle layer, and the fibrous outer layer. The muscle layer, called the detrusor muscle, consists of fibers arranged in inner and outer longitudinal layers in a middle circular layer. This arrangement allows the bladder to expand and contract according to the amount of urine it holds.

   Nursing Process: Assessment

   Patient Need: Physiological Integrity

7. Answer: 2

   Rationale: The urinary bladder is posterior to the symphysis pubis and serves as a storage site for urine. In males, the bladder lies immediately in front of the rectum; in females, the bladder lies in front of the vagina and the uterus. The size of the bladder varies with the amount of urine it contains. In healthy adults, the bladder holds about 300–500 mL of urine before internal pressure rises and signals the need to empty the bladder through micturition (also called urination and voiding). However, the bladder can hold more than twice that amount if necessary. Openings for the ureters and the urethra are inside the bladder.

   Nursing Process: Assessment

   Patient Need: Physiological Integrity

8. Answer: 4

   Rationale: Oliguria means voiding scant amounts of urine. Hematuria means blood in the urine. Nocturia means excessive urination at night. Polyuria means voiding excessive amounts of urine.

   Nursing Process: Assessment

   Patient Need: Physiological Integrity

9. Answer: 4

   Rationale: The ketone level should be negative. The color of urine should be light straw to amber yellow. The pH range is 4.5–8.0. WBCs should be 3–4.

   Nursing Process: Assessment

   Patient Need: Physiological Integrity

Chapter 27

Terms Matching

1. F
2. K
3. P
4. J
5. N
6. A
7. S
8. B
9. E
10. R
11. O
12. D

13. L
14. U
15. V
16. M
17. H
18. C
19. Q
20. G
21. I
22. T

Focused Study

1. Surgery may be indicated for recurrent UTI if diagnostic testing indicates calculi, structural anomalies, or strictures that contribute to the risk of infection. Stones, or calculi, in the renal pelvis or in the bladder are an irritant and provide a matrix for bacterial colonization. Treatment may include surgical removal of a large calculus from the renal pelvis or cystoscopic removal of bladder calculi. Percutaneous ultrasonic pyelolithotomy or extracorporeal shock wave lithotripsy may be used instead of surgery to crush and remove stones.

   Ureteroplasty, surgical repair of a ureter, may be indicated for structural abnormality or stricture of a ureter. This may be combined with a ureteral reimplantation if vesicoureteral reflux is present. The patient returns from these surgeries with an indwelling urinary catheter (Foley or suprapubic) and a ureteral stent (a thin catheter inserted into the ureter to provide for urine flow and ureteral support), which remains in place for three to five days.

   A number of surgical procedures, ranging from simple resection of noninvasive tumors to removal of the bladder and surrounding structures, are used to treat urinary tract tumors. Transurethral tumor resection may be performed by excision, *fulguration* (destruction of tissue using electric sparks generated by a high-frequency current), or *laser photocoagulation* (use of light energy to destroy abnormal tissue). Laser surgery carries the lowest risk of bleeding and perforation of the bladder wall. Following cystoscopic tumor resection, patients are checked at three-month intervals for tumor recurrence. Recurrences may develop anywhere in the urinary tract, including the renal pelvis, ureter, or urethra.

   Cystectomy, surgical removal of the bladder, is necessary to treat invasive cancers. Partial cystectomy may be done to remove a solitary lesion; however, radical cystectomy is the standard treatment for invasive tumors. The bladder and adjacent muscles and tissues are removed. In men, the prostate and seminal vessels are also removed, resulting in impotence. In women, a total hysterectomy and bilateral salpingo-oophorectomy (removal of the uterus, fallopian tubes, and ovaries) accompanies the procedure, causing sterility. At the time of surgery, a urinary diversion is created to provide for urine collection and drainage.

   Surgical procedures to remove tumors involving other portions of the urinary tract vary according to the site and stage of the tumor. When the distal ureter is involved, the tumor may be resected and the ureter implanted into the opposite ureter to provide for drainage. A proximal ureteral tumor necessitates removal of the ureter and kidney on the affected side.

   Surgery may be required when urination cannot be effectively managed using more conservative measures. *Rhizotomy*, or destruction of the nerve supply to the detrusor muscle or the external sphincter, may be used for patients with hyperreflexia or spasticity. Urinary diversion is another surgical technique used when conservative management fails. Implantation of an artificial sphincter may be useful for some patients with neurogenic bladder.

   Surgery may be used to treat stress incontinence associated with cystocele or urethrocele and overflow incontinence associated with an enlarged prostate gland.

   Suspension of the bladder neck, a technique that brings the angle between the bladder and urethra closer to normal, is effective in treating stress incontinence associated with urethrocele in 80%–95% of patients. A laparoscopic, vaginal, or abdominal approach may be used to perform this surgery.

   Prostatectomy, using either the transurethral or suprapubic approach, is indicated for the patient who is experiencing overflow incontinence as a result of an enlarged prostate gland and urethral obstruction.

   Other surgical procedures of potential benefit in the treatment of incontinence include implantation of an artificial sphincter, formation of a urethral sling to elevate and compress the urethra, and augmentation of the bladder with bowel segments to increase bladder capacity.

2.
   - Intravenous pyelography (IVP) is used to evaluate for structural or functional abnormalities, such as vesicoureteral reflux of the kidneys, ureters, and bladder.
   - Voiding cystourethrography may be ordered to detect structural or functional abnormalities of the bladder and urethral strictures. This test has a lower risk of allergic response to the contrast dye than does IVP.
   - Cystoscopy may be used to diagnose conditions such as prostatic hypertrophy, urethral strictures, bladder calculi, tumors, polyps or diverticula, and congenital abnormalities. A tissue biopsy may be obtained during the procedure and other interventions performed (for example, stone removal or stricture dilation).
   - Manual pelvic or prostate examinations are done to assess for structural changes of the genitourinary tract, such as prostatic enlargement, cystocele, or rectocele.

3. *Urinary Tract Infection:* Pathogens usually enter the urinary tract by ascending from the mucous membranes of the perineal area into the lower urinary

tract. Bacteria that have colonized the urethra, vagina, or perineal tissues are the usual source of infection (Porth & Matfin, 2009). From the bladder, bacteria may continue to ascend the urinary tract, eventually infecting the *parenchyma* (functional tissue) of the kidneys. Hematogenous spread of infection to the urinary tract is rare. Infections introduced in this manner are usually associated with previous damage or scarring of the urinary tract. Bacteria introduced into the urinary tract may cause asymptomatic bacteriuria or an inflammatory response with manifestations of UTI. Asymptomatic bacteriuria is commonly found in pregnant women, the elderly, and patients with diabetes mellitus or patients who have an indwelling urinary catheter (Lin & Fajardo, 2008).

Urinary tract infections can be categorized in several ways. Anatomically, UTIs may affect the lower or upper urinary tract. Lower urinary tract infections include *urethritis*, inflammation of the urethra; *prostatitis*, inflammation of the prostate gland; and *cystitis*, inflammation of the urinary bladder. The most common upper urinary tract infection is pyelonephritis, inflammation of the kidney and renal pelvis. The infection may involve superficial tissues such as the bladder mucosa or may invade other tissues such as prostate or renal tissues. Epidemiologically, UTIs are identified as community-acquired or catheter-associated.

Urinary Calculi: Three factors contribute to urolithiasis: supersaturation, nucleation, and lack of inhibitory substances in the urine.

When the concentration of an insoluble salt in the urine is very high (that is, when the urine is supersaturated), crystals may form. Usually, these crystals disperse and are eliminated because the bonds holding them together are weak. However, a nucleus of crystals may develop stable bonds to form a stone. More often, crystals form around an organic matrix, or mucoprotein nucleus, to become a stone. The stimulus required to initiate crystallization in supersaturated urine may be minimal. Ingesting a meal high in insoluble salt or decreased fluid intake as occurs during sleep allows the concentration to increase to the point where precipitation occurs and stones are formed and grow. When fluid intake is adequate, no stone growth occurs. The acidity or alkalinity of the urine and the presence or absence of calculus-inhibiting compounds also affect lithiasis.

Most kidney stones (70%–80%) are *calcium stones*, composed of calcium oxalate and/or calcium phosphate. These stones are generally associated with high concentrations of calcium in the blood or urine. *Uric acid stones* develop when the concentration of uric acid in urine is high. They are more common in men and may be associated with gout. Genetic factors contribute to the development of uric acid stones and calcium stones. *Struvite* (magnesium ammonium phosphate) *stones* are associated with UTI caused by urease-producing bacteria such as *Proteus*. These stones can grow to become very large, filling the renal pelvis and calyces. They often are called *staghorn stones* because of their shape. *Cystine stones* are rare and are associated with a genetic defect.

Urinary Tract Tumor: Most urinary tract malignancies arise from epithelial tissue. Transitional epithelium lines the entire tract from the renal pelvis through the urethra. Carcinogenic breakdown products of certain chemicals and from cigarette smoke are excreted in the urine and stored in the bladder, possibly causing a local influence on abnormal cell development. Squamous cell carcinoma of the urinary tract occurs less frequently than transitional epithelial cell tumors.

Urinary tract tumors begin as nonspecific cellular alterations that develop into flat or papillary lesions. These lesions may be either superficial or invasive. Most bladder tumors are papillary lesions (*papillomas*), a polyplike structure attached by a stalk to the bladder mucosa. Papillomas are generally superficial, noninvasive tumors that bleed easily and frequently recur (Fauci et al., 2008). They rarely progress to become invasive, and the prognosis for recovery is good.

Urinary Retention: Either mechanical obstruction of the bladder outlet or a functional problem can cause urinary retention. *Benign prostatic hypertrophy (BPH)* is a common cause; difficulty initiating and maintaining urine flow is often the presenting complaint in men with BPH. Fecal impaction may be a contributing factor in urinary retention, particularly in older adults and immobile patients. Acute inflammation associated with infection or trauma of the bladder, the urethra, or perineal tissues may also interfere with micturition. Scarring due to repeated urinary tract infection can lead to urethral stricture and a mechanical obstruction. Bladder calculi may also obstruct the urethral opening from the bladder.

Surgery, particularly abdominal and pelvic surgery, may disrupt detrusor muscle function, leading to urine retention. Drugs also may interfere with its function. Anticholinergic medications such as atropine, glycopyrrolate (Robinul®), propantheline bromide (Pro-Banthine®), and scopolamine hydrochloride (Transderm-Scōp®) can lead to acute urinary retention and bladder distention. Many other drug groups have anticholinergic side effects and may cause urinary retention. Among these are antianxiety agents such as diazepam (Valium®), antidepressant and tricyclic drugs such as imipramine (Tofranil®), antiparkinsonian drugs, antipsychotic agents, and some sedative/hypnotic drugs. In addition, antihistamines common in over-the-counter cough, cold, allergy, and sleep-promoting drugs have anticholinergic effects and may interfere with bladder emptying. Diphenhydramine (Benadryl®) is an example of a nonprescription antihistamine.

Voluntary urinary retention (particularly common among nurses!) may lead to overfilling of the bladder and a loss of detrusor muscle tone.

Neurogenic Bladder: Bladder filling and emptying are controlled by the central nervous system (CNS). This neurologic control can be disrupted at any level: the cerebral cortex (voluntary impulses), the micturition center of the midbrain, the spinal cord tracts, or the peripheral nerves of the bladder itself.

Urinary Incontinence: Urinary continence requires input from the CNS, a bladder able to expand and contract, and sphincters that maintain a urethral pressure higher than that in the bladder. Intact cognition, mobility, motivation, and manual dexterity also are necessary to maintain continence. Mechanically, incontinence results when the pressure in the urinary bladder exceeds urethral resistance, allowing urine to escape. Any condition causing higher-than-normal bladder pressure or reduced urethral resistance may result in incontinence. Relaxation of the pelvic musculature, disruption of cerebral and nervous system control, and disturbances of the bladder and its musculature are common contributing factors.

Incontinence may be an acute, self-limited disorder, or it may be chronic. The causes may be congenital or acquired, reversible or irreversible. Congenital disorders associated with incontinence include *epispadias* (absence of the upper wall of the urethra) and *meningomyelocele* (a neural tube defect in which a portion of the spinal cord and its surrounding meninges protrude through the vertebral column). CNS or spinal cord trauma, stroke, and chronic neurologic disorders such as multiple sclerosis and Parkinson's disease are examples of acquired, irreversible causes of incontinence. Reversible causes include acute confusion, medications such as diuretics and sedatives, prostatic enlargement, vaginal and urethral atrophy, UTI, and fecal impaction.

Incontinence is commonly categorized as stress incontinence, urge incontinence (also known as overactive bladder), overflow incontinence, and functional incontinence. Table 27–7 summarizes each type with its physiological cause and associated factors. *Mixed incontinence*, with elements of both stress and urge incontinence, is common. *Total incontinence* is loss of all voluntary control over urination, with urine loss occurring without stimulus and in all positions. Incontinence is associated with an increased risk for falls, fractures, pressure ulcers, urinary tract infection, and depression. It contributes to the stress of caregivers and often is a factor in institutionalizing the patient.

4. **Female**
   - Short, straight urethra
   - Proximity of urinary meatus to vagina and anus
   - Sexual intercourse
   - Use of diaphragm and spermicidal compounds for birth control
   - Pregnancy

Male
   - Uncircumcision
   - Prostatic hypertrophy

Both Female and Male
   - Aging
   - Urinary tract obstruction
   - Neurogenic bladder dysfunction
   - Vesicoureteral reflux
   - Genetic factors
   - Catheterization
   - Anal intercourse

Case Study

1. *Explain cystitis.* Cystitis, inflammation of the urinary bladder, is the most common UTI. The infection tends to remain superficial, involving the bladder mucosa. The mucosa becomes hyperemic (red) and may hemorrhage. The inflammatory response causes pus to form. This process causes the classic manifestations associated with cystitis. Typical presenting symptoms of cystitis include dysuria (painful or difficult urination), urinary frequency and urgency (a sudden, compelling need to urinate), and nocturia (voiding two or more times at night). In addition, the urine may have a foul odor and appear cloudy (*pyuria*) or bloody (hematuria) because of mucus, excess white cells in the urine, and bleeding of the inflamed bladder wall. Suprapubic pain and tenderness also may be present.

2. *What can occur if cystitis is left untreated?* Cystitis is usually uncomplicated and readily responds to treatment. When left untreated, however, the infection can ascend to involve the kidneys. Severe or prolonged infection may lead to sloughing of bladder mucosa and ulcer formation. Chronic cystitis can lead to bladder stones.

3. *Why does cystitis occur more frequently in adult females?* Cystitis in adult females usually results from colonization of the bladder by bacteria normally found in the lower gastrointestinal tract. These bacteria gain entry by ascending the short, straight female urethra. In addition to the risk factors listed on page 784, personal hygiene practices and voluntary urinary retention can contribute to the risk for UTI in women.

4. *List the manifestations of cystitis.*
   - Dysuria
   - Pyuria
   - Frequency
   - Hematuria
   - Urgency
   - Suprapubic discomfort
   - Nocturia

Short Answers

Fill in the table regarding manifestations of acute pyelonephritis. Give examples of each.

Urinary	Systemic
Urinary frequency	Vomiting
Dysuria	Diarrhea
Pyuria	Acute fever
Hematuria	Shaking chills
Flank pain	Malaise
Costovertebral tenderness	

NCLEX-RN® Review Questions

1. **Answer: 4**
   Rationale: Catheter-associated UTIs often involve other gram-negative bacteria such as *Proteus*, *Klebsiella*, *Serratia*, and *Pseudomonas*. UTI affects approximately 12.8 million women (13.3%) in the United States annually. The incidence of UTI in men is significantly lower, affecting about 2 million men (2.3%) annually. Community-acquired urinary tract infections (UTIs) are common in young women and are unusual in men under the age of 50. Most community-acquired UTIs are caused by *Escherichia coli*, a common gram-negative enteral bacteria.
   Nursing Process: Evaluation
   Patient Need: Health Promotion and Maintenance

2. **Answer: 1**
   Rationale: The anatomic area below the urethra is not sterile. The remaining statements are correct.
   Nursing Process: Evaluation
   Patient Need: Physiological Integrity

3. **Answer: 2**
   Rationale: Stress incontinence is the loss of urine associated with increased intra-abdominal pressure during sneezing, coughing, or lifting. Quantity of urine lost is usually small. Urge incontinence is the involuntary loss of urine. Overflow incontinence is the inability to empty the bladder, resulting in overdistention and frequent loss of small amounts of urine. Functional incontinence results from physical, environmental, or psychosocial causes.
   Nursing Process: Assessment
   Patient Need: Physiological Integrity

4. **Answer: 1**
   Rationale: The correct statement is "These drugs are used along with hygiene practices to prevent recurrent urinary tract infection (UTI). Take as directed, even when no symptoms are present." The following is a list of health education information for the patient and family in regards to anti-infectives.
   • Drink six to eight glasses of water or fluid per day while taking these drugs.
   • Take the drug with meals or food to reduce gastric effects; however, avoid milk products because they may interfere with absorption.
   • Trimethoprim should not be taken during pregnancy. Contact your physician before attempting to become pregnant.
   • Contact your doctor if you develop any of the following symptoms: chest pain, difficulty breathing, cough, chills, and fever; numbness and tingling or weakness of the extremities; rash or pruritus (itching).
   • If you are taking an oral suspension of nitrofurantoin, rinse your mouth thoroughly after each dose to avoid staining the teeth.
   • Nitrofurantoin turns the urine brown. This is not harmful and subsides when the drug is discontinued.
   • If you are taking trimethoprim along with phenytoin (Dilantin®) or a related anticonvulsant, contact your doctor if you become sedated or begin to stagger.
   Nursing Process: Evaluation
   Patient Need: Health Promotion and Maintenance

5. **Answer: 1**
   Rationale: Nursing care for the patient with urolithiasis is directed at providing for comfort during acute renal colic, assisting with diagnostic procedures, ensuring adequate urinary output, and teaching the patient information necessary to prevent future stone formation.
   • Collect and strain all urine, saving any stones.
   • Report stone passage to the physician and bring the stone in for analysis.
   • Report to physician any changes in the amount or character of urine output.
   • Increase fluid intake to 2500–3500 mL per day.
   • Follow recommended dietary guidelines.
   • Maintain activity level to prevent urinary stasis and bone resorption.
   • Take medications as prescribed.
   Nursing Process: Planning
   Patient Need: Health Promotion and Maintenance

6. **Answer: 2**
   Rationale: An estimated 70,980 new cases of bladder cancer were diagnosed in the United States in 2009, and 14,330 people died as a result of the disease. The incidence of bladder cancer is nearly four times higher in men than it is in women and about twice as high in white men as it is in black men (ACS, 2009). Cigarette smoking is the primary risk factor for bladder cancer. Most people who develop bladder cancer are over age 60.
   Nursing Process: Assessment
   Patient Need: Health Promotion and Maintenance

7. **Answer: 2**
   Rationale: The following table identifies possible food and fluid modifications with regard to uroliathisis.

Foods high in oxalate	Asparagus, beer and colas, beets, cabbage, celery, chocolate and cocoa, fruits, green beans, nuts, tea, tomatoes

Purine-rich foods	Goose, organ meats, sardines and herring, venison; moderate consumption of beef, chicken, crab, pork, salmon, veal
Acidifying foods	Cheese, cranberries, eggs, grapes, meat and poultry, plums and prunes, tomatoes, whole grains
Alkalinizing foods	Legumes, green vegetables, rhubarb, fruit (except as noted above), flour, milk and milk products

Nursing Process: Planning
Patient Need: Health Promotion and Maintenance

8. Answer: 4
Rationale: It is inappropriate to apply the bag with an opening no more than 3–4 mm wider than the outside of the stoma. All of the following are appropriate when providing urinary stoma care:
 • Gather all supplies: a clean, disposable pouch; a liquid skin barrier or barrier ring; 4×4 gauze squares; a stoma guide; an adhesive solvent; clean gloves; and a clean washcloth.
 • Assess knowledge, learning needs, ability, and willingness to assist with procedure. Explain the procedure as needed.
 • Use standard precautions.
 • Remove old pouch, pulling it away from the skin gently. Use warm water or adhesive solvent to loosen the seal if necessary.
 • Assess the stoma. Normally, the stoma is bright red and appears moist. Report a dark purple, black, or very pale stoma to the physician. Slight bleeding with cleansing is normal, especially in the immediate postoperative period.
 • Prevent urine flow during cleaning by placing a rolled gauze square or tampon over the stoma opening.
 • Cleanse skin around the stoma with soap and water, rinse, and pat or air-dry.
 • Use the stoma guide to determine the correct size for the bag opening and/or protective ring seal. Trim the bag or seal as needed.
 • Apply skin barrier; allow to dry.
 • Apply the bag with an opening no more than 1–2 mm wider than the outside of the stoma. Allow no wrinkles or creases where the bag comes in contact with the skin.
 • Connect the bag to the urine-collection device. Dispose of old pouch, used supplies, and gloves appropriately. Wash hands.
 • Chart procedure, including stoma appearance and response of the patient.
Nursing Process: Implementation
Patient Need: Safe, Effective Care Environment

9. Answer: 4
Rationale: Teach measures to prevent UTI to older adults, and to all patients, particularly to young sexually active women. Encourage patients to maintain a generous fluid intake of 2.0–2.5 quarts per day, increasing intake during hot weather or strenuous activity. Decrease fluid intake after the evening meal to reduce nocturia. Discuss the need to avoid voluntary urinary retention, emptying the bladder every three to four hours. Older adults might use behavioral techniques such as scheduled toileting, habit training, and bladder training to reduce the frequency of incontinence. Instruct women to cleanse the perineal area from front to back after voiding and defecating. Teach to void before and after sexual intercourse to flush out bacteria introduced into the urethra and bladder.
Nursing Process: Planning
Patient Need: Health Promotion and Maintenance

Chapter 28

Terms Matching
1. G
2. M
3. Q
4. I
5. N
6. U
7. B
8. W
9. A
10. O
11. D
12. T
13. E
14. V
15. F
16. J
17. L
18. R
19. C
20. K
21. H
22. S
23. P

Focused Study
1. Hemodialysis uses the principles of diffusion and ultrafiltration to remove electrolytes, waste products, and excess water from the body. Blood is taken from the patient via a vascular access and is pumped to the dialyzer. The porous membranes of the dialyzer unit allow small molecules such as water, glucose, and electrolytes to pass through, but block larger molecules such as serum proteins and blood cells. The dialysate, a solution of approximately the same composition and temperature as normal extracellular fluid, passes along the other side of the membrane. Small solute molecules move freely across the membrane by diffusion. The direction of movement for any substance is determined by the concentrations of that substance in the blood and the dialysate. Electrolytes and waste products such as urea and

creatinine diffuse from the blood into the dialysate. If something must be added to the blood, such as calcium to replace depleted stores, it can be added to the dialysate to diffuse into the blood. Excess water is removed by creating a higher hydrostatic pressure of the blood moving through the dialyzer than of the dialysate, which flows in the opposite direction. This process is known as ultrafiltration.

Initially, patients with acute renal failure (ARF) typically undergo hemodialysis for three to four hours daily, then three or four sessions per week as indicated. Hemodialysis is not used if the patient is hemodynamically unstable (for example, with hypotension or low cardiac output).

Continuous Renal Replacement Therapy: Patients with ARF may be unable to tolerate hemodialysis and rapid fluid removal if their cardiovascular status is unstable (for example, due to trauma, major surgery, or heart failure). Continuous renal replacement therapy (CRRT) (also called sustained renal replacement therapy) is a hemofiltration procedure that allows more gradual fluid and solute removal. In CRRT, blood is continuously circulated through a highly porous hemofilter for a period of 8–12 or more hours. A large central catheter usually is used to provide venous access. Excess water and solutes such as electrolytes, urea, creatinine, uric acid, and glucose drain into a collection device. During CCRT, fluid is replaced with normal saline or a balanced electrolyte solution as needed. This slower process helps maintain hemodynamic stability and avoid complications associated with rapid changes in ECF composition.

CRRT is typically performed in an intensive care unit or a specialized nephrology unit. A double-lumen venous catheter is used for most types of CRRT. Strict aseptic technique is vital in caring for vascular access sites to reduce the risk of infection.

Vascular Access: Acute or temporary vascular access for hemodialysis or CRRT usually is gained by inserting a double-lumen catheter into the subclavian, jugular, or femoral vein. The double-lumen catheter has a central partition separating the blood withdrawal side of the catheter from the return side. Blood is drawn into the catheter through small openings in the proximal portion of the catheter and returned to circulation through an opening in the distal end of the catheter to avoid withdrawing the blood that has just been dialyzed.

For longer-term vascular access, an *arteriovenous (AV) fistula* is created. In preparation for fistula formation, the nondominant arm is not used for venipuncture or blood pressure measurement during renal failure. The fistula is created by surgical anastomosis of an artery and vein, usually the radial artery and cephalic vein. It takes about a month for the fistula to mature so that it can be used for taking and replacing blood during dialysis. A functional AV fistula has a palpable pulsation and a bruit on auscultation. Venipunctures and blood pressures are avoided on the arm with the fistula.

In chronic renal failure, an *arteriovenous graft* is most often used for vascular access. The graft, a tube made of Gore-Tex®, is surgically implanted and connects the artery and the vein. Blood flows through the graft from the artery to the vein. Occasionally, an *external AV shunt* connecting a peripheral artery with a peripheral vein is used for vascular access.

The rate of complications and mortality associated with catheter access is higher than that with AV fistulas or grafts. Ideally, an AV fistula or graft is created as soon as the potential need for long-term renal replacement therapies is identified. Localized AV fistula, graft, or shunt problems can occur, however. Infection and clotting, or thrombosis, are the most common shunt problems. Aneurysms may also develop. Both infection and thrombosis can lead to systemic complications such as septicemia and embolization. These local complications may cause the fistula or graft to fail, necessitating development of a new site. The psychologic impact of AV fistula or graft failure is significant, often causing depression and low self-esteem in the patient.

Peritoneal Dialysis: In peritoneal dialysis, the highly vascular peritoneal membrane serves as the dialyzing surface. Warmed sterile dialysate is instilled through a catheter and inserted into the peritoneal cavity. Metabolic waste products and excess electrolytes diffuse into the dialysate while it remains in the abdomen. Water movement is controlled using dextrose as an osmotic agent to draw it into the dialysate. The fluid is then drained out of the peritoneal cavity by gravity into a sterile bag. This process of dialysate infusion, dwell time of the solution in the abdomen, and drainage is repeated at prescribed intervals.

Because excess fluid and solutes are removed more gradually in peritoneal dialysis, compared to other dialysis procedures, it poses less risk for the unstable patient; however, this slower rate of metabolite removal can be a disadvantage in ARF. Peritoneal dialysis increases the risk for developing peritonitis. It is contraindicated for patients who have had recent abdominal surgery, significant lung disease, or peritonitis.

2. Polycystic kidney disease, a hereditary disease characterized by formation of fluid-filled cysts and massive kidney enlargement, affects both children and adults. This disease has two forms: The autosomal dominant form affects primarily adults; the autosomal recessive form is present at birth (Porth & Matfin, 2009). Autosomal recessive polycystic kidney disease is rare. It usually is diagnosed prenatally or in infancy. Renal failure generally develops during childhood, necessitating kidney transplant or dialysis. Autosomal dominant polycystic kidney disease (ADPKD) is relatively common, affecting 1 in every 400–1000 people and

accounting for approximately 4.5% of patients with ESRD in the United States (Fauci et al., 2008; NKUDIC, 2009).

3.
- Renal ultrasonography is the diagnostic procedure of choice for polycystic kidney disease.
- A computed tomography (CT) scan of the kidney may be used to detect cystic disease at an earlier stage when there is a positive family history.
- Genetic testing for ADPKD type 1 and type 2 is available and is particularly important when a family member is being considered as a potential kidney donor.

4. Risk factors for *acute renal artery thrombosis* (formation of a blood clot in the renal artery) include severe abdominal trauma, vessel trauma from surgery or angiography, aortic or renal artery aneurysms, and severe aortic or renal artery atherosclerosis. Emboli from the left side of the heart can travel via the aorta to occlude the renal artery. Emboli may form as a result of atrial fibrillation (irregular and uncoordinated electrical activity of the atria), after myocardial infarction, as vegetative growths on heart valves associated with bacterial endocarditis, or from fatty plaque in the aorta.

Case Study

1. *"Why didn't my husband have any signs or symptoms until the last few days?"* Renal tumors are often silent with few manifestations. The classic triad of symptoms—gross hematuria, flank pain, and a palpable abdominal mass—is seen in only about 10% of people with renal cell carcinoma. Hematuria, often microscopic, is the most consistent symptom. Systemic manifestations include fever without infection, fatigue, and weight loss.

2. *"What tests might the physician order to determine whether Brent has a renal tumor?"* Hematuria is often the only initial manifestation of renal cancer; its presence indicates a need for further diagnostic studies, including the following:
   - Renal ultrasonography to detect renal masses and differentiate cystic kidney disease from renal carcinoma
   - A CT scan of the abdomen to determine tumor density, local extension of the tumor, and regional lymph node or vascular involvement (Figure 28–3)
   - A chest x-ray, a bone scan, an MRI, and liver function studies to identify potential metastases

3. *"What is the treatment of choice for a renal tumor?"* Radical nephrectomy is the treatment of choice for stage I or II kidney tumors. In a radical nephrectomy, the adrenal gland, upper ureter, fat and fascia surrounding the kidney, as well as the entire kidney, are removed. Regional lymph nodes may also be resected. Although nephrectomy can be done using a laparoscopic approach, laparotomy primarily is used for radical nephrectomy.

Short Answers

List possible manifestations associated with each of the following electrolyte imbalances.

Electrolyte Imbalance	Manifestations
Hyperkalemia	Irritability
	Nausea
	Diarrhea
	Abdominal cramping
	Cardiac dysrhythmias
	ECG changes
Hyponatremia	Nausea
	Vomiting
	Headache
	Lethargy
	Confusion
	Seizure
	Coma
Hyperphosphatemia	Hyperreflexia
	Paresthesias
	Tetany

NCLEX-RN® Review Questions

1. Answer: 2, 3

   Rationale: Glomerular disorders and diseases are the leading cause of chronic kidney disease in the United States. Hematuria, proteinuria, and hypertension often are early manifestations of glomerular disorders. Acute poststreptococcal glomerulonephritis (also called acute proliferative glomerulonephritis) is the most common primary glomerular disorder. Diabetes mellitus, hypertension, and SLE are common causes of secondary glomerulonephritis

   Nursing Process: Assessment

   Patient Need: Physiological Integrity

2. Answer: 4

   Rationale: The progression to end-stage renal disease (ESRD) tends to occur more rapidly in blacks and in men. Polycystic kidney disease is slowly progressive. Symptoms usually develop by age 40 to 50. Common manifestations include flank pain, microscopic or gross hematuria (blood in the urine), proteinuria (proteins in the urine), and polyuria and nocturia because the concentrating ability of the kidney is impaired. Urinary tract infection and renal calculi are common because cysts interfere with normal urine drainage. Most patients develop hypertension from disruption of renal vessels. The kidneys become palpable, enlarged, and knobby. Symptoms of renal insufficiency and chronic renal failure typically develop by age 60 to 70.

   Nursing Process: Assessment

   Patient Need: Physiological Integrity

3. Answer: 4

   Rationale: A daily protein intake is limited to 0.6 g/kg of body weight, or approximately 40 g/day for an average male patient. Water intake of 1–2 L per day is generally recommended to maintain water balance.

Sodium is restricted to 2 g per day initially. Potassium intake is limited to less than 60–70 mEq/day (normal intake is about 100 mEq/day) (McPhee et al., 2008).

Nursing Process: Planning

Patient Need: Health Promotion and Maintenance

4. Answer: 4

Rationale: Serum triglyceride levels increase with peritoneal dialysis. For the patient who is not a candidate for renal transplantation or who has had a transplant failure, dialysis is life-sustaining. Hemodialysis for ESRD typically is done three times a week for a total of 9–12 hours. Patients on long-term dialysis have a higher risk for complications and death than does the general population.

Nursing Process: Planning

Patient Need: Health Promotion and Maintenance

5. Answer: 4

Rationale: Major trauma or surgery, infection, hemorrhage, severe heart failure, severe liver disease, and lower urinary tract obstruction are risk factors for ARF.

Nursing Process: Assessment

Patient Need: Physiological Integrity

6. Answer: 3

Rationale: Diabetes mellitus is the leading cause of CKD, followed by hypertension, glomerulonephritis, and cystic kidney disease (USRDS, 2008). The incidence of CKD and ESRD is significantly higher in people aged 65 and older. People of Hispanic origin have a higher incidence of CKD and ESRD than do non-Hispanics. Men are more likely to be affected by CKD and ESRD than are women.

Nursing Process: Evaluation

Patient Need: Health Promotion and Maintenance

7. Answer: 1

Rationale: The donor kidney is placed in the lower abdominal cavity of the recipient, and the renal artery, vein, and ureter are anastomosed. Kidney transplant improves both survival and quality of life for the patient with ESRD. Most transplanted kidneys are obtained from deceased donors; however, transplants from living donors are increasing. Hypertension is a possible complication of a kidney transplant.

Nursing Process: Evaluation

Patient Need: Health Promotion and Maintenance

8. Answer: 1

Rationale: The course of acute renal failure due to ATN typically includes three phases: initiation, maintenance, and recovery.

Nursing Process: Assessment

Patient Need: Physiological Integrity

Chapter 29

Terms Matching

1. N
2. D
3. F
4. A
5. K
6. B
7. I
8. O
9. H
10. L
11. J
12. C
13. M
14. G
15. E

Focused Study

1. The contraction and relaxation of the heart constitutes one heartbeat and is called the cardiac cycle. Ventricular filling is followed by ventricular systole, a phase during which the ventricles contract and eject blood into the pulmonary and systemic circuits. Systole is followed by a relaxation phase known as diastole, during which the ventricles refill, the atria contract, and the myocardium is perfused. Normally, the complete cardiac cycle occurs about 70–80 times per minute, measured as the heart rate.

2. The sympathetic and parasympathetic nervous systems are the primary mechanisms that regulate blood pressure. Stimulation of the sympathetic nervous system causes vasoconstriction of the arterioles and increases blood pressure. Parasympathetic stimulation causes vasodilation of the arterioles, which lowers blood pressure.

   Baroreceptors and chemoreceptors are located in the aortic arch, the carotid sinus, and other large vessels. They are sensitive to pressure and chemical changes and cause reflex sympathetic stimulation, which results in vasoconstriction, increased heart rate, and increased blood pressure.

   The kidneys help maintain blood pressure by excreting or conserving sodium and water. When blood pressure decreases, the kidneys initiate the renin–angiotensin mechanism. This results in vasoconstriction and the release of the hormone aldosterone from the adrenal cortex, increasing sodium ion reabsorption and water retention. In addition, pituitary release of antidiuretic hormone promotes renal reabsorption of water. The net result is an increase in blood volume and a consequent increase in cardiac output and blood pressure.

   Temperature may affect peripheral resistance: Cold causes vasoconstriction, and warmth produces vasodilation.

   Many chemicals, hormones, and drugs influence blood pressure by affecting cardiac output (CO) and/or pulmonary vascular resistance (PVR). For example, epinephrine causes vasoconstriction and increased heart rate; prostaglandins dilate blood vessel diameter; endothelin, a chemical released by the inner lining of vessels, is a potent vasoconstrictor;

nicotine causes vasoconstriction; and alcohol and histamine cause vasodilation.

Dietary factors such as intake of salt, saturated fats, and cholesterol elevate blood pressure by affecting blood volume and vessel diameter.

3. Red blood cells have a life span of approximately 120 days. Old or damaged red blood cells are lysed by phagocytes in the spleen, liver, bone marrow, and lymph nodes. The process of red blood cell destruction is called hemolysis. Phagocytes save and reuse amino acids and iron from heme units in the lysed red blood cells. Most of the heme unit is converted to bilirubin.

4. Ask about family members with health problems affecting the cardiovascular system, such as high blood pressure, high cholesterol levels, leukemia, or early onset coronary artery disease. Depending on the racial and ethnic background of the patient, ask about any family members with sickle cell anemia or thalassemia. During the physical assessment, assess for manifestations that may indicate a genetic disorder. If data are found to indicate genetic risk factors or alterations, ask about genetic testing and refer for appropriate genetic counseling and evaluation.

Case Study

1. *What is an electrocardiogram (ECG)?* An electrocardiogram (ECG) is a graphic record of the heart's activity. An ECG converts the electrical impulses it receives into a series of waveforms that represent cardiac depolarization and repolarization. ECG waveforms and patterns are examined to detect dysrhythmias as well as myocardial damage, the effects of drugs, and electrolyte imbalances.

2. *How are ECG waveforms recorded?* ECG waveforms are recorded by a heated stylus on heat-sensitive paper. The paper is marked at standard intervals that represent time and voltage or amplitude. Each small box is 1 mm². The recording speed of the standard ECG is 25 mm/sec, so each small box represents 0.04 second. Five small boxes horizontally and vertically make one large box, equivalent to 0.20 second. Five large boxes represent 1 full second. Measured vertically, each small box represents 0.1 millivolt (mV).

3. *The experienced nurse who works in cardiovascular testing has been asked to interpret Mr. Drake's ECG results. What six steps are used to interpret an ECG?* (1) Determine rate, (2) determine regularity, (3) assess P wave, (4) assess P to QRS relationship, (5) determine interval durations, and (6) identify abnormalities.

4. *Mr. Drake is preparing for the stress test. About what should the nurse educate Mr. Drake prior to the test?* The nurse should tell Mr. Drake to wear comfortable shoes for walking on the treadmill and to avoid food, fluids, and smoking for two to three hours before the test. The nurse should assess for events that contraindicate the tests, such as recent myocardial infarction, severe or unstable angina, controlled

dysrhythmias, congestive heart failure, or recent pulmonary embolism.

5. *During the stress test, Mr. Drake complains of chest pain. What are some common ways that patients describe chest pain?* Pressure; tightness; crushing, burning, or aching quality; heaviness; dullness; "heartburn" or indigestion

6. *With further testing, the physician determines that Mr. Drake's heart rate is 92 beats per minute and his stroke volume is 40 mL/beat. Calculate Mr. Drake's cardiac output.* Heart rate (HR) × Stroke volume (SV) = Cardiac output (CO). 92 beats per minute × 40 mL per beat = 3680 mL, or 3.68 liters per minute. The average cardiac output is 4–8 liters per minute.

7. *Mr. Drake has blood drawn to determine his lipid levels. His cholesterol is 392 mg/dL, and triglycerides are 210 mg/dL. What are normal values?* His cholesterol level should be 140–200 mg/dL, and triglycerides should be 40–190 mg/dL. His cholesterol and triglycerides levels are elevated.

Short Answers

Fill in the blanks noting the significance of each age-related change in the patient.

Age-Related Change	Significance
Myocardium: ↓ *efficiency and contractibility* *Sinus node:* ↑ *in thickness of shell surrounding the node and* ↓ *in the number of pacemaker cells*	CO decreases with physiological stress; resulting tachycardia lasts longer.
Left ventricle: Slight hypertrophy, prolonged isometric contraction phase and relaxation time; ↑ *time for diastolic filling and systolic emptying cycle*	Stroke volume may increase to compensate for tachycardia, leading to increased blood pressure.
Valves and blood vessels: Elongated and dilated aorta, thicker and more rigid valves, and increase in resistance to peripheral blood flow by 1% per year	Blood pressure increases to compensate for increased peripheral resistance and decreased CO.
Bone marrow: ↓ *ability of bone marrow to respond to need for increased RBCs, WBCs, and platelets*	Anemia may result.

Blood vessels:
Tunica intima: fibrosis, calcium and lipid accumulation, cellular proliferation
Tunica media: thins, elastin fibers calcify; increase in calcium results in stiffening. Baroreceptor function is impaired and peripheral resistance increases.

As a result of age-related changes, the systolic blood pressure rises. Decreased arterial elasticity results in vascular changes in the heart, kidneys, and pituitary gland. Decreased baroreceptor function results in postural hypotension. Vessels in the head, neck, and extremities are more prominent.

Inefficient vasoconstriction, decreased CO, and reduced muscle mass and subcutaneous tissue lead to a reduced ability to respond to cold temperatures.

With a decrease in blood pressure and changes in blood vessel walls, tissue perfusion may be inadequate, leading to edema, inflammation, pressure ulcers, and changes in effects of medications.

Immune system: Impaired function of B and T lymphocytes; ↓ *production of antibodies*

Risk for infection increases, with decreased manifestations of an actual infection.

Incidence of cancers increase.

NCLEX-RN® Review Questions

1. Answer: 3
   Rationale: The heart wall consists of three layers of tissue: the epicardium, the myocardium, and the endocardium. The epicardium covers the entire heart and great vessels and then folds over to form the parietal layer that lines the pericardium and adheres to the heart surface. The myocardium, which is the middle layer of the heart wall, consists of specialized cardiac muscle cells (myofibrils) that provide the bulk of contractile heart muscle. The endocardium, which is the innermost layer, is a thin membrane composed of three layers; the innermost layer is made up of smooth endothelial cells that line the inside of the heart's chambers and great vessels. The pericardium encases the heart and anchors it to surrounding structures, forming the pericardial sac. The outermost layer is the parietal pericardium, and the visceral pericardium (or epicardium) adheres to the heart surface.
   Nursing Process: Assessment
   Patient Need: Physiological Integrity

2. Answer: 2
   Rationale: The right ventricle receives deoxygenated blood from the right atrium and pumps it through the pulmonary artery to the pulmonary capillary bed for oxygenation. The right atrium receives deoxygenated blood from the veins of the body. The left atrium receives freshly oxygenated blood from the lungs through the pulmonary veins. The superior vena cava returns blood from the body area above the diaphragm, the inferior vena cava returns blood from the body below the diaphragm, and the coronary sinus drains blood from the heart.
   Nursing Process: Evaluation
   Patient Need: Physiological Integrity

3. Answer: 2
   Rationale: The greater the volume, the greater the stretch of the cardiac muscle fibers and the greater the force with which the fibers contract to accomplish emptying. This principle is called Starling's law of the heart. The other choices in the question are not correct.
   Nursing Process: Assessment
   Patient Need: Physiological Integrity

4. Answer: 3
   Rationale: The cellular action potential serves as the basis for electrocardiography (ECG), a diagnostic test of cardiac function. The SA node acts as the normal "pacemaker" of the heart, usually generating an impulse 60–100 times per minute. The sinoatrial (SA) node is located at the junction of the superior vena cava and right atrium. The electrical stimulus increases the permeability of the cell membrane, which creates an action potential (electrical potential).
   Nursing Process: Assessment
   Patient Need: Physiological Integrity

5. Answer: 1, 3, 5
   Rationale: The stimulus for red blood cell production is tissue hypoxia. The hormone erythropoietin is released by the kidneys in response to hypoxia. It stimulates the bone marrow to produce RBCs. Coronary artery disease, emphysema, and pneumonia may result in tissue hypoxia. The body would produce more red blood cells in response. Renal failure and cirrhosis would not result in increased red blood cell production.
   Nursing Process: Assessment
   Patient Need: Physiological Integrity

6. Answer: 3
   Monocytes are phagocytic cells that mature into macrophages. Neutrophils are active phagocytes. Immature neutrophils are called bands. Basophils and eosinophils increase in number during allergic reactions.
   Nursing Process: Assessment
   Patient Need: Physiological Integrity

Chapter 30

Terms Matching

1. Q
2. D
3. B
4. G
5. M

6. I
7. K
8. P
9. A
10. C
11. H
12. N
13. E
14. F
15. O
16. J
17. L

Focused Study

1. The two main coronary arteries—the left and the right—supply blood, oxygen, and nutrients to the myocardium. They originate in the root of the aorta, just outside the aortic valve. The left main coronary artery divides to form the anterior descending and circumflex arteries. The anterior descending artery supplies the anterior interventricular septum and the left ventricle, including the apex of the heart. The circumflex branch supplies the lateral wall of the left ventricle. The right coronary artery supplies the right ventricle and forms the posterior descending artery. The posterior descending artery supplies the posterior portion of the heart.

2. Total serum cholesterol is elevated in the patient with hyperlipidemia. A lipid profile includes triglyceride, HDL, and LDL levels and enables calculation of the ratio of HDL to total cholesterol. The ratio should be at least 1:5, with 1:3 being the ideal ratio. Elevated lipid levels are associated with an increased risk of atherosclerosis. In patients with a strong family history of premature coronary heart disease (CHD) or familial hypercholesterolemia, lipoprotein (a) also may be measured. Elevated levels of Lp(a) may independently increase the risk of CHD. Other subsets of blood lipids may also be measured in selected patients.

   C-reactive protein is a serum protein associated with inflammatory processes. Recent evidence suggests that elevated blood levels of this protein may be predictive of CHD.

   Ankle-brachial blood pressure index is an inexpensive, noninvasive test for peripheral vascular disease that may be predictive of CHD. The systolic blood pressure in the brachial, posterior tibial, and dorsalis pedis arteries is measured by Doppler. An ABI of < 0.9 in either leg indicates the presence of peripheral arterial disease and is a significant risk for CHD.

   Exercise ECG testing assesses the cardiac response to increased workload induced by exercise. The test is considered "positive" for CHD if myocardial ischemia is detected on the ECG; the patient develops chest pain; or the test is stopped due to excess fatigue, dysrhythmias, or other symptoms before the predicted maximal heart rate is achieved.

   EBCT is a diagnostic test that creates a three-dimensional image of the heart and coronary arteries that can reveal coronary artery calcification and other abnormalities. A coronary artery calcium score can be calculated from this test, providing additional important information in the diagnosis of CHD. This noninvasive test requires no special preparation and can identify patients who are at risk for developing myocardial ischemia.

   Myocardial perfusion imaging evaluates myocardial blood flow and perfusion, both at rest and during stress testing. Perfusion imaging studies are costly and therefore are not recommended for routine CHD risk assessment.

3. Nitrates such as nitroglycerin and longer-acting nitrate preparations are used to treat acute anginal attacks and to prevent angina. Sublingual nitroglycerin is the drug of choice to treat acute angina. It acts within one to two minutes, decreasing myocardial work and oxygen demand through venous and arterial dilation, which in turn reduce preload and afterload. It may also improve myocardial oxygen supply by dilating collateral blood vessels and reducing stenosis. Longer-acting nitroglycerin preparations (oral tablets, ointments, or transdermal patches) are used to prevent attacks of angina, not to treat an acute attack.

   Beta blockers such as propranolol, metoprolol, nadolol, and atenolol are considered first-line drugs to treat stable angina. They block the cardiac-stimulating effects of norepinephrine and epinephrine, preventing anginal attacks by reducing heart rate, myocardial contractility, and blood pressure, thus reducing myocardial oxygen demand. Beta blockers may be used alone or combined with other medications to prevent angina. Beta blockers are contraindicated for patients with asthma or severe COPD because they may cause severe bronchospasm. They are not used in patients with significant bradycardia, or AV conduction blocks, and are used cautiously in heart failure. Beta blockers are not used to treat Prinzmetal's angina because they may make it worse.

   Calcium channel blockers such as verapamil, diltiazem, and nifedipine reduce myocardial oxygen demand and increase myocardial blood and oxygen supply. These medications lower blood pressure, reduce myocardial contractility, and lower the heart rate, thereby decreasing myocardial oxygen demand. They are also potent coronary vasodilators, effectively increasing oxygen supply. They are used for long-term prophylaxis. These drugs are not usually prescribed in the initial treatment of angina. They are used cautiously in patients with dysrhythmias, heart failure, or hypotension.

   The patient with angina is at risk for myocardial infarction because of significant narrowing of the coronary arteries. Low-dose aspirin is often prescribed to reduce the risk of platelet aggregation and thrombus formation.

4.
- Assess for verbal and nonverbal signs of pain. Document the characteristics and intensity of the pain using a standard pain scale. Verify nonverbal indicators of pain with the patient. Rationale: Frequent and careful pain assessment allows early intervention to reduce the risk of further damage. Pain is a subjective experience; its expression may vary with location and intensity, previous experiences, and cultural and social background. A pain scales provide an objective tool for measuring pain and a way to assess pain relief or reduction.
- Administer oxygen at 2–5 L/min per nasal cannula. Rationale: Supplemental oxygen increases oxygen supply to the myocardium, decreasing ischemia and pain.
- Promote physical and psychologic rest. Provide information and emotional support. Rationale: Rest decreases cardiac workload and sympathetic nervous system stimulation, promoting comfort. Information and emotional support help decrease anxiety and provide psychologic rest.
- Titrate intravenous nitroglycerin as ordered to relieve chest pain, maintaining a systolic blood pressure greater than 100 mmHg. Rationale: Nitroglycerin decreases chest pain by dilating peripheral vessels, reducing cardiac work, and dilating coronary vessels, including collateral channels, thereby improving blood flow to ischemic tissue.
- Administer 2–4 mg morphine by intravenous push for chest pain as needed. Rationale: Morphine is an effective narcotic analgesic for chest pain. It decreases pain and anxiety, acts as a venodilator, and decreases the respiratory rate. The resulting reduction in preload and sympathetic nervous system stimulation reduces cardiac work and oxygen consumption.

Case Study

1. *What are some modifiable and nonmodifiable risk factors for coronary heart disease (CHD)?* Age is a nonmodifiable risk factor for CHD. Over 50% of heart attack victims are 65 and older; 80% of deaths due to myocardial infarction occur in this age group. Gender and genetic factors also are nonmodifiable risk factors for CHD. Compared to women, men are affected by CHD at an earlier age. A family history of CHD in a male first-degree relative younger than age 55 or a female first-degree relative younger than 65 years is identified as a risk factor for CHD (National Cholesterol Education Program [NCEP], 2002). Modifiable risk factors include lifestyle and pathologic conditions that predispose the patient to developing CHD. Disease conditions that contribute to CHD include hypertension, diabetes mellitus, hyperlipidemia, and metabolic syndrome. Although these conditions are not a matter of choice, they are modifiable risk factors that can often be controlled through medication, weight control, diet, and exercise.

Cigarette smoking, obesity, physical inactivity, and a poor diet are other modifiable risk factors.

2. *What are atheromas?* Atheromas are complex lesions in the arterial walls that consist of lipids, fibrous tissue, collagen, calcium, cellular debris, and capillaries. These calcified lesions can ulcerate or rupture, stimulating thrombosis. The vessel lumen may be rapidly occluded by the thrombus, or it may embolize to occlude a distal vessel.

3. *What are characteristics of metabolic syndrome?* Characteristics of metabolic syndrome include abdominal obesity; abnormal blood lipids (low HDL, high triglycerides); hypertension; elevated fasting blood glucose; clotting tendency; and inflammatory factors.

4. *Mr. Baldwin received training on how to perform cardiopulmonary resuscitation (CPR) 10 months ago. He asks the nurse to refresh his memory about how to perform CPR.* Mr. Baldwin can be referred to a CPR course to help refresh his memory. Also, the nurse should provide him with the procedure for CPR, as follows:

   1. Assess for responsiveness; shake the patient and shout.
   2. Call for help. Dial 911 (if outside the healthcare facility) or initiate the institutional code or cardiac arrest procedure.
   3. Open the airway using the head-tilt, chin-lift maneuver. Simultaneously press down on the forehead with one hand while lifting the chin upward with the other hand.
   4. Check for breathing; look and listen. Inspect the chest for rise and fall with respirations; listen and feel for air movement through the nose or mouth. This step should take no more than 10 seconds.
   5. If not breathing, begin rescue breathing using a pocket mask, mouth shield, or bag-valve mask. Administer two breaths (one second per breath), observing for rise of the chest with each breath.
   6. Check the carotid or femoral artery for a pulse ($\leq$ 10 sec).
   7. If a pulse is present, continue rescue breathing, administering 8–10 breaths per minute, until help arrives or spontaneous respirations resume. Recheck the carotid pulse every two minutes.
   8. If no pulse is present, analyze rhythm and defibrillate or if arrest was not witnessed or automated external defibrillator (AED) is unavailable, initiate external cardiac compressions. Place on a firm surface. Position the heel of one hand in the center of the chest between the nipples (child and adult) with the other hand on top and the fingers either interlocked or extended.
   9. Initiate hard and fast cardiac compressions, pressing straight down to depress the sternum 1.5–2 inches, keeping the elbows locked and positioning the shoulders directly over the hands. Release pressure completely between compressions but do not lift the hands from the chest.

10. Compress the chest at a rate of approximately 100 times per minute. With one- or two-rescuer CPR, provide two breaths after every 30 compressions. Assess the pulse after five complete cycles of 30 compressions and two breaths; continue CPR until help arrives.

5. *Mr. Baldwin's mother states, "I quit smoking three months ago. Will that have any effect on my lipid levels?" How should the nurse respond?* When patients stop smoking, it improves their HDL levels, lowers their LDL levels, and reduces the blood's tendency to clot.

6. *Mr. Baldwin requests information about how eating fish can reduce his mother's risk factors.* Certain cold-water fish (for example, tuna, salmon, and mackerel) contain high levels of omega-3 fatty acids, which help raise HDL levels and decrease serum triglycerides, total serum cholesterol, and blood pressure.

7. *Mr. Baldwin's mother requests information about how exercise can reduce her risk factors.* Regular physical exercise reduces the risk for CHD in several ways. It lowers VLDL, LDL, and triglyceride levels, and it raises HDL levels. Regular exercise lowers blood pressure and insulin resistance. Patients are encouraged to participate in at least 30 minutes of moderate-intensity physical activity five or six days each week. To achieve weight loss and prevent weight gain, 60–90 minutes of moderate-intensity exercise daily is recommended (U.S. Department of Health & Human Services, 2005).

Care Plan Critical-Thinking Activity

1. Synchronized cardioversion delivers direct electrical current synchronized with Ms. Vasquez's heart rhythm. Synchronization of the shock with the QRS complex prevents ventricular fibrillation by avoiding current delivery during the vulnerable period of repolarization. Cardioversion is usually done as an elective procedure to treat supraventricular tachycardia, atrial fibrillation, atrial flutter, or hemodynamically stable ventricular tachycardia.

2. The patient is lightly sedated with diazepam prior to this procedure because the procedure can induce anxiety. Diazepam is thought to help relieve pain and may induce some amnesia.

3. Ms. Vasquez's history of rheumatic fever may indicate that she has an increased risk for heart failure due to changes that occur to the heart as a result of the infection.

Short Answers

Fill in the blanks regarding dietary recommendations to reduce CHD risk.

Nutrient	Recommendation
Calories	Adjusted to attain/maintain desirable body weight
Total fat	25%–35% of total calories
• Saturated fats	< 7% of total calories
• Polyunsaturated fat	Up to 10% of total calories
• Monounsaturated fat	Up to 20% of total calories
• Cholesterol	< 200 mg/day
Carbohydrate (primarily complex carbohydrates such as whole grains, fruits, and vegetables)	50%–60% of total calories
Dietary fiber	20–30 g/day
Protein	About 15% of total calories

NCLEX-RN® Review Questions

1. Answer: 2

   Rationale: The patient with coronary heart disease (CHD) may be asymptomatic. CHD is caused by impaired blood flow to the myocardium. CHD affects 13.2 million people in the United States and causes more than 500,000 deaths annually. Accumulation of atherosclerotic plaque in the coronary arteries is the usual cause of CHD.

   Nursing Process: Evaluation

   Patient Need: Physiological Integrity

2. Answer: 3

   Rationale: High HDL is not associated with metabolic syndrome. Characteristics of metabolic syndrome include abdominal obesity; abnormal blood lipids (low HDL, high triglycerides); hypertension; elevated fasting blood glucose; clotting tendency; and inflammatory factors.

   Nursing Process: Assessment

   Patient Need: Physiological Integrity

3. Answer: 3

   Rationale: The patient should keep sublingual tablets in their original amber glass bottle to protect them from heat, light, and moisture. Patients should replace their supply every six months. If the first nitrate dose does not relieve angina within five minutes, the patient should take a second dose. After five more minutes, the patient may take a third dose if needed. If the pain is unrelieved or lasts 20 minutes or longer, the patient should seek medical assistance immediately. The patient should carry a supply of nitroglycerin tablets. He or she should dissolve sublingual nitroglycerin tablets under the tongue or between the upper lip and gum. The patient should not eat, drink, or smoke until the tablet is completely dissolved. The patient should rotate ointment or transdermal patch application sites. He or she should apply to a hairless area and spread ointment evenly without rubbing or massaging. The patient should remove the patch or residual ointment at bedtime daily and apply a fresh dose in the morning.

   Nursing Process: Planning

   Patient Need: Physiological Integrity

4. Answer: 1, 3, 5

   Rationale: Dissecting or ruptured aortic or ventricular aneurysm, valve disorders, and inflammatory myocardial disorders are examples of cardiac causes of sudden cardiac death. Choking, cerebral hemorrhage, and pulmonary embolism are noncardiac causes of sudden cardiac death.

Nursing Process: Assessment

Patient Need: Physiological Integrity

5. Answer: 3

Rationale: Cardiopulmonary resuscitation: Assess for responsiveness; shake the patient and shout. Open the airway using the head-tilt, chin-lift maneuver. Check the carotid or femoral artery for a pulse ($\leq$ 10 sec). With one- or two-rescuer CPR, provide two breaths after every 30 compressions. Assess the pulse after five complete cycles of 30 compressions and two breaths; continue CPR until help arrives.

Nursing Process: Implementation

Patient Need: Physiological Integrity

6. Answer: 4

Rationale: Ischemia, which is deficient blood flow to tissue, may be caused by partial obstruction of a coronary artery, a coronary artery spasm, or a thrombus. The AV nodal delay allows the atria to contract and delivers an extra bolus of blood to the ventricles before they contract (the atrial kick). Angina pectoris, or angina, is chest pain that results from reduced coronary blood flow, which causes a temporary imbalance between myocardial blood supply and demand. Aberrant (abnormal) impulses may originate outside normal conduction pathways and cause ectopic beats.

Nursing Process: Assessment

Patient Need: Physiological Integrity

7. Answer: 2

Rationale: MI usually affects the left ventricle because it is the major "workhorse" of the heart; its muscle mass and oxygen demands are greater. MI occurs when blood flow to a portion of cardiac muscle is completely blocked, which results in prolonged tissue ischemia and irreversible cell damage. MIs are described by the damaged area of the heart. Risk factors for MI are the same as those for coronary heart disease: age, gender, heredity, race, smoking, obesity, hyperlipidemia, hypertension, diabetes, sedentary lifestyle, and diet, among others.

Nursing Process: Assessment

Patient Need: Physiological Integrity

Chapter 31

Terms Matching

1. S
2. C
3. H
4. N
5. T
6. K
7. D
8. A
9. Q
10. R
11. E
12. O
13. J
14. F
15. B
16. P
17. M
18. L
19. I
20. G

Focused Study

1. *Stage A:* Patients at high risk for developing heart failure but without structural heart disease or symptoms of heart failure (patients with hypertension, CHD, diabetes, obesity, metabolic syndrome; patients who have a family history of cardiomyopathy; or patients who are taking cardiotoxic drugs)

   Stage B: Patients with structural heart disease but no manifestations of heart failure (patients with previous MI, asymptomatic valve disease, or left ventricular dysfunction)

   Stage C: Patients with structural heart disease and current or prior symptoms of heart failure (shortness of breath, fatigue, decreased exercise tolerance)

   Stage D: Refractory heart failure (patients with manifestations of heart failure at rest despite aggressive treatment)

2. Acute infective endocarditis: sudden onset with spiking fever and chills; manifestations of heart failure; caused by *Staphylococcus aureus;* usually occurs in previously normal heart; associated with intravenous drug use, infected intravenous sites; rapid valve destruction

   Subacute infective endocarditis: gradual onset of febrile illness with cough, dyspnea, arthralgias, and abdominal pain; caused by *Streptococcus viridans*, enterococci, gram-negative and gram-positive bacilli, fungi, or yeasts; usually occurs in damaged or deformed hearts; associated with dental work, invasive procedures, and infections; valve destruction leads to regurgitation; embolization of friable vegetations

3.

	Dilated	Hypertrophic	Restrictive
Causes	Usually idiopathic; may be secondary to chronic alcoholism or myocarditis	Hereditary; may be secondary to chronic hypertension	Usually secondary to amyloidosis, radiation, or myocardial fibrosis
Clinical Manifestations	Heart failure Cardiomegaly Dysrhythmias S_3 and S_4 gallop; murmur of mitral regurgitation	Dyspnea, anginal pain, syncope Left ventricular hypertrophy Dysrhythmias Loud S_4 Sudden death	Dyspnea, fatigue Right-sided heart failure Mild to moderate cardiomegaly S_3 and S_4 Mitral regurgitation murmur

4. • Assess apical pulse before administering medication. Withhold digitalis and notify the physician if heart rate is below 60 beats per minute and/or the patient has developed any manifestations of decreased cardiac output. Record apical rate on medication record.
   • Evaluate ECG for scooped ST segment, AV block, bradycardia, and other dysrhythmias.
   • Report manifestations of digitalis toxicity: anorexia, nausea, vomiting, abdominal pain, weakness, vision changes, and new-onset dysrhythmias.
   • Assess potassium, magnesium, calcium, and serum digoxin levels before giving digitalis. Hypokalemia can precipitate toxicity even when the serum digitalis level is in the "normal" range.
   • Carefully monitor patients with renal insufficiency or renal failure and older adults for digitalis toxicity.
   • Prepare to administer digoxin immune fab (Digibind®) for digoxin toxicity.

Case Study

1. *What is heart failure?* Heart failure develops when the heart cannot effectively fill or contract with adequate strength to function as a pump to meet the needs of the body. As a result, cardiac output falls, leading to decreased tissue perfusion.

2. *What are the causes of heart failure?* Causes of impaired myocardial function include coronary heart disease, cardiomyopathies, rheumatic fever, and infective endocarditis. Causes of increased cardiac workload include hypertension, valve disorders, anemias, and congenital heart defects. Causes of acute noncardiac conditions include volume overload, hyperthyroidism, fever and infection, and massive pulmonary embolus.

3. *What are some clinical manifestations associated with left-sided heart failure?* The manifestations of left-sided heart failure result from pulmonary congestion and decreased cardiac output. Fatigue and activity intolerance are common early manifestations. Dizziness and syncope also may result from decreased cardiac output. Pulmonary congestion causes dyspnea, shortness of breath, and cough. The patient may develop orthopnea, prompting use of two or three pillows or a recliner for sleeping. Cyanosis from impaired gas exchange may be noted. Upon auscultation of the lungs, inspiratory crackles and wheezes may be heard in lung bases. An S_3 gallop may be present, reflecting the heart's attempts to fill an already distended ventricle.

4. *What are the complications of heart failure?* The compensatory mechanisms initiated in heart failure can lead to complications in other body systems. Congestive hepatomegaly and splenomegaly caused by engorgement of the portal venous system results in increased abdominal pressure, ascites, and gastrointestinal problems. With prolonged right-sided heart failure, liver function may be impaired. Myocardial distention can precipitate dysrhythmias, further impairing cardiac output. Pleural effusions and other pulmonary problems may develop. Major complications of severe heart failure are cardiogenic and acute pulmonary edema.

5. *How is heart failure diagnosed?* Diagnosis of heart failure is based on the history, physical examination, and diagnostic findings.
   • Atrial natriuretic factor (ANF), also called atrial natriuretic hormone (ANH), and B-type natriuretic peptide (BNP) are hormones released by the heart muscle in response to changes in blood volume. Blood levels of these hormones increase in heart failure; however, BNP levels may be elevated in women and in people over age 60 who do not have heart failure. Therefore, an elevated BNP cannot be used alone to diagnosis heart failure (Hunt et al., 2005).
   • Serum electrolytes are measured to evaluate fluid and electrolyte status. Serum osmolality may be low due to fluid retention. Sodium, potassium, and chloride levels provide a baseline for evaluating the effects of treatment; serum calcium and magnesium are measured as well.
   • Urinalysis, blood urea nitrogen (BUN), and serum creatinine are obtained to evaluate renal function.
   • Liver function tests, including ALT, AST, LDH, serum bilirubin, and total protein and albumin levels, are obtained to evaluate possible effects of heart failure on liver function.
   • Thyroid function tests, including TSH and TH levels, are obtained because both hyperthyroidism and hypothyroidism can be a primary or a contributing cause of heart failure (Hunt et al., 2005).
   • In acute heart failure, arterial blood gases (ABGs) are drawn to evaluate gas exchange in the lungs and tissues.
   • A chest x-ray may show pulmonary vascular congestion and cardiomegaly in heart failure.
   • Electrocardiography is used to identify ECG changes associated with ventricular enlargement and to detect dysrhythmias, myocardial ischemia, or infarction.
   • Echocardiography with Doppler flow studies are performed to evaluate left ventricular function. Either transthoracic echocardiography or transesophageal echocardiography may be used. See Chapter 29 for more information and the nursing implications of these tests.
   • Radionuclide imaging is used to evaluate ventricular function and size.

6. *Mr. Hacking's physician states that she wants a Swan-Ganz catheter to be placed. The student nurse requests information about this catheter and an explanation as to how it can be used to monitor Mr. Hacking's condition.* The pulmonary artery catheter is a flow-directed, balloon-tipped catheter first used in the early 1970s. The PA catheter is often called a Swan-Ganz catheter, named after the physicians who developed it. The PA catheter is used to evaluate left ventricular and overall cardiac function. The PA catheter is inserted into a central vein, usually the internal jugular or subclavian vein, and threaded into the right atrium. A small balloon at the tip of the catheter allows the catheter to be drawn into the right ventricle and from there into the pulmonary artery. The inflated balloon carries the catheter forward until the balloon wedges in a small branch of pulmonary vasculature. Once in place, the balloon is deflated and multiple lumens of the catheter allow measurement of pressures in the right atrium, pulmonary artery, and left ventricle. The normal PA pressure is around 25/10 mmHg; normal mean pulmonary artery pressure is about 15 mmHg. Pulmonary artery pressure is increased in left-sided heart failure.

7. *Mr. Hacking's physician writes an order for the nurse to administer fosinopril (Monopril®). The student nurse requests information about what type of medication this is and how it works.* Fosinopril (Monopril®) is an ACE inhibitor. ACE inhibitors interrupt the conversion of angiotensin I to angiotensin II by inhibiting the enzyme that mediates the conversion. Angiotensin II causes intense vasoconstriction, increasing afterload and ventricular wall stress and increasing preload and ventricular dilation. It also stimulates aldosterone and ADH production, causing fluid retention. ACE inhibitors block this RAAS activity, decreasing cardiac work and increasing cardiac output. ACE inhibitors reduce the progression and manifestations of heart failure, thus reducing the number and frequency of hospital admissions, decreasing mortality rates, and preventing cardiac complications.

Care Plan Critical-Thinking Activity

1. This will help evaluate the effectiveness of the interventions used to treat her case of mitral valve prolapse.
2. Energy drinks, some carbonated beverages (soda), coffee, tea, chocolate, and some medications (for example, Excedrin®)
3. Mitral valve prolapse increases the patient's risk for developing bacterial endocarditis. Progressive worsening of regurgitation can lead to heart failure. Thrombi may form on prolapsed valve leaflets; embolization may cause transient ischemic attacks.

Crossword Puzzle

question	term answer
The force needed to eject blood into the circulation	AFTERLOAD
The ability of the heart to increase cardiac output to meet demand is the _____ reserve	CARDIAC
The volume of blood ejected with each heartbeat is the _____ volume	STROKE
The volume of blood in the ventricles prior to contraction	PRELOAD
The amount of blood that returns to the ventricles	VENOUS

The ventricular filling time	DIASTOLE
When the _____ nervous system is stimulated, the heart rate and contractility increase	SYMPATHETIC

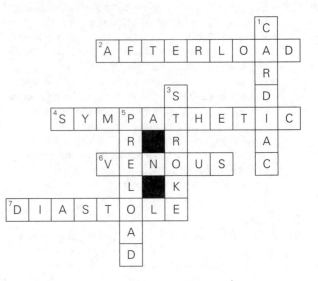

NCLEX-RN® Review Questions

1. Answer: 1
   Rationale: An advantage of a prosthetic heart valve is its long-term durability. Advantages of biologic tissue valves include the fact that they have a low incidence of thromboembolism, no long-term anticoagulation is required, and they are quiet.
   Nursing Process: Planning
   Patient Need: Physiological Integrity
2. Answer: 4
   Rationale: Home activity guidelines for a patient with heart failure include eating six small meals a day, not lifting heavy objects, using laxatives or stool softeners, and beginning a graded exercise program. The patient should be advised to spread out meals and activities. The patient should avoid straining and should avoid constipation and straining during bowel movements. The patient should plan to walk at home twice a day at a comfortable, slow pace for the first couple of weeks and then gradually increase the distance and pace.
   Nursing Process: Planning
   Patient Need: Health Promotion and Maintenance
3. Answer: 4
   Rationale: Diet restrictions for valvular disease are enacted to reduce fluid retention. Patients with valvular disease should notify all of their healthcare providers about valve disease. The patient should allow for adequate rest to prevent fatigue. The patient should immediately report any evidence of bleeding to the healthcare provider.
   Nursing Process: Evaluation
   Patient Need: Physiological Integrity

4. Answer: 2

Rationale: Stress the relationship between effective diabetes management and reduced risk of heart failure. Teach patients about coronary heart disease, the primary cause of heart failure. Discuss the importance of monitoring weight daily, which is an objective way to monitor fluid balance. Routinely screen patients for elevated blood pressure and refer patients to a primary care provider as indicated. Discuss the importance of effectively managing hypertension to reduce future risk for heart failure. Patients should take their medication as ordered by their physician.

Nursing Process: Assessment

Patient Need: Health Promotion and Maintenance

5. Answer: 1

Rationale: In cardiogenic pulmonary edema, the contractility of the left (not the right) ventricle is severely impaired. Pulmonary edema is a medical emergency. Immediate treatment for acute pulmonary edema focuses on restoring effective gas exchange and reducing fluid and pressure in the pulmonary vascular system. The patient often is restless and highly anxious, although severe hypoxia may cause confusion or lethargy.

Nursing Process: Evaluation

Patient Need: Physiological Integrity

6. Answer: 3

Rationale: The peak incidence of rheumatic fever is in children aged 5 to 15, not in adults. Rheumatic heart disease frequently damages the heart valves and is a major cause of mitral and aortic valve disorders. Rheumatic fever is a systemic inflammatory disease caused by an abnormal immune response to pharyngeal infection by group A beta-hemolytic streptococci. Rheumatic fever and rheumatic heart disease are significant public health problems in many developing countries.

Nursing Process: Evaluation

Patient Need: Health Promotion and Maintenance

Chapter 32

Terms Matching

1. C
2. E
3. F
4. H
5. X
6. O
7. M
8. J
9. U
10. R
11. V
12. P
13. I
14. T
15. N
16. G
17. L
18. S
19. A
20. Q
21. Y
22. B
23. D
24. K
25. W

Focused Study

1.
- Sympathetic nervous system stimulation of α- and β-adrenergic receptors, resulting in vasoconstriction and increased cardiac output.
- Altered function of the renin–angiotensin–aldosterone system and its responsiveness to factors such as sodium intake and overall fluid volume. The renin–angiotensin–aldosterone system affects vasomotor tone and salt and water excretion. Chronically high levels of angiotensin II lead to arteriolar remodeling, which permanently increases SVR.
- Other chemical mediators of vasomotor tone and blood volume, such as atrial natriuretic peptide, also play a role by affecting vasomotor tone and sodium and water excretion. Vascular endothelium produces hormones that can result in vasoconstriction.
- The interaction between insulin resistance, hyperinsulinemia and endothelial function may be a primary cause of hypertension. Excess insulin has several effects that may contribute to hypertension: (1) sodium retention by the kidneys, (2) increased sympathetic nervous system activity, (3) hypertrophy of vascular smooth muscle, and (4) changes in ion transport across cell membranes (Huether & McCance, 2008).

2. Doppler ultrasonography or a duplex Doppler ultrasound can be performed to identify specific locations of incompetent valves. This test is particularly useful before surgery to identify valves that allow reflux of blood from the femoral, popliteal, or peripheral deep veins into the superficial veins. The Trendelenburg test can be performed to determine the underlying cause of superficial venous insufficiency. The leg is elevated; then an elastic tourniquet is placed around the distal thigh. The varicosities are observed as the patient stands. When valves of the deep veins are incompetent, the veins remain flat upon standing; they rapidly distend when the superficial venous valves are the underlying cause.

3.
- Monitor intake and output in addition to weight each day or each week. Use the same scale at the same time of the day and weigh the patient in a similar clothing to ensure accurate weight measurements. Intake and output records and short-term changes in weight reflect fluid balance. Measures of fluid balance permit evaluation of the effectiveness of interventions such as restricted sodium intake and diuretic therapy.

- Discuss the rationale for restricted sodium intake if ordered. Teach ways to maintain the recommended sodium restriction and assist in choosing foods that are low in sodium. Sodium causes retention of extracellular water; restricting dietary sodium may help prevent additional fluid accumulation in interstitial spaces.
- During acute episodes of lymphedema, assess the affected extremity daily for increased edema. Measure the girth of the extremity using a consistent technique. The size of the affected extremity provides a measure of the effectiveness of ordered interventions and progression of the disorder.

4. The edema begins distally, progressing up the limb to involve the entire extremity. Initial edema is soft and pitting; with chronic congestion, subcutaneous tissues become fibrotic, causing thick, rough skin and a woody texture of the limb. When contrasted with venous disorders, the edema associated with venous disorders is softer and the skin often is hyperpigmented with evidence of stasis dermatitis. Lymphedema generally is painless, although the limb may feel heavy.

Case Studies

Case Study 1

1. *What factors influence arterial blood pressure?* Blood flow, peripheral vascular resistance, and blood pressure, all of which influence arterial circulation, are in turn influenced by the following factors:
   - The sympathetic and parasympathetic nervous systems are the primary mechanisms that regulate blood pressure. Stimulation of the sympathetic nervous system exerts a major effect on peripheral resistance by causing vasoconstriction of the arterioles, thereby increasing blood pressure. Parasympathetic stimulation causes vasodilation of the arterioles, which lowers blood pressure.
   - Baroreceptors and chemoreceptors in the aortic arch, carotid sinus, and other large vessels are sensitive to pressure and chemical changes and cause reflex sympathetic stimulation, which results in vasoconstriction, increased heart rate, and increased blood pressure.
   - The kidneys help maintain blood pressure by excreting or conserving sodium and water. When blood pressure decreases, the kidneys initiate the renin–angiotensin mechanism. This stimulates vasoconstriction, which results in the release of the hormone aldosterone from the adrenal cortex, increasing sodium ion reabsorption and water retention. In addition, pituitary release of antidiuretic hormone promotes renal reabsorption of water. The net result is an increase in blood volume and a consequent increase in cardiac output and blood pressure.
   - Temperatures may also affect peripheral resistance: Cold causes vasoconstriction, whereas warmth

produces vasodilation. Many chemicals, hormones, and drugs influence blood pressure by affecting cardiac output and/or peripheral vascular resistance. For example, epinephrine causes vasoconstriction and increased heart rate; prostaglandins dilate blood vessel diameter; endothelin, a chemical released by the inner lining of vessels, is a potent vasoconstrictor; nicotine causes vasoconstriction; and alcohol and histamine cause vasodilation.
   - Dietary factors such as intake of salt, saturated fats, and cholesterol elevate blood pressure by affecting blood volume and vessel diameter.
   - Race, gender, age, weight, time of day, position, exercise, and emotional state may also affect blood pressure. These factors influence the arterial pressure. Although it is much lower than arterial blood pressure, systemic venous pressure is also influenced by factors such as blood volume, venous tone, and right atrial pressure.

2. *Explain peripheral vascular resistance (PVR) and mean arterial pressure (MAP).* Peripheral vascular resistance (PVR) refers to the opposing forces, or impedance, to blood flow as the arterial channels become more distant from the heart. Peripheral vascular resistance is determined by the following factors:
   - Blood viscosity: The greater the viscosity, or thickness, of the blood, the greater its resistance to moving and flowing.
   - Length of the vessel: The longer the vessel, the greater the resistance to blood flow.
   - Diameter of the vessel: The smaller the diameter of a vessel, the greater the friction against the walls of the vessel and, thus, the greater the impedance to blood flow.

   Blood pressure is the force exerted against the walls of the arteries by the blood as it is pumped from the heart. Blood pressure is most accurately referred to as mean arterial pressure (MAP). The highest pressure exerted against the arterial walls at the peak of ventricular contraction (systole) is called the systolic blood pressure. The lowest pressure exerted during ventricular relaxation (diastole) is the diastolic blood pressure.

   Mean arterial blood pressure is regulated mainly by cardiac output (CO) and peripheral vascular resistance (PVR), as represented in the formula MAP = CO 3 PVR. For clinical use, the MAP may be estimated by calculating the diastolic blood pressure plus one-third of the pulse pressure (the difference between the systolic and diastolic blood pressure).

3. *What are some common clinical manifestations found in patients experiencing hypertensive emergencies?* Patients with hypertensive emergencies typically experience clinical manifestations that occur with a rapid onset. Patients can experience blurred vision, papilledema, systolic pressure greater than 180 mmHg, diastolic pressure greater than 120 mmHg, headache, confusion, motor deficits, and sensory deficits.

Case Study 2

1. *Discuss the manifestations of primary hypertension.*
   The early stages of primary hypertension typically are asymptomatic, marked only by elevated blood pressure. Blood pressure elevations are initially transient but eventually become permanent. When symptoms do appear, they are usually vague. Headache, usually in the back of the head and neck, may be present upon awakening, subsiding during the day. Other signs and symptoms result from target organ damage and may include nocturia, confusion, nausea and vomiting, and visual disturbances. Examination of the retina of the eye may reveal narrowed arterioles, hemorrhages, exudates, and papilledema.

2. *Explain the complications of primary hypertension.*
   Sustained hypertension affects the cardiovascular, neurologic, and renal systems. The rate of atherosclerosis accelerates, increasing the risk for coronary heart disease and stroke. The workload of the left ventricle increases, which may lead to ventricular hypertrophy. The increased workload of the left ventricle increases the risk for coronary heart disease, dysrhythmias, and heart failure. The diastolic blood pressure is a significant cardiovascular risk factor until age 50; the systolic pressure then becomes the more important factor contributing to cardiovascular risk (NHLBI, 2004). Most deaths due to hypertension result from coronary heart disease and acute myocardial infarction or heart failure.

   Accelerated atherosclerosis associated with hypertension increases the risk for cerebral infarction (stroke). Increased pressure in the cerebral vessels can lead to development of microaneurysms and an increased risk for cerebral hemorrhage. Hypertensive encephalopathy, a syndrome characterized by extremely high blood pressure, altered level of consciousness, increased intracranial pressure, papilledema, and seizures may develop. Its etiology is unclear.

   Hypertension also can lead to nephrosclerosis and renal insufficiency. Proteinuria and microscopic hematuria develop, as well as signs of chronic renal failure. Compared to whites, African Americans experience hypertensive kidney disease more frequently.

3. *Briefly summarize the lifestyle changes Ms. Drake should enact to help control her hypertension.*
   Ms. Drake should maintain a normal body weight. She should be eating a diet rich in fruits, vegetables, and low-fat dairy products. She should reduce her sodium, cholesterol, and total and saturated fat intake. Because she is a woman and is not overweight, she should limit her alcohol intake to no more than 1/2 oz. per day. She should engage in aerobic exercise for 30 minutes most days of the week. She should stop smoking and use stress management techniques such as relaxation therapy.

Short Answers

Fill in the information regarding arterial ulcers and venous ulcers.

Factor	Arterial Ulcers	Venous Ulcers
Location	Toes, feet, shin	Over medial or anterior ankle
Ulcer appearance	Deep, pale	Superficial, pink
Skin appearance	Normal to atrophic, pallor upon elevation of extremities, rubor with extremities are dependent	Brown discoloration, stasis dermatitis, cyanotic extremities with dependency
Skin temperature	Cool	Normal
Edema	Absent or mild	May be significant
Pain	Usually severe, intermittent claudication, pain at rest	Usually mild, aching pain
Gangrene	May occur	Does not occur
Pulses	Decreased or absent	Normal

NCLEX-RN® Review Questions

1. Answer: 2
   Rationale: The systolic blood pressure is felt as the peripheral pulse and is heard as Korotkoff's sounds during blood pressure measurement. In healthy adults, the average systolic pressure is less than 120 mmHg. During diastole, or cardiac relaxation and filling, elastic arterial walls maintain a minimum pressure, which is the diastolic blood pressure, to maintain blood flow through the capillary beds. The average diastolic pressure in a healthy adult is less than 80 mmHg. The difference between the systolic and diastolic pressure, normally about 40 mmHg, is known as the pulse pressure. The mean arterial pressure (MAP) is the average pressure in the arterial circulation throughout the cardiac cycle.
   Nursing Process: Assessment
   Patient Need: Physiological Integrity

2. Answer: 3
   Rationale: The mean arterial pressure (MAP) is the average pressure in the arterial circulation throughout the cardiac cycle. It can be calculated using the formula [systolic BP + 2 (diastolic BP)] / 3.
   Nursing Process: Assessment
   Patient Need: Physiological Integrity

3. Answer: 1
   Rationale: Implement interventions to reduce the risk of aneurysm rupture: Maintain bed rest with legs flat (not elevated), maintain a calm environment and implement measures to reduce psychologic stress, instruct patient

to prevent straining during defecation and to avoid holding his or her breath while moving, and administer beta blockers and antihypertensives as prescribed.

Nursing Process: Implementation

Patient Need: Physiological Integrity

4. Answer: 3

Rationale: Raynaud's disease has no identifiable cause. Raynaud's phenomenon occurs secondary to another disease (for example, collagen vascular diseases such as scleroderma and rheumatoid arthritis), other known causes of vasospasm, or long-term exposure to cold or machinery. Raynaud's disease affects primarily young women between the ages of 20 and 40. Raynaud's disease is characterized by episodes of intense vasospasm in the small arteries and arterioles of the fingers and sometimes the toes. Raynaud's disease has been called the "blue-white-red" disease because affected digits initially turn blue as blood flow is reduced due to vasospasm, then white as circulation is more severely limited, and finally very red as the fingers are warmed and the spasm resolves.

Nursing Process: Assessment

Patient Need: Physiological Integrity

5. Answer: 2

Rationale: Complications of varicose veins include venous insufficiency and stasis ulcers. Because elastic stockings inhibit blood flow through small superficial vessels, they should be removed once each day for at least 30 minutes. Prolonged standing, the force of gravity, lack of leg exercise, and incompetent venous valves all weaken the muscle-pumping mechanism, which reduces venous blood return to the heart. Varicose veins may be asymptomatic, but most cause manifestations such as severe aching leg pain, leg fatigue, leg heaviness, itching, or feelings of heat in the legs.

Nursing Process: Planning

Patient Need: Physiological Integrity

6. Answer: 1

Rationale: Obesity is a modifiable risk factor for hypertension. Age, race, and family history are nonmodifiable risk factors.

Nursing Process: Planning

Patient Need: Physiological Integrity

7. Answer: 2

Rationale: Lymphangitis, inflammation of the lymph vessels draining an infected area of the body, is characterized by a red streak along the inflamed vessels, pain, heat, and swelling. Fever and chills also may be present. Enlargement of the lymph nodes is referred to as lymphadenopathy.

Lymphangiography uses injected contrast media to illustrate lymphatic vessels on x-rays. This is a diagnostic test that will not cure the patient. The patient does not need to force fluids. The infection needs to be treated with antibiotics.

Nursing Process: Implementation

Patient Need: Physiological Integrity

Chapter 33

Terms Matching

1. S
2. C
3. E
4. J
5. R
6. A
7. H
8. L
9. P
10. N
11. B
12. O
13. I
14. F
15. Q
16. M
17. D
18. G
19. K

Focused Study

1. Ferrous sulfate (Feosol®, Fer-In-Sol®), ferrous gluconate (Fergon®, Ferralet®, Fertinic®), iron dextran injection (Imferon®), iron polysaccharide, iron sucrose (Venofer®), sodium ferric gluconate (Ferrlecit®). Education: Gastrointestinal side effects may be reduced by taking iron with food; iron should not be taken with milk because absorption will be decreased; stools may be dark green or black; fluids and fiber should be increased to decrease constipation.

2.
   • Hypertension
   • Headache, tinnitus, blurred vision
   • Plethora: dark redness of the lips, feet, ears, fingernails, and mucous membranes
   • Splenomegaly (polycythemia vera)
   • Severe pruritus, extremity pain
   • Weight loss, night sweats
   • Gastrointestinal bleeding
   • Intermittent claudication

3. Obvious hemorrhage from incisions; oozing of blood from punctures, intravenous catheter sites; purpura, petechiae, bruising; cyanosis of extremities; gastrointestinal bleeding or hemorrhage; dyspnea, tachypnea, bloody sputum; tachycardia, hypotension; hematuria, oliguria, acute renal failure; manifestations of increased intracranial pressure such as decreased level of consciousness and papillary, motor, and sensory changes; changes in mental status

4.

Feature or Manifestation	Hodgkin's Disease	Non-Hodgkin's Lymphoma
Lymphadenopathy	Localized to a single node or chain; often cervical, subclavicular, or mediastinal	Multiple peripheral nodes; nodes of the mesentery often involved
Spread	Orderly and continuous	Diffuse and unpredictable
Extranodal involvement	Rare	Early and common
Bone marrow involvement	Uncommon	Common
Fever, night sweats, weight loss	Common	Uncommon until disease is extensive
Other manifestations	Fatigue, pruritus, splenomegaly; anemia, neutrophilia	Abdominal pain, nausea, vomiting; dyspnea, cough; CNS symptoms; lymphocytopenia

Case Study

1. *What are the different types of anemias.* The different types of anemias include iron-deficiency anemia, vitamin B_{12} deficiency anemia, folic acid deficiency anemia, sickle cell anemia, thalassemia, and aplastic anemia.
2. *What are some dietary sources of heme and nonheme iron?* Sources of heme iron include beef, pork loin, chicken, turkey, egg yolk, veal, clams, and oysters. Sources of nonheme iron include dried fruits, bran flakes, brown rice, greens, whole-grain breads, oatmeal, and dried beans.
3. *What are some common causes of iron-deficiency anemia?* Jonathan's mother may have dietary deficiencies due to a vegetarian diet or inadequate protein intake. She may unable to absorb adequate amounts of iron due to gastric surgery, chronic diarrhea, or other malabsorption problems. She may have increased metabolic requirements due to pregnancy or lactation. Bleeding may result in iron-deficiency anemia. She may have developed this because she has gastrointestinal bleeding, excessive blood loss due to menstruation, or blood loss from her urine.
4. *Which population is most at risk for developing ALL?* ALL affects primarily children and young adults; leukemic cells may infiltrate CNS.
5. *What are the associated clinical manifestations of ALL?* Common clinical manifestations include recurrent infections, bleeding, pallor, bone pain, weight loss, sore throat, fatigue, night sweats, and weakness.
6. *Jonathan has been scheduled for a chest x-ray to rule out pneumonia. How may pneumonia be related to ALL?* The manifestations of ALL result from neutropenia and thrombocytopenia. Decreased neutrophils lead to recurrent severe infections such as pneumonia, septicemia, abscesses, and mucous membrane ulceration.
7. *The nurse studies Jonathan's laboratory results and determines that his platelet count is low. What problems may arise because of this?* The manifestations of thrombocytopenia include petechiae, purpura, and ecchymoses; epistaxis; hematomas; hematuria; and gastrointestinal bleeding.
8. *The physician spoke with Jonathan and his mother about how ALL is treated. Which medications are typically used?* Daunorubicin (Cerubidine®, an antitumor antibiotic) *with* vincristine (Oncovin®, a plant alkaloid) with prednisone with asparaginase (Elspar®)

Care Plan Critical-Thinking Activity

1. Ice acts as a vasoconstrictor to help control bleeding. Manual pressure may be used to occlude bleeding vessels and help stop the bleeding.
2. Depending on the severity of the clotting factor deficit, even minor trauma can lead to serious bleeding episodes. He should be advised to participate in safer activities (for example, noncontact sports such as swimming and golf).
3. Information that may be available includes emergency contact numbers, physician's name and phone number, disease, allergies, current medications, and blood type.

Short Answers

List three conditions that may result in disseminated intravascular coagulation (DIC).

Tissue Damage	Vessel Damage	Infections
1. Trauma	1. Aortic aneurysm	1. Bacterial infection or sepsis
2. Obstetric complications: septic abortion, abruptio placentae, amniotic fluid embolus, retained dead fetus	2. Acute glomerulonephritis	2. Viral or fungal infections
3. Neoplasms: acute leukemia, adenocarcinomas	3. Hemolytic uremic syndrome	3. Parasitic or rickettsial infection

Other possible answers: hemolysis and fat embolism

NCLEX-RN® Review Questions

1. Answer: 3
   Rationale: Inadequate dietary iron intake also contributes to anemia in the older adult. Iron deficiency anemia is the most common type of anemia. The body cannot synthesize hemoglobin without iron. Iron deficiency anemia results in fewer numbers of RBCs.
   Nursing Process: Evaluation
   Patient Need: Physiological Integrity

2. Answer: 4
Rationale: Dried fruits are a source of nonheme iron. Sources of heme iron include beef, pork loin, chicken, turkey, egg yolk, veal, clams, and oysters.
Nursing Process: Planning
Patient Need: Health Promotion and Maintenance

3. Answer: 2
Rationale: The caregiver should provide medications for pain or nausea 30 minutes before meals. The caregiver should also provide rest periods before meals, liquids with different textures and tastes, and mouth care before and after meals.
Nursing Process: Evaluation
Patient Need: Physiological Integrity

4. Answer: 3
Rationale: The Ann Arbor Staging System is used to assess the extent and severity of lymphomas. In stage III, there is involvement of lymph node regions or structures on both sides of the diaphragm.

The other stages are stage I, involvement of a single lymph node region or lymphoid structure (for example, spleen, thymus, or lymphoid tonsillar tissue); stage II, involvement of two or more lymph node regions on the same side of the diaphragm; and stage IV, involvement of an extranodal site (not proximal or contiguous with an involved node) such as the liver, lung or pleura, bone or bone marrow, or skin.
Nursing Process: Assessment
Patient Need: Physiological Integrity

5. Answer: 3
Rationale: Teach measures to prevent or relieve nausea and vomiting, which include the following: eating soda crackers and sucking on hard candy; eating soft, bland foods that are cold or at room temperature; avoiding unpleasant odors; and getting fresh air. Crackers and hard candy often relieve queasiness. The other measures enhance appetite and promote nutritional intake.
Nursing Process: Planning
Patient Need: Health Promotion and Maintenance

6. Answer: 2
Rationale: In aplastic anemia, the bone marrow fails to produce all three types of blood cells (red blood cells, white blood cells, and platelets), which leads to pancytopenia. Manifestations of aplastic anemia include fatigue, pallor, progressive weakness, exertional dyspnea, headache, and ultimately tachycardia and heart failure. Aplastic anemia also may occur with viral infections such as mononucleosis, hepatitis C, and HIV disease. Aplastic anemia is rare.
Nursing Process: Planning
Patient Need: Physiological Integrity

7. Answer: 2
Rationale: Secondary polycythemia occurs when erythropoietin levels are elevated. In primary polycythemia, RBC production is increased. In relative polycythemia, the total RBC count is normal. In relative polycythemia, the hematocrit is elevated because of increased cell concentration.

Nursing Process: Evaluation
Patient Need: Physiological Integrity

8. Answer: 1
Rationale: Restrict visitors because they may expose the patient to infectious illnesses. Provide oral hygiene after every meal. Ensure meticulous handwashing among all people who come in contact with the patient. Infection is the major cause of death in patients with leukemia. Mucous membranes are especially susceptible to breakdown and infection as a result of tissue damage from chemotherapy or radiation. Maintain protective isolation as indicated. These precautions minimize exposure to bacterial, viral, and fungal pathogens.
Nursing Process: Implementation
Patient Need: Physiological Integrity

Chapter 34

Terms Matching
1. L
2. C
3. E
4. K
5. B
6. I
7. A
8. H
9. G
10. D
11. J
12. F

Focused Study
1. The pharynx, a funnel-shaped passageway about 5 inches (13 cm) long, extends from the base of the skull to the level of the C_6 vertebra. The pharynx serves as a passageway for both air and food. It is divided into three regions: the nasopharynx, the oropharynx, and the laryngopharynx. The nasopharynx serves only as a passageway for air. Masses of lymphoid tissue are located in the mucosa high in the posterior wall; tissues trap and destroy infectious agents entering with the air. The auditory tubes open into the nasopharynx, connecting it with the middle ear. The oropharynx lies behind the oral cavity and extends from the soft palate to the level of the hyoid bone. It serves as a passageway for air and food. An upward rise of the soft palate prevents food from entering the nasopharynx during swallowing. The laryngopharynx, extending from the hyoid bone to the larynx, serves as a passageway for food and air. The larynx is about 2 inches (5 cm) long. It provides an airway, routes air and food into the proper passageway, and contains the vocal cords. As long as air is moving through the larynx, its inlet is open; however, the inlet closes during swallowing. The larynx is framed by the thyroid, the cricoid, and the epiglottis cartilages. The thyroid cartilage is formed by the fusion of two cartilages; the fusion point is visible as the Adam's

apple. The cricoid cartilage lies below the thyroid cartilage. The epiglottis normally projects upward to the base of the tongue; however, during swallowing, the larynx moves upward and the epiglottis tips to cover the opening to the larynx. If anything other than air enters the larynx, a cough reflex expels the foreign substance before it can enter the lungs. This protective reflex does not work if the person is unconscious.

2. During the physical assessment, assess for any manifestations that might indicate a genetic disorder. If data are found to indicate genetic risk factors or alterations, ask about genetic testing and refer for appropriate genetic counseling and evaluation. During the health assessment interview, ask about family members with health problems affecting respiratory function. In addition, ask about a family history of emphysema, asthma, cystic fibrosis, or lung cancer.

- Deficiency of alpha$_1$-antitrypsin is caused by a mutation of a gene located on chromosome 14. Deficiency of this protein leaves the lung susceptible to emphysema.
- Asthma, a disease that affects more than 5% of the population, is an inheritable disease with a number of genes responsible.
- Cystic fibrosis is the most common fatal genetic disease in the United States today. All gene defects result in defective transport of chloride and sodium by epithelial cells. As a result, the amount of sodium chloride is increased in body secretions. Thick mucus is produced that clogs the lungs, leads to infection, and blocks pancreatic enzymes from reaching the intestines to digest food.
- A familial history of lung cancer increases the risk of developing lung cancer, and small-cell lung cancer has a definite genetic component. In addition, researchers have found that lung cancer patients who never smoked are more likely than smokers to have one of two genetic mutations linked to the disease.

3.

Age-Related Change	Significance
• ↓ elastic recoil of lungs during expiration because of less elastic collagen and elastin • Calcification of the costal cartilage and weakening of the intercostal muscles • Loss of skeletal muscle strength in the thorax and diaphragm; flattening of the diaphragm • Alveoli that are less elastic and more fibrotic and that have fewer functional capillaries • Less effective cough • PO$_2$ reduced as much as 15% by age 80	The older adult often has an increased anterior-posterior chest diameter, with kyphosis and barrel chest. There is a reduction in vital capacity and an increase in residual volume, with decreased effectiveness in coughing up phlegm or sputum. All of these changes greatly increase the risk of respiratory infections, especially if the person becomes immobile. Also, with these changes, respiratory infections are more difficult to treat.

4. A bronchoscopy is the direct visualization of the larynx, trachea, and bronchi through a bronchoscope to identify lesions, remove foreign bodies and secretions, obtain tissue for biopsy, and improve tracheobronchial drainage. The bronchoscope is passed through the nose or mouth into the trachea. During the test, a catheter brush or biopsy forceps can be passed to obtain secretions or tissue for examination for cancer. The test is done in the hospital and may be done at the bedside, in a special procedure room, or in the surgical suite.

The following are associated nursing interventions:
- Assess for pregnancy and hypersensitivity to anesthetics, antibiotics, iodine, or contract dyes; if present, notify the physician.
- Tell the patient not to eat or drink fluids for 8–12 hours before the test.
- Remove dentures, contact lenses, and jewelry.
- Assess and record vital signs.
- Administer ordered premedications.
- After the procedure, assess for complications (laryngeal edema, bronchospasm, pneumothorax, cardiac dysrhythmias, and bleeding).
- Monitor for manifestations of respiratory difficulty (dyspnea, decreased breath sounds, decreased O$_2$ saturation) and hemoptysis (bloody sputum).
- Assess that the gag reflex is present before beginning food or fluids.
- Instruct the patient not to smoke for six to eight hours after the procedure, as smoking may cause coughing and bleeding.
- Tell the patient that it is normal to have some blood-tinged sputum, hoarseness, and/or a sore throat, but to notify the physician of any bleeding, pain, or respiratory difficulty.

Case Study

1. *What are some factors that affect ventilation and respiration?* Many factors affect ventilation and respiration. They include changes in volume and capacity; air pressures; oxygen, carbon dioxide, and hydrogen ion concentrations in the blood; airway resistance, lung compliance and elasticity; and alveolar surface tension.

2. *Where are the sinuses, and what is the purpose of sinuses?* The nasal cavity is surrounded by paranasal sinuses, located in the frontal, sphenoid, ethmoid, and maxillary bones. Sinuses lighten the skull, assist in speech, and produce mucus that drains into the nasal cavities to help trap debris.

3. *What is the difference between inspiratory reserve volume (IRV) and expiratory reserve volume (ERV)?* IRV is the amount of air (approximately 2000 to 3100 mL) that can be inhaled forcibly over the tidal volume. ERV is the amount of air that can be forced out over the tidal volume (approximately 1000 mL).

4. *What are some implications of changes in the patient's breathing pattern?* Damage to the brainstem from a stroke or head injury may result in tachypnea or bradypnea. Bradypnea is seen with some

circulatory disorders and lung disorders and as a side effect of some medications. Tachypnea is seen in atelectasis, pneumonia, asthma, pleural effusion, pneumothorax, congestive heart failure, and anxiety and in response to pain. Apnea, cessation of breathing that lasts from a few seconds to a few minutes, may occur after a stroke or head trauma, as a side effect of some medications, or after airway obstruction.

5. *What are the different characteristics of vesicular, bronchovesicular, and bronchial breath sounds?*

Type of Breath Sound	Characteristics
Vesicular	• Soft, low-pitched, gentle sounds • Sound heard over all areas of the lungs except the major bronchi • A 3:1 ratio for inspiration and expiration, with inspiration lasting longer than expiration
Bronchovesicular	• Medium pitch and intensity of sounds • A 1:1 ratio, with inspiration and expiration being equal in duration • Sound heard anteriorly over the primary bronchus on each side of the sternum and posteriorly between the scapulae
Bronchial	• Loud, high-pitched sounds • A gap between inspiration and expiration • A 2:3 ratio for inspiration and expiration, with expiration longer than inspiration • Sound heard over the manubrium

6. *How does the patient's trachea location change when the patient has a pleural effusion, pneumothorax, or atelectasis?* The trachea is normally midline. The trachea shifts to the unaffected side in pleural effusion and pneumothorax and shifts to the affected side in atelectasis.

Short Answers

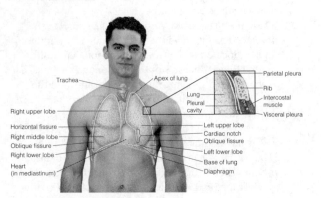

Figure 34–3 ■ The lower respiratory system, showing the location of the lungs, the mediastinum, and layers of visceral and parietal pleura.

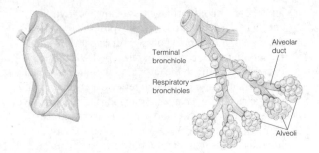

Figure 34–4 ■ Respiratory bronchi, bronchioles, alveolar ducts, and alveoli.

NCLEX-RN® Review Questions

1. Answer: 2
   Rationale: The left lung is smaller and has two lobes, whereas the right lung has three lobes. The laryngopharynx extends from the hyoid bone to the larynx. The parietal pleura lines the thoracic wall and mediastinum. During expiration, carbon dioxide is expelled.
   Nursing Process: Planning
   Patient Need: Physiological Integrity

2. Answer: 1
   Rationale: There are 12 pairs of ribs, and all of them articulate with the thoracic vertebrae. Anteriorly, the first seven ribs articulate with the body of the sternum. The eighth, ninth, and tenth ribs articulate with the cartilage immediately above the ribs. The eleventh and twelfth ribs are called floating ribs because they are unattached.
   Nursing Process: Assessment
   Patient Need: Physiological Integrity

3. Answer: 3
   Rationale: During expiration, the inspiratory muscles relax, the diaphragm rises, the ribs descend, and the lungs recoil. During inspiration, the diaphragm contracts and flattens out to increase the vertical diameter of the thoracic cavity. Expiration is primarily a passive process that occurs as a result of the elasticity of the lungs. A single inspiration lasts for about 1–1.5 seconds, whereas expiration lasts for about 2–3 seconds.
   Nursing Process: Evaluation
   Patient Need: Physiological Integrity

4. Answer: 3
   Rationale: A bronchoscopy is a direct visualization of the larynx, trachea, and bronchi. A pulmonary angiography identifies pulmonary emboli, tumors, aneurysms, vascular changes associated with emphysema, and pulmonary circulation. Arterial blood gases are conducted to evaluate alterations in acid–base balances. Pulse oximetry is used to evaluate or monitor the oxygen saturation of the blood. A thoracentesis, when done for diagnostic purposes, is conducted to obtain a specimen of pleural fluid.
   Nursing Process: Evaluation
   Patient Need: Physiological Integrity

5. Answer: 1

    Rationale: Dullness is heard in patients with atelectasis, lobar pneumonia, and pleural effusion. Retraction of intercostal spaces may be seen in asthma, not pneumothorax. Bulging of intercostal spaces may be seen in pneumothorax, not asthma. Bilateral chest expansion is decreased (not increased) in emphysema.

    Nursing Process: Assessment

    Patient Need: Physiological Integrity

6. Answer: 3

    Rationale: The lower respiratory tract includes the pleura. The upper respiratory tract includes the nose, trachea, and sinuses.

    Nursing Process: Assessment

    Patient Need: Physiological Integrity

7. Answer: 1

    Rationale: The upper respiratory tract includes the larynx. The lower respiratory tract includes the lungs, bronchi, and rib cage.

    Nursing Process: Assessment

    Patient Need: Physiological Integrity

Chapter 35

Terms Matching

1. C
2. H
3. L
4. J
5. F
6. M
7. D
8. B
9. A
10. E
11. G
12. I
13. K

Focused Study

1. Nasal mucous membranes appear red or erythematous and boggy. Swollen mucous membranes, local vasodilation, and secretions cause nasal congestion. Clear, watery secretions lead to coryza, profuse nasal discharge. Sneezing and coughing are common. Sore throat is common and may be the initial symptom. Systemic manifestations of acute viral upper respiratory infection infrequently include low-grade fever, headache, malaise, and muscle aches. Symptoms generally last for a few days up to two weeks.

2. Phenylephrine (Neo-Synephrine®), phenylpropanolamine (Comtrex®, Ornade, Triaminic®), pseudoephedrine (Sudafed®, Actifed®) The patient and family should be educated as follows:

    • Do not use more than the recommended dose.

    • Check with the healthcare provider before taking decongestants if you are taking any prescription medications or are being treated for high blood pressure or heart disease.

    • Use nasal sprays for no more than three to five days. Chronic use may lead to rhinitis medicamentosa, a rebound phenomenon of drug-induced nasal irritation and inflammation.

    • Increase fluid intake to relieve mouth dryness.

    • Stop the drugs if nervousness, shakiness, or difficulty sleeping occur.

    • Keep in mind that in some states, drugs containing pseudoephedrine may require a prescription or may be kept behind the counter to reduce its use in preparing methamphetamine.

3. Reye's syndrome is a rare but potentially fatal complication of influenza. Although it is more likely to affect children, it also has been identified in older adults. It is most often associated with influenza B virus. Reye's syndrome develops within two to three weeks after the onset of influenza. It has a 30% mortality rate. Hepatic failure and encephalopathy develop rapidly in patients with Reye's syndrome.

4.

    • Men are affected more than four times as often as women.

    • Cancer of the larynx usually develops between ages 50 and 70.

    • Tobacco use is the major risk factor for laryngeal cancer. The risk of developing laryngeal cancer is significantly greater in smokers than in nonsmokers.

    • Alcohol consumption is a significant cofactor in increasing the risk.

    • Other risk factors include poor nutrition, human papillomavirus infection, exposure to asbestos and other occupational pollutants, and race (African American).

Case Study

1. *Explain the pathophysiology of sleep apnea.* During sleep, all skeletal muscle tone decreases except the diaphragm. Skeletal tone is significantly decreased during rapid eye movement sleep. There is a loss of normal pharyngeal muscle tone, which permits the pharynx to collapse during inspiration as pressure in the airways becomes negative in relation to atmospheric pressure. Also during sleep, gravity pulls the tongue against the posterior pharyngeal wall, causing further obstruction. Obesity, changes in skeletal muscle tone, or changes in soft tissue that decrease inspiratory tone (for example, having a relatively large tongue in a relatively small oropharynx) also contribute to the problem. Airflow obstruction causes the oxygen saturation, PO_2, and pH to fall and the PCO_2 to rise in the patient's body. This progressive asphyxia causes brief arousal from sleep, which restores airway patency and airflow. Sleep can be severely fragmented as these episodes may occur hundreds of times each night.

2. *List the manifestations of obstructive sleep apnea.*
- Loud, cyclic snoring
- Periods of apnea lasting 15–120 seconds during sleep
- Gasping or choking during sleep
- Restlessness, thrashing during sleep
- Daytime fatigue and sleepiness
- Morning headache
- Personality changes, depression
- Intellectual impairment
- Impotence
- Hypertension

3. *Review the risk factors associated with obstructive sleep apnea.*
- Male gender
- Increasing age
- Obesity
- Large neck circumference (> 17 inches in men and > 16 inches in women)
- Use of central nervous system depressants

4. *How is obstructive sleep apnea typically diagnosed?*
The diagnosis of obstructive sleep apnea is based on polysomnography, an overnight sleep study. Several variables are recorded during the study, including the following:
- Electroencephalogram and measurements of ocular activity and muscle tone
- Recordings of ventilatory activity and airflow
- Continuous arterial oxygen saturation readings
- Heart rate

5. *Review the nonsurgical methods used to treat obstructive sleep apnea.* Mild to moderate obstructive sleep apnea may be treated through weight reduction, abstinence from alcohol, improved nasal patency, and avoidance of the supine position for sleep. Although weight reduction often cures the disorder, maintaining optimal weight is difficult. Oral appliances designed to keep the mandible and tongue forward also may be prescribed.

Nasal continuous positive airway pressure (CPAP) is the treatment of choice for obstructive sleep apnea. Positive pressure generated by an air compressor and administered through a tight-fitting nasal mask splints the pharyngeal airway, preventing collapse and obstruction. With proper training, this device is well tolerated by the patient. Nasal airways can become dry and irritated with CPAP, so an in-line humidifier or a room humidifier is recommended. A newer device, the BiPap® ventilator, delivers higher pressures during inhalation and lower pressures during expiration, providing less resistance to exhaling.

6. *Review the surgical methods for treating obstructive sleep apnea.* Tonsillectomy and adenoidectomy may help relieve upper airway obstruction in some patients. Excision of obstructive tissue from the soft palate, uvula, and posterior lateral pharyngeal wall may be accomplished by uvulopalatopharyngoplasty (UPPP). Although only about 50% of these surgeries are successful in treating sleep apnea, UPPP is useful in selected cases. In severe cases, tracheostomy may be performed to bypass the area of obstruction.

7. *Identify common nursing diagnoses that may be used in the plan of care for Mr. Smith.*
- *Fatigue* related to interrupted sleep patterns
- *Ineffective Breathing Pattern* related to obstruction of upper airway during sleep
- *Impaired Gas Exchange* related to altered lung ventilation during obstructive episodes
- *Disturbed Sleep Pattern* related to repeated apneic episodes
- *Risk for Injury* related to daytime somnolence and altered judgment
- *Risk for Sexual Dysfunction* related to impotence resulting from sleep apnea

Care Plan Critical-Thinking Activity

1. Ice-cold fluids may be easier to swallow than hot or room-temperature beverages and may provide a local analgesic effect.
2. Ms. Wunderman should avoid citrus fruits such as oranges, grapefruits, and lemons. Spicy food may irritate her throat. Foods served at a high temperature may cause pain. She should avoid chips and crunchy, hard foods after the surgery. It is recommended that she avoid these types of foods for at least one week.

Short Answers
Identify how laryngeal tumors are staged.

Stage 0	• Carcinoma *in situ*
	• No lymph node involvement or metastasis
Stage I	• Tumor confined to site of origin with normal vocal cord mobility
	• No lymph node involvement or metastasis
Stage II	• Tumor involves adjacent tissues
	• No lymph node involvement or metastasis
Stage III	• Tumor confined to larynx with fixation of vocal cords; immediately surrounding supraglottic tissues may be involved
	• No lymph node involvement or a single positive node on the side of the tumor
	• No metastasis
Stage IV	• Massive tumor that extends beyond boundaries of larynx to involve surrounding tissues
	• Single or multiple lymph nodes may be involved
	• Distant metastasis may be present

NCLEX-RN® Review Questions

1. Answer: 2
Rationale: The patient should blow his or her nose with both nostrils open to prevent infected matter from being forced into the eustachian tubes. The patient should use disposable tissues to cover his or her mouth and nose while coughing or sneezing to reduce airborne spread of the virus. The patient should wash his or her hands frequently, especially after coughing or sneezing, to limit viral transmission. The patient should limit use of nasal

decongestants to every four hours for only a few days at a time to prevent rebound effect.

Nursing Process: Evaluation

Patient Need: Physiological Integrity

2. Answer: 4

Rationale: Influenza types A, B, and C are found in humans.

Nursing Process: Assessment

Patient Need: Physiological Integrity

3. Answer: 3

Rationale: The patient should avoid straining during bowel movements, vigorous coughing, and strenuous exercise. The patient should apply ice or cold compresses to the nose to decrease swelling, promote comfort, and prevent bleeding. The patient should avoid blowing the nose for 24–48 hours after nasal packing is removed to prevent complications. Encourage the patient to rest for two to three days after surgery to reduce the risk of bleeding.

Nursing Process: Planning

Patient Need: Health Promotion and Maintenance

4. Answer: 1

Rationale: Water sports are contraindicated with a permanent tracheostomy. The patient should increase fluid intake to maintain mucosal moisture and loosen secretions. The patient should shield the stoma with a stoma guard to prevent particulate matter from entering the lower respiratory tract. The patient should use a humidifier or vaporizer to add humidity to inspired air.

Nursing Process: Evaluation

Patient Need: Health Promotion and Maintenance

5. Answer: 3

Rationale: Polyps are usually bilateral and have a stemlike base, which makes them fairly moveable. Polyps form in areas of dependent mucous membrane and present as pale, edematous masses that are covered with mucous membrane. Nasal polyps are benign grapelike growths of the mucous membrane that lines the nose. Polyps may be asymptomatic, although large polyps may cause nasal obstruction, rhinorrhea, and loss of sense of smell.

Nursing Process: Planning

Patient Need: Physiological Integrity

6. Answer: 2

Rationale: CPAP is used continuously throughout the night, not intermittently. Using the CPAP intermittently would not be effective for the patient's condition. Effective sleep apnea management depends on the patient's willingness to participate in care. The nurse should provide teaching about the following topics: the importance of using CPAP continuously at night, the relationship of alcohol and sedatives to sleep apnea, the need for an alcohol treatment program or Alcoholics Anonymous as indicated, the relationship between obesity and sleep apnea, and the importance of maintaining moist mucous membranes through adequate fluid intake.

Nursing Process: Planning

Patient Need: Health Promotion and Maintenance

Chapter 36

Terms Matching

1. F
2. L
3. A
4. K
5. H
6. D
7. B
8. J
9. C
10. E
11. G
12. I
13. N
14. M

Focused Study

1. The nurse should educate the patient about the following:
   • Increase fluid intake to keep mucus thin and meet increased needs related to fever.
   • Use over-the-counter analgesics and cough preparations containing dextromethorphan for symptom relief.
   • Understand the use and effects of any prescribed medications.
   • Recognize the importance of smoking cessation (as appropriate).

2. A number of defense mechanisms help maintain this sterile environment. Infectious particles trapped by the mucous membranes of the nose are removed by sneezing, while those deposited in the nasopharynx usually are swallowed or expectorated. Reflex closure of the epiglottis and the branching bronchial tree present anatomic barriers to entry of microorganisms and other possible contaminants. The cilia and mucus that line the respiratory tract and the cough reflex serve to trap and eliminate foreign matter that enters the lower respiratory tract. Organisms that make it past these barriers usually are rapidly phagocytized in the alveolus by resident macrophages; then they are attacked by the inflammatory and immune defenses of the body.

3. Manifestations of a lung abscess typically develop about two weeks after the precipitating event. The onset may be either acute or insidious. Early clinical manifestations are those of pneumonia: productive cough, chills and fever, pleuritic chest pain, malaise, and anorexia. The patient's temperature may be significantly elevated—103°F (39.4°C) or higher. When the abscess ruptures, the patient may expectorate large amounts of foul-smelling, purulent, and possibly blood-streaked sputum. Breath sounds are often diminished, and crackles may be auscultated in the region of the abscess. A dull sound may be noted upon percussion over the affected area.

4.
- General health and nutritional status, including intake of specific nutrients such as vitamin D (lack of vitamin D is associated with a higher risk of developing active tuberculosis)
- Presence of a chronic disease such as silicosis, diabetes, alcoholism, or HIV infection; past history of a gastrectomy
- History of a positive tuberculin test
- Medications such as corticosteroids or other immunosuppressive drugs
- Living and social situation
  - Natural light and ventilation in the home
  - Access to clean water, cooking facilities, grocery stores, and other services
  - Possible exposure to infected people (for example, sharing a household with someone with active TB, living in crowded facilities, being homeless, participating in senior activities frequently, and volunteering at residential care facilities or other institutional settings)
  - Access to health care

Case Study

1. *What are some other clinical manifestations of acute bacterial pneumonia?* The patient may exhibit diminished breath sounds, and fine crackles may be heard over the affected area of lung. A pleural friction rub may be audible. If the involved area is large and gas exchange is impaired, dyspnea and cyanosis may be noted.

2. *What are some differences in the way Ms. Sutter might present if she were older?* As an older adult, she may have atypical manifestations of pneumonia, with little cough, scant sputum, and minimal evidence of respiratory distress. Fever, tachypnea, and altered mentation or agitation could be the primary presenting symptoms.

3. *Ms. Sutter is diagnosed with pneumococcal pneumonia. What is the pathophysiology of this infection?* It is caused by *Streptococcus pneumoniae*. These bacteria reside in the upper respiratory tract of up to 70% of adults. The bacteria may be spread by direct person-to-person contact via droplets. In many cases, infection results from aspiration of resident bacteria. In the lower respiratory tract, the inflammatory response initiated by these organisms produces alveolar edema and the formation of exudate. As alveoli and respiratory bronchioles fill with serous exudate, blood cells, fibrin, and bacteria, consolidation of lung tissue occurs. The lower lobes of the lungs are usually affected because of gravity. Consolidation of a large portion of an entire lung lobe is known as lobar pneumonia. This is the typical pattern for pneumococcal pneumonia.

Bronchopneumonia is patchy consolidation involving several lobules. Other bacterial pneumonias often present with patchy involvement of bronchopneumonia; pneumococcal pneumonia may also follow this pattern. The process resolves when macrophages predominate, digesting and removing inflammatory exudate from the infected lung.

4. *What are some diagnostic tests that were likely used to determine that Ms. Sutter has pneumococcal pneumonia?*
- A chest x-ray is obtained to determine the extent and pattern of lung involvement. Fluid, infiltrates, consolidated lung tissue, and atelectasis appear as densities on the film.
- A CT scan provides a more detailed image of pulmonary tissue and may be used when the chest x-ray is not diagnostic.
- A sputum gram stain quickly identifies the infecting organisms as gram-positive or gram-negative bacteria. Antibiotic therapy can then be directed at the predominant type of organism until culture and sensitivity results are obtained.
- Sputum culture and sensitivity is ordered to identify the infecting organism and to determine the most effective antibiotic therapy. When obtaining sputum for culture, it is important to obtain secretions from the lower respiratory tract, not the mouth and nasal passages.
- Complete blood count (CBC) with white blood cell (WBC) differential shows an elevated WBC ($11,000/mm^3$ or higher) with increased circulating immature leukocytes in response to the infectious process. Changes in white blood cells are minimal in viral and other pneumonias.
- Serology testing, blood tests to detect antibodies to respiratory pathogens, may be used to identify the infecting organism when blood and sputum cultures are negative.
- Pulse oximetry, a noninvasive method of measuring arterial oxygen saturation, is ordered to continuously monitor gas exchange. Normally, the SaO_2 is 95% or higher. An SaO_2 of less than 95% may indicate impaired alveolar gas exchange.
- Arterial blood gases (ABGs) may be ordered to evaluate gas exchange. Respiratory secretions or pleuritic pain can interfere with alveolar ventilation. Alveolar inflammation can interfere with gas exchange across the alveolar-capillary membrane, especially when exudate or consolidation is present. An arterial oxygen tension (PO_2) of less than 75–80 mmHg indicates impaired gas exchange or alveolar ventilation. See Chapter 36 for more information about gas transport, arterial blood gases, and normal or expected values.
- Fiberoptic bronchoscopy may be done to obtain a sputum specimen or to remove secretions from the bronchial tree.

5. *Who should receive the pneumococcal pneumonia vaccine?* The vaccine is recommended for people who have a high risk of adverse outcome from bacterial pneumonias: people over age 65; individuals with chronic cardiac or respiratory conditions, diabetes mellitus, alcoholism, or other chronic diseases; and immunocompromised people.

A one-time revaccination is recommended for selected populations, including people over age 65 who were immunized more than five years previously and before age 65, people with chronic renal failure or immunosuppressive conditions, and people receiving chemotherapy with selected agents.

6. *Who should not receive the influenza vaccine?* Because the vaccine contains egg protein, it is not recommended for people who have a severe allergy to eggs or who have previously experienced a severe hypersensitivity response to the vaccine.

Care Plan Critical-Thinking Activity

1. Small cell lung carcinomas can synthesize bioactive products and hormones such as adrenocorticotropic hormones (ACTH), antidiuretic hormone (ADH), a parathormone-like hormone, and gastrin-releasing peptide. The nurse would not be surprised to find that the patient has a positive fluid balance due to increased levels of ADH.
2. Nicotine patches, nicotine gum, medications used to block nicotine receptors, counseling, and hypnosis; educating Mr. Mueller about the hazards of continuing to smoke

Short Answers

Fill in the blanks regarding the surgeries used to treat lung cancer.

Procedure	Description	Used for
Laser bronchoscopy	Bronchoscopy-guided laser used to resect tumor	Tumors localized in a main bronchus
Mediastinoscopy	Visualization of the mediastinum using an endoscope passed through a suprasternal incision	Evaluation and biopsy of a mediastinal tumor and lymph nodes
Thoracotomy	Incision into the chest wall	Access to the lung and thoracic cavity for surgery
Wedge resection	Removal of a small section of peripheral lung tissue	Small peripheral lung tumors
Segmental resection	Removal of an individual bronchovascular segment of a lobe	Peripheral lung tumor with no evidence of extension to the chest wall or metastasis
Sleeve resection (bronchoplastic reconstruction)	Resection of a section of a major bronchus with reconstruction of remaining normal bronchus	Small lesion of a major bronchus
Lobectomy	Removal of a single lung lobe	Tumors confined to a single lobe
Pneumonectomy	Removal of an entire lung	Widespread tumor throughout the lung, tumor that involves the main bronchus, or tumor fixed to the hilum

NCLEX-RN® Review Questions

1. Answer: 2
   Rationale: Bacteria, viruses, fungi, protozoa, and other microbes can lead to infectious pneumonia. Inflammation of the lung parenchyma (the respiratory bronchioles and alveoli) is known as pneumonia. Noninfectious causes of pneumonia include aspiration of gastric contents and inhalation of toxic or irritating gases. The most common causative organism for community-acquired pneumonia is *Streptococcus pneumoniae* (also called pneumococcus), a gram-positive bacterium.
   Nursing Process: Evaluation
   Patient Need: Physiological Integrity
2. Answer: 4
   Rationale: The infective agent responsible for SARS is a coronavirus not previously identified in humans. The incubation period for SARS is generally 2–7 days, although it may be as long as 10 days in some people. Fever higher than 100.4°F (38°C) is typically the initial manifestation of the disease. The primary population affected by SARS is previously healthy adults aged 25 to 70 years.
   Nursing Process: Evaluation
   Patient Need: Physiological Integrity
3. Answer: 3
   Rationale: A previously healed tuberculosis lesion may be reactivated. Primary or secondary tuberculosis lesions may affect other body systems such as the kidneys, the genitalia, bone, and the brain. Worldwide, TB continues to be a significant health problem. *Mycobacterium tuberculosis* is a relatively slow-growing, slender, rod-shaped, acid-fast organism with a waxy outer capsule that increases its resistance to destruction.
   Nursing Process: Planning
   Patient Need: Physiological Integrity
4. Answer: 4
   Rationale: Tuberculosis is not spread by touching inanimate objects, so no special precautions are required for eating utensils. Patient teaching for ways to limit transmitting the disease to others includes to

cough and expectorate into tissues, dispose of tissues properly by placing them in a closed bag, and wear a mask if you are sneezing or unable to control respiratory secretions.

Nursing Process: Planning

Patient Need: Health Promotion and Maintenance

5. Answer: 3

Rationale: Histoplasmosis, an infectious disease caused by *Histoplasma capsulatum*, is the most common fungal lung infection in the United States. The organism is found in the soil and is linked to exposure to bird droppings and bats. Initial chest x-rays are nonspecific; later ones show areas of calcification. Infection occurs when the spores are inhaled and reach the alveoli.

Nursing Process: Evaluation

Patient Need: Physiological Integrity

6. Answer: 2

Rationale: Preprocedure fasting or sedation is not required for a thoracentesis. Verify the presence of a signed informed consent for the procedure. Position the patient upright and leaning forward with arms and head supported on an anchored overbed table. Administer a cough suppressant if indicated.

Nursing Process: Implementation

Patient Need: Physiological Integrity

Chapter 37

Terms Matching

1. C
2. E
3. J
4. B
5. D
6. H
7. N
8. K
9. P
10. M
11. I
12. L
13. O
14. A
15. F
16. G

Focused Study

1. Aging affects pulmonary ventilation as well as gas exchange. The number of alveoli decrease, and emphysematous changes reduce the surface area for gas exchange. Alveoli become less elastic, causing increased air trapping and dead space. For most older adults who remain active, these changes have minimal effect on exercise tolerance and activities of daily living. When combined with lung disease, however, age-related pulmonary changes increase the patient's risk for developing respiratory failure.

2. Theophylline (Bronkotabs®, Quibron®, Slo-Phyllin®, Theolair®, Theo-Dur®), aminophylline (Somophyllin)

Monitor the patient for manifestations of toxicity. Anorexia, nausea, vomiting, restlessness, insomnia, cardiac dysrhythmias, and seizures are early manifestations. Other manifestations include epigastric pain, hematemesis, diarrhea, headache, irritability, muscle twitching, palpitations, tachycardia, flushing, and circulatory failure.

3. Leukotriene modifiers are used for maintenance therapy in adults and in children over the age of 12 as an alternative to inhaled corticosteroid therapy. They are not used to treat an acute attack.

Montelukast (Singulair®), Zafirlukast (Accolate®), Zileuton (Zyflo®)

4. Pursed-lip and diaphragmatic breathing techniques help minimize air trapping and fatigue. Pursed-lip breathing helps maintain open airways by maintaining positive pressures longer during exhalation. Teach the patient to do the following:
• Inhale through the nose with the mouth closed.
• Exhale slowly through pursed lips, as though whistling or blowing out a candle, making exhalation twice as long as inhalation.

Diaphragmatic, or abdominal, breathing helps conserve energy by using the larger and more efficient muscles of respiration. Teach the patient to do the following:
• Place one hand on the abdomen and the other on the chest.
• Inhale, concentrating on pushing the abdominal hand outward while the chest hand remains still.
• Exhale slowly while the abdominal hand moves inward and the chest hand remains still.

Several different coughing techniques may be useful. For the controlled cough technique, teach the patient to do the following:
• After prescribed bronchodilator treatment, inhale deeply and hold breath briefly.
• Cough twice—the first time to loosen mucus, the second time to expel secretions.
• Inhale by sniffing to prevent mucus from moving back into deep airways.
• Rest. Avoid prolonged coughing to prevent fatigue and hypoxemia.

For "huff" coughing, teach the patient to do the following:
• Inhale deeply while leaning forward.
• Exhale sharply with a "huff" sound to help keep airways open while mobilizing secretions.

Case Study

1. *Summarize the triggers of asthma.* Childhood asthma is most often linked to inhalation of allergens such as pollen, animal dander, or household dust. Patients with allergic asthma often have a history of other allergies. Environmental pollutants such as tobacco smoke and irritant gases can provoke asthma. Exposure to

secondhand smoke as a child is associated with a higher risk for and increased severity of asthma. Agents found in the workplace, such as noxious fumes and gases, chemicals, and dusts, may cause occupational asthma. Respiratory infections (viral infections in particular) are a common internal stimulus for an asthmatic attack. Exercise-induced asthma attacks also are common. Loss of heat or water from the bronchial surface may contribute to exercise-induced asthma. Exercising in cold, dry air increases the risk of an asthma attack in susceptible people. Emotional stress is a significant etiologic factor for attacks in as many as half of the patients with asthma. Common pharmacologic triggers include aspirin and other NSAIDs, sulfites, and beta-blockers.

2. *List the clinical manifestations associated with acute asthma.*
   - Chest tightness
   - Cough
   - Dyspnea
   - Wheezing
   - Tachypnea and tachycardia
   - Anxiety and apprehension

3. *Explain how to use a metered-dose inhaler and a dry powder inhaler.* Proper use of a metered-dose inhaler is as follows:
   - Firmly insert a charged metered-dose inhaler canister into the mouthpiece unit or spacer.
   - Remove mouthpiece cap. Shake canister vigorously for three to five seconds.
   - Exhale slowly and completely.
   - When a spacer is being used, hold the canister upside down, place the mouthpiece in the mouth, and close the lips around it. When no spacer is used, hold the mouthpiece directly in front of the mouth.
   - Press and hold the canister down while inhaling deeply and slowly for three to five seconds.
   - Hold breath for 10 seconds, release pressure on the container, remove from mouth, and exhale. Wait 20–30 seconds before repeating the procedure for a second puff.
   - Rinse the mouth after using the inhaler to minimize systemic absorption and drying of the mucous membranes.
   - Rinse the inhaler mouthpiece and spacer after use; store in a clean location.

   Proper use of a dry powder inhaler is as follows:
   - Keep the inhaler and medication in a clean, dry location. Do not refrigerate or store in a humid place such as the bathroom.
   - Remove the cap and hold the inhaler upright. Inspect to make sure the mechanism is clean and the mouthpiece is clear.
   - If necessary, load the dose into the inhaler and follow the manufacturer's directions.
   - Hold the inhaler level with the mouthpiece, end facing down.
   - Breathe slowly and completely. Tilt head back slightly.
   - Place the mouthpiece in the mouth with the teeth over the mouthpiece. Seal the lips around the mouthpiece. Do not block the inhaler with the tongue.
   - Breathe in rapidly and deeply through the mouth for two to three seconds to activate the flow of medication.
   - Remove the inhaler from the mouth and hold breath for 10 seconds.
   - Exhale slowly through pursed lips to allow the medication to enter distal airways. To prevent clogging, do not exhale into the inhaler mouthpiece.
   - Rinse mouth or brush teeth after using the inhaler to prevent the medication from leaving a bad taste. This also prevents a yeast infection if a corticosteroid medication is used.
   - Store the inhaler in a clean, sealed plastic bag; do not wash the inhaler unless directed to do so by the manufacturer. The mouthpiece should be cleaned weekly using a dry cloth.

4. *Discuss methods that can be used to prevent asthma attacks.* Asthma attacks often can be prevented by avoiding allergens and environmental triggers. Modifying the home environment by controlling dust, removing carpets, covering mattresses and pillows to reduce dust mite populations, and installing air filtration systems may be useful. Pets may need to be removed from the household. Eliminating all tobacco smoke in the home is vital. Wearing a mask that retains humidity and warm air during exercise in cold weather may help prevent attacks of exercise-induced asthma. Early treatment of respiratory infections is vital to prevent asthma exacerbations.

5. *What is the underlying pathophysiology of asthma?* The airways are in a persistent state of inflammation. During symptom-free periods, airway inflammation in asthma is subacute or quiet. Even during these periods, however, inflammatory cells such as eosinophils, neutrophils, and lymphocytes may be found in airway tissues and edema may be present. An acute inflammatory response, during which time resident inflammatory cells interact with inflammatory mediators, cytokines, and additional infiltrating inflammatory cells, may be triggered by a variety of factors. Common triggers for an acute asthma attack include exposure to allergens, respiratory tract infection, exercise, inhaled irritants, and emotional upsets.

6. *What is status asthmaticus?* It is severe, prolonged asthma that does not respond to routine treatment. Without aggressive therapy, status asthmaticus can lead to respiratory failure with hypoxemia, hypercapnia, and acidosis. Endotracheal intubation, mechanical ventilation, and aggressive drug treatment may be necessary to sustain life.

7. *What diagnostic tests can be used to diagnose asthma?*
   - Pulmonary function tests are used to evaluate the degree of airway obstruction. Pulmonary function testing done before and after use of an aerosolized bronchodilator helps determine the reversibility of airway obstruction. Airway reversibility is a cardinal sign seen on pulmonary function testing in

asthma. The residual volume (RV) of the lungs may be increased and vital capacity decreased or normal even during periods of remission. The forced expiratory volume (FEV_1) and peak expiratory flow rate (PEFR), commonly referred to as peak flow, are the most valuable pulmonary function studies used to evaluate the severity of an asthma attack and the effectiveness of treatment measures.

- Challenge or bronchial provocation testing uses an inhaled substance such as methacholine or histamine with PFTs to confirm the diagnosis of asthma by detecting airway hyperresponsiveness.
- Arterial blood gases (ABGs) are drawn during an acute attack to evaluate oxygenation, carbon dioxide elimination, and acid–base status. ABGs initially show hypoxemia with a low PO_2 and mild respiratory alkalosis with an elevated pH and low PCO_2 due to tachypnea. Severe airflow obstruction causes significant hypoxemia and respiratory acidosis, indicative of respiratory failure and the need for mechanical ventilation.
- Skin testing may be done to identify specific allergens if an allergic trigger is suspected for asthma attacks.

Care Plan Critical-Thinking Activity

1. Mrs. Adamson has an increased risk for reduced cardiac output. Urinary output can help the nurse determine how well Mrs. Adamson's kidneys are being perfused. Her kidneys are being perfused well if her cardiac output is sufficient, and her urinary output will remain at 30 mL or greater per hour.

Short Answers

Fill in the blanks regarding the stepwise approach to asthma management in adults.

Step/Disease Severity	Preferred Treatment	Alternative or As-Needed Treatment
Step 1 Mild Intermittent	No daily medication needed	Use systemic corticosteroids for severe exacerbations.
Step 2 Mild Persistent	Low-dose inhaled corticosteroids	Use cromolyn, leukotriene modifier, nedocromil, or sustained release theophylline.
Step 3 Moderated Persistent	Low- to moderate-dose inhaled corticosteroids *and* long-acting inhaled beta2-agonist	Increase inhaled corticosteroid dose *or* combine inhaled corticosteroid with leukotriene modifier or theophylline.
Step 4 Severe Persistent	High-dose inhaled corticosteroid *and* long-acting inhaled beta2-agonist	Add systemic corticosteroid.

NCLEX-RN® Review Questions

1. Answer: 1

   Rationale: In a patient with cystic fibrosis, the secretions in the affected organs become thick and viscous, obstructing glands and ducts. There is excess mucus production in the respiratory tract with impaired ability to clear secretions and progressive chronic obstructive pulmonary disease. The patient develops pancreatic enzyme deficiency and impaired digestion. There is an abnormal elevation of sodium and chloride concentrations in sweat.

   Nursing Process: Assessment
   Patient Need: Physiological Integrity

2. Answer: 2

   Rationale: It is a state of partial or total lung collapse and airlessness. The most common cause of atelectasis is obstruction of the bronchus that ventilates a segment of lung tissue. It can be an acute or chronic condition. The primary therapy for atelectasis is prevention.

   Nursing Process: Assessment
   Patient Need: Physiological Integrity

3. Answer: 1

   Rationale: Inhalation using a metered-dose inhaler should be for only three to five seconds. Other patient teaching for using a metered-dose inhaler includes the following: Firmly insert a charged metered-dose inhaler (MDI) canister into the mouthpiece unit or spacer (if used), remove mouthpiece cap, and shake canister vigorously for 3–5 seconds; exhale slowly and completely; when a spacer is used, hold the canister upside down, place the mouthpiece in the mouth, and close the lips around it; when no spacer is used, hold the mouthpiece directly in front of the mouth, press and hold the canister down while inhaling deeply and slowly for 3–5 seconds, hold breath for 10 seconds, release pressure on the container, remove from mouth, and exhale; wait 20–30 seconds before repeating the procedure for a second puff; rinse the mouth after using the inhaler to minimize systemic absorption and drying of the mucous membranes; rinse the inhaler mouthpiece and spacer after use; and store in a clean location.

   Nursing Process: Implementation
   Patient Need: Physiological Integrity

4. Answer: 2

   Rationale: When using a dry powder inhaler, the inhaler should be held with the mouthpiece end facing down, not up. Other patient teaching for using a dry powder inhaler includes the following: Keep the inhaler and medication in a clean, dry location; do not refrigerate or store in a humid place such as the bathroom; remove the cap and hold the inhaler upright; inspect the inhaler to make sure the mechanism is clean and the mouthpiece is clear; if necessary, load the dose into the inhaler and follow manufacturer's directions; hold the inhaler level with the mouthpiece end facing down; breathe slowly and completely; tilt the head back slightly; place the mouthpiece in the mouth with the teeth over the

mouthpiece; seal the lips around the mouthpiece; do not block the inhaler with the tongue; breathe in rapidly and deeply through the mouth for 2–3 seconds to activate the flow of medication; remove the inhaler from the mouth and hold breath for 10 seconds; exhale slowly through pursed lips to allow the medication to enter distal airways; do not exhale into the inhaler mouthpiece to prevent clogging; rinse mouth or brush teeth after using the inhaler to prevent the medication from leaving a bad taste and to prevent a yeast infection if a corticosteroid medication is being used; store the inhaler in a clean, sealed plastic bag; do not wash the inhaler unless directed to do so by the manufacturer; and clean the mouthpiece weekly using a dry cloth.
Nursing Process: Evaluation
Patient Need: Physiological Integrity

5. Answer: 3
Rationale: The patient should be taught to perform the "huff" coughing technique. The patient should increase fluid intake to at least 2500 mL per day and should have a humidifier at bedside. Head of bed should be elevated to at least 30 degrees at all times. The nurse should assess the patient's respiratory status and level of consciousness every one to two hours until stable, then at least every five hours.
Nursing Process: Assessment
Patient Need: Physiological Integrity

Chapter 38

Terms Matching
1. D
2. G
3. B
4. I
5. C
6. E
7. A
8. F
9. H

Focused Study
1. The primary manifestations of altered function of the musculoskeletal system are pain and limited mobility. Specific descriptors of the pain, its location, and its nature are important. Other significant information includes associated manifestations such as fever; fatigue; and changes in weight, rash, and/or swelling.
2. Collect information about the patient's lifestyle, including type of employment, ability to carry out activities of daily living (ADL) and provide self-care, exercise or participation in sports, use of alcohol or drugs, and nutrition. Explore past injuries and measures to self-treat pain [such as over-the-counter (OTC) medications, prescribed medications, application of heat or cold, splinting, wrapping, or rest].
3. The musculoskeletal system is composed of bones of the skeletal system, cartilage (a connective tissue),

ligaments, tendons, and skeletal muscles and joints. The bones serve as the framework for the body and for the attachment of muscles, tendons, and ligaments. Innervated by the nervous system, contraction and relaxation of muscles permit movement at joints.

4.

Abduction	Move limb away from body midline
Adduction	Move limb toward body midline
Extension	Straighten limbs at joint
Flexion	Bend limbs at joint
Dorsiflexion	Bend ankle to bring top of foot toward shin
Plantar flexion	Straighten ankle to point toes down
Pronation	Turn forearm to place palm down
Supination	Turn forearm to place palm up
Eversion	Turn out
Inversion	Turn in
Circumduction	Move in circle
Internal rotation	Move inward on a central axis
External rotation	Move outward on a central axis
Protraction	Move forward and parallel to ground

Case Study
1. *Bones are classified by which shapes?* Long bones, short bones, flat bones, and irregular bones
2. *Summarize bone remodeling in adults.* Although the bones of adults do not normally increase in length and size, constant remodeling of bones, as well as repair of damaged bone tissue, occurs throughout life. In the bone remodeling process, bone resorption and bone deposit occur at all periosteal and endosteal surfaces. Hormones and forces that put stress on the bones regulate this process, which involves a combined action of the osteocytes, osteoclasts, and osteoblasts. Bones that are in use—and are therefore subjected to stress—increase their osteoblastic activity to increase ossification (the development of bone). Bones that are inactive undergo increased osteoclast activity and bone resorption.
3. *What are the different types of joints?* Joints may be classified by function as synarthroses, amphiarthroses, or diarthroses.

Short Answers
Fill in the table below regarding the functional classification of joints.

Type	Description	Examples
Synarthrosis	Immovable joint	Skull sutures Epiphyseal plates Joint between first rib and manubrium of sternum

Amphiarthrosis	Slightly moveable joint	Vertebral joints Joint of the symphysis pubis
Diarthrosis	Freely moveable joint	Joints of the extremities Shoulder joints Hip joints

NCLEX-RN® Review Questions

1. Answer: 4
   Rationale: The tissues and structures of the musculoskeletal system perform many functions, including support, protection, and movement. The musculoskletal system is composed of bones of the skeletal system, cartilage (a connective tissue), ligaments, tendons, and skeletal muscles and joints. The bones serve as the framework for the body and for the attachment of muscles, tendons, and ligaments. The musculoskeletal system has two subsystems: (1) the bones and joints of the skeleton and (2) the skeletal muscles.
   Nursing Process: Evaluation
   Patient Need: Health Promotion and Maintenance

2. Answer: 2
   Rationale: The human skeleton is made up of 206 bones. Bones store minerals and serve as a site for blood cell formation. Bones of the skeletal system are divided into the axial skeleton (skull, thorax, and vertebrae) and the appendicular skeleton (shoulders, arms, pelvic girdle, and legs). Bones form the body's structure and provide support for soft tissues. They protect vital organs from injury and serve to move body parts by providing points of attachment for muscles.
   Nursing Process: Assessment
   Patient Need: Physiological Integrity

3. Answer: 2
   Rationale: Long bones are longer than they are wide.
   Nursing Process: Assessment
   Patient Need: Physiological Integrity

4. Answer: 4
   Rationale: Short bones, also called cuboid bones, include the bones of the wrist and ankle.
   Nursing Process: Assessment
   Patient Need: Physiological Integrity

5. Answer: 1
   Rationale: The three types of muscle tissue in the body are skeletal muscle, smooth muscle, and cardiac muscle.
   Nursing Process: Assessment
   Patient Need: Physiological Integrity

6. Answer: 3
   Rationale: The body has approximately 600 skeletal muscles.
   Nursing Process: Assessment
   Patient Need: Physiological Integrity

7. Answer: 4
   Rationale: Synovial joints are freely moveable, allow many kinds of movements, and are found at all articulations of the limb. Amphiarthrosis joints are

slightly moveable. Cartilaginous joints are immobile. Fibrous joints permit little or no movement.
   Nursing Process: Assessment
   Patient Need: Physiological Integrity

8. Answer: 3
   Rationale: Abduction is to move the limb away from the body midline.
   Nursing Process: Assessment
   Patient Need: Physiological Integrity

9. Answer: 2
   Rationale: A lateral, S-shaped curvature of the spine is called scoliosis.
   Nursing Process: Assessment
   Patient Need: Physiological Integrity

10. Answer: 3
    Rationale: Numbness and burning in the fingers during Phalen's test may indicate carpal tunnel syndrome.
    Nursing Process: Assessment
    Patient Need: Physiological Integrity

Chapter 39

Terms Matching
1. E
2. K
3. G
4. O
5. A
6. M
7. N
8. F
9. J
10. B
11. L
12. C
13. I
14. H
15. D

Focused Study

1. The nursing care of a patient with a repetitive use injury focuses on relieving pain, teaching about the disease process and treatment, and improving physical mobility.
   Acute Pain: Swelling and nerve inflammation cause pain in the patient with a repetitive use injury.
   • Ask the patient to rate the pain on a scale of 0–10 (with 10 being the most severe pain) before and after any intervention. This facilitates objective assessment of the effectiveness of the chosen pain relief strategy.
   • Encourage the use of immobilizers. Splinting maintains joint alignment and prevents pain due to movement of inflamed tissues.
   • Teach the patient to apply ice and/or heat as prescribed. Ice causes vasoconstriction and decreases the pooling of blood in the inflamed area. Ice may also numb the tender area. Heat decreases swelling by increasing venous return.

- Encourage use of NSAIDs as prescribed. NSAIDs decrease swelling by inhibiting prostaglandins.
- Explain why treatment should not be abruptly discontinued. Abrupt discontinuation of treatment may cause reinflammation of the injured area.

    Impaired Physical Mobility: Joint pain and swelling can limit range of motion of the affected joint.

- Suggest interventions to alleviate pain (such as using an immobilizer and taking pain medications). If the joint is pain-free, the patient will be more likely to take an active role in therapy.
- Refer to a physical therapist for exercises. The physical therapist can assist the patient with exercise to prevent joint stiffness.
- Suggest consultation with an occupational therapist. Occupational therapy can help the patient learn new ways to perform tasks to prevent recurring symptoms.

2. Nursing interventions for patients with a cast include the following:
- Perform frequent neurovascular assessments.
- Palpate the cast for "hot spots" that may indicate the presence of underlying infection.
- Promptly report increased or severe pain, changes in neurovascular status, or a hot spot or drainage on the cast.

    Nursing interventions for patients in traction include the following:

- Maintain the pulling force and direction of the traction:
    a. Keep in mind that in most instances, the patient's weight provides countertraction.
    b. Center the patient on the bed; maintain body alignment with the direction of pull.
    c. Do not wedge the patient's foot or place it flush with the footboard of the bed.
    d. Ensure that weights hang freely and do not touch the floor.
    e. Ensure that nothing is lying on or obstructing the ropes.
    f. Do not allow the knots at the end of the rope to come in contact with the pulley.
- Perform neurovascular assessments frequently.
- Assess for common complications of immobility, including pressure ulcer formation, renal calculi, deep venous thrombosis, pneumonia, paralytic ileus, and loss of appetite.
- If a problem is detected, assist in repositioning. Stabilize the fracture site during repositioning.
- Teach the patient and family about the type of traction and its purpose.

For skin traction:
    a. Frequently assess skin, bony prominences, and pressure points for evidence of pressure, shearing, or pending breakdown.
    b. Protect pressure sites with padding and protective dressings as indicated.
    c. Remove weights only if intermittent traction has been ordered to alleviate muscle spasm.

For skeletal traction:
    a. Never remove the weights.

    b. Frequently assess pin insertion sites and provide pin site care per policy.
    c. Report signs of infection at the pin sites, such as redness, drainage, and increased tenderness.

Nursing interventions for patients with internal fixation include the following:
- Frequently assess type, location, and severity of pain. Report pain that is increasing in severity, is unexpected, or is unrelieved by prescribed analgesia.
- Perform neurovascular assessments frequently, promptly reporting any change in pulses, color, temperature, capillary refill, or movement or sensation of the affected extremity.

Assess the following:
    a. Amount, color, and odor of drainage on dressing and in wound drain device (for example, Hemovac, Jackson-Pratt).
    b. Bowel sounds
    c. Lung sounds
- Administer medications such as analgesics and antibiotics per physician's orders.
- In hip fractures, place an abductor pillow between patient's legs to prevent dislocation of the hip joint.
- Arrange for physical and occupational therapy as ordered.
- Assist with weight-bearing program if ordered.
- Encourage early mobilization, coughing, and deep breathing as appropriate to help prevent complications.

3. Fracture healing progresses over four phases: hematoma formation, fibrocartilaginous callus formation, bony callus formation, and remodeling.

    A hematoma forms between the fractured bone ends and around the bone surfaces. Fractured bone surfaces and fragments are deprived of oxygen and nutrients, leading to localized necrosis. Cellular necrosis heightens the inflammatory response and release of inflammatory mediators. In turn, these chemicals cause vasodilation and edema. Fibroblasts, lymphocytes, and macrophages migrate to the fracture site. Fibroblasts in the hematoma form a fibrin meshwork. Lymphocytes and macrophages wall off the area, localizing and containing the inflammation.

    Within 48 hours, fibroblasts and new capillaries growing into the fracture form granulation tissue that gradually replaces the hematoma. Phagocytes remove cell debris. Osteoblasts (bone-forming cells) migrate to the fracture site, where they build a web of collagen fibers from both sides of the fractured bone. Chondroblasts lay down patches of cartilage as a base for bone growth. This fibrocartilaginous callus connects bone fragments, splinting the fracture and maintaining bone alignment. However, it cannot yet support weight bearing.

    The third stage of fracture healing, bony callus formation, begins three to four weeks after the injury and continues for two to three months. Osteoblasts continue to form collagen fibers and bone matrix, which are gradually mineralized with calcium and mineral salts. Osteoclasts migrate to the repair site to remove damaged and excess bone in the callus. Fibrocartilagenous callus is gradually replaced with spongy bone. This process progresses from the outer surface of the bone toward the fracture site.

In the final phase of healing, remodeling, excess callus is removed and new bone is laid down along the fracture line. As the bone heals and again is subjected to the mechanical stress of everyday use, osteoblasts and osteoclasts remodel the repair site along the lines of force. Spongy bone is replaced by compact bone, and the remodeled area closely resembles the original unbroken bone.

4. Potential complications of an amputation include infection, delayed healing, chronic stump pain and phantom pain, and contractures.

Case Study

1. *Define* strain *and* sprain. A strain is a stretching injury to a muscle or a muscle-tendon unit caused by mechanical overloading. A muscle that is forced to extend past its elasticity will develop microscopic tears. A sprain is a stretch and/or tear of one or more ligaments surrounding a joint. Forces going in opposite directions cause the ligament to overstretch and/or tear. The ligaments may be partially or completely torn.

2. *Give examples of how a strain or sprain could occur.* A person lifting heavy objects without bending the knees or a sudden acceleration/deceleration, as in a motor vehicle crash, can cause strains. Coming down awkwardly on a knee or an ankle after jumping or turning the ankle or knee during walking or running also may cause a sprain.

3. *What are the manifestations of a strain and a sprain?* The manifestations of a strain include pain, limited motion, muscle spasms, swelling, and possible muscle weakness. Severe strains that partially or completely tear the muscle or tendon can be disabling with significant bleeding, swelling, and bruising around the muscle. Manifestations include loss of the functional ability of the joint, a feeling of a "pop" or tear, discoloration, pain, and rapid swelling. Motion increases the joint pain. The intensity of the manifestations of a sprain depend on the severity.

4. *Explain RICE therapy.* The goal of the initial stage of treating soft tissue trauma is to reduce swelling and pain. Patients should follow a regimen of rest, ice, compression, and elevation (RICE) for the first 24–48 hours.

RICE therapy for musculoskeletal injuries is as follows:

Rest	• Decrease regular activities of daily living and exercise as needed. • Limit weight bearing on the injured extremity for 48 hours. • If you use a cane or crutch to avoid weight bearing, use it on the uninjured side so that you can lean away from and relieve weight on the injured leg.
Ice	• To avoid cold injury or frostbite, apply an ice pack to the injured area for no more than 20 minutes at a time, four to eight times a day. • An ice bag, a cold pack, a plastic bag filled with crushed ice and wrapped in a towel, or a bag of frozen peas may be used.
Compression	• Compression often helps reduce swelling. • Examples of compression bandages include Ace™ wraps, special boots, air casts, and splints.
Elevation	• Keep the injured extremity elevated on a pillow above heart level to help reduce swelling and pain.

Short Answers

Fill in the table regarding the manifestations of fractures.

Manifestation	Pathophysiology
Deformity	Abnormal position of bones secondary to fracture and muscles pulling on fractured bone
Swelling	Edema from localization of serous fluid and bleeding
Pain/tenderness	Muscle spasm, direct tissue trauma, nerve pressure, movement of fractured bone
Numbness	Nerve damage or nerve entrapment
Guarding	Pain
Crepitus	Grating of bones or entrance of air into an open fracture. *Note:* Do not manipulate the extremity to elicit crepitus; doing so may cause additional damage.
Hypovolemic shock	Blood loss or associated injuries
Muscle spasms	Muscle contraction near the fracture
Ecchymosis	Extravasation of blood into the subcutaneous tissue

NCLEX-RN® Review Questions

1. Answer: 2
   Rationale: The manifestations of a strain include pain, limited motion, muscle spasms, swelling, and possible muscle weakness. Common sites for a muscle strain are the lower back and the hamstring muscle in the back of the thigh. Severe strains that partially or completely tear the muscle or tendon can be disabling with significant bleeding, swelling, and bruising around the muscle. A sprain is a stretch and/or tear of one or more ligaments surrounding a joint.
   Nursing Process: Assessment
   Patient Need: Physiological Integrity

2. Answer: 1
   Rationale: The *R* in RICE stands for rest. RICE stands for rest, ice, compression, and elevation.

Nursing Process: Implementation
Patient Need: Physiological Integrity

3. Answer: 1
Rationale: A dislocation is an injury in which the ends of bones are displaced out of their normal position and joint articulation is lost.
Nursing Process: Diagnosis
Patient Need: Physiological Integrity

4. Answer: 4
Rationale: Two basic mechanisms produce fractures: direct force and indirect force. Fractures vary in severity according to the location and type of fracture. A fracture occurs when the bone is subjected to more kinetic energy than it can absorb. Any of the 206 bones in the body can be fractured.
Nursing Process: Diagnosis
Patient Need: Physiological Integrity

5. Answer: 1
Rationale: Compartment syndrome usually develops within the first 48 hours of injury, when edema is at its peak. Compartment syndrome occurs when pressure in this confined space constricts and entraps the structures. Acute compartment syndrome may result from hemorrhage and edema in the compartment after a fracture or from a crush injury or from external compression of the limb by a cast that is too tight. Muscles, nerves, and blood vessels of the extremities are enclosed by a fibrous membrane or fascia. The fascia, which is nonexpendable, supports these tissues.
Nursing Process: Evaluation
Patient Need: Physiological Integrity

6. Answer: 2
Rationale: Types of traction are as follows:
• In skeletal traction, the pulling force is applied directly through pins inserted into the bone. Local, spinal, or general anesthetic is provided during pin placement. One or more pulling forces may be applied with skeletal traction. Skeletal traction allows more weight to be used to maintain the proper anatomic alignment. The risk of infection is greater, however, and it may cause more discomfort. The weights used for skeletal traction are not removed by the nurse.
• Skin traction (also called straight traction) is used to control muscle spasms and to immobilize a part of the body during transport or before surgery, with traction exerting its grabbing and pulling force through the patient's skin. Skin traction is noninvasive and is relatively comfortable for the patient. The most common type of skin traction is Buck's traction, used to immobilize the leg before surgery to repair a hip or proximal femur fracture. Buck's traction uses traction tape or a foam boot applied to the lower leg and attached to a free-hanging weight to immobilize the leg.
• Balanced suspension traction involves more than one force of pull to raise and support the injured extremity off the bed and maintain its alignment.

Balanced suspension traction increases mobility while maintaining bone position. It also makes it easier to change linen and perform back care.
• Manual traction is applied by physically pulling on the extremity. Manual traction often is used to reduce a fracture or dislocation.
Nursing Process: Implementation
Patient Need: Physiological Integrity

7. Answer: 1
Rationale: A cast is a rigid device applied to immobilize the injured bones and promote healing. The cast immobilizes the joint above and the joint below the fractured bone so that the bone will not move during healing. A plaster cast may require up to 48 hours to dry, whereas a fiberglass cast dries within an hour. Casts are applied on patients who have relatively stable fractures. The cast must be allowed to dry before any pressure is applied to it.
Nursing Process: Evaluation
Patient Need: Physiological Integrity

8. Answer: 4
Rationale: Education for the patient and family:
• The cast dries from the inside out; do not use a blow dryer to speed drying; do not cover the cast while it is drying.
• A sensation of warmth during drying is normal.
• Do not put anything into the cast.
• Keep the cast clean and dry; use plastic wrap as needed to protect it.
• If the cast is made of fiberglass, dry it with a blow dryer on the cool setting if it becomes wet.
• Notify your doctor immediately if you develop increased pain, coolness, changes in color, increased swelling, and/or loss of sensation.
• Use a blow dryer on the cool setting to relieve itching by blowing cool air into the cast.
• A sling may be used to distribute the weight of the cast evenly around the neck. Do not roll the sling; this can impair circulation to the neck.
• If crutches are used, arrange for physical therapist to teach correct crutch walking.
• When the cast is removed, an oscillating cast saw will be used. It is noisy, and you will feel its vibration; however, a guard prevents it from penetrating past the depth of the cast.
Nursing Process: Implication
Patient Need: Physiological Need

9. Answer: 1
Rationale: The following guidelines may help preserve the amputated part until it can be surgically reattached:
• Keep the person in a prone position with the legs elevated.
• Apply firm pressure to the bleeding area using a towel or an article of clothing.
• Wrap the amputated part in a clean cloth. If possible, soak the cloth in saline (such as contact lens solution).

• Put the amputated part in a plastic bag and put the bag on ice. Do not let the amputated part come in direct contact with the ice or water.
• Send the amputated part to the emergency department with the injured person and make sure the emergency personnel know what it is.

Nursing Process: Implementation
Patient Need: Physiological Integrity

Chapter 40

Terms Matching

1. C
2. H
3. J
4. P
5. D
6. I
7. T
8. A
9. M
10. K
11. E
12. S
13. Q
14. L
15. G
16. B
17. R
18. U
19. N
20. O

Focused Study

1. Surgical procedures can provide dramatic results for patients with significant chronic pain and loss of joint function associated with osteoarthritis. Although elective surgical procedures are frequently avoided in older adults, even they can benefit significantly if they do not have a chronic medical condition that contraindicates surgery.

    An arthroscopy is a surgical procedure in which an arthroscope (a thin tube that is lighted and has a camera on one end) is inserted into a joint. The procedure may be done to diagnose the type of arthritis or to perform debridement by smoothing rough cartilage and flushing out the joint to remove debris. Although arthroscopic debridement and lavage of involved joints have been used, arthroscopy has not proven effective in the treatment of knee OA (Gutierrez, 2008). It may be useful to remove large pieces of debris or repair a torn cartilage.

    An osteotomy, an incision into or transection of the bone, may be performed to realign an affected joint, particularly when significant bony overgrowth or osteophyte formation has occurred. This procedure may also be used to shift the joint load toward areas of less severely damaged cartilage. Although osteotomy does not halt the process of OA, it may have a

beneficial effect on joint function and pain, delaying the need for a joint replacement by several years.

    A joint arthroplasty is the reconstruction or replacement of a joint. Arthroplasty is usually indicated when the patient has severely restricted joint mobility and pain at rest. Pain is virtually eliminated, and the function of the joint is generally improved. Arthroplasty may involve partial joint replacement or reshaping of the bones of a joint. For most patients with OA, both surfaces of the affected joint are replaced with prosthetic parts in a procedure known as a total joint replacement. Joints that may be replaced include the hip, knee, shoulder, elbow, ankle, and wrist and joints of the fingers and toes.

    In a total joint replacement, some or all of the synovium, cartilage, and bone on both sides of the joint are removed. A metallic prosthesis is inserted to replace one joint surface (generally the load end, or distal portion, of a weight-bearing joint). The other joint surface is replaced by a silicone-lined ceramic or plastic prosthesis.

    Most prosthetic joints are uncemented, that is, made of porous ceramic and metal components inserted so that they fit tightly into existing bone. The implant is secured by new bone growth into the prosthesis, a process that requires approximately six weeks. Although a longer non-weight-bearing period is necessary initially until the prosthesis is fixed in place by the bony growth, the implant appears to have a longer useful life span than cemented prostheses. In a cemented joint replacement, methyl methacrylate (a pliable polymer that hardens to hold the prosthesis in place) is used to secure the prosthesis to existing bone. Although the patient is able to resume normal activities more rapidly following a cemented joint replacement, methyl methacrylate initiates an inflammatory response, and the joint eventually loosens.

• In a total hip replacement, the articular surfaces of the acetabulum and femoral head are replaced. The entire head of the femur and part of the femoral neck are removed and replaced with a prosthesis. The acetabulum is remodeled, and a prosthesis of high-molecular-weight polyethylene is inserted. The success rate for total hip replacement is reported to be greater than 90%. Approximately 233,000 total hip replacements are done each year in the United States; most are for treatment of OA (CDC, 2008). Most hip replacements last 10–15 years, after which a second joint replacement, called a revision, can be performed. Potential problems associated with a total hip replacement include blood clots in leg veins, dislocation within the prosthesis, loosening of joint components from surrounding bone, and infection. If recurrent or ineffectively treated, these complications may necessitate removal of the prosthesis, resulting in severe shortening of the extremity and an unstable hip joint.

- Total knee replacement is performed when the patient has intractable pain and x-ray films show evidence of arthritis of the knee. More than 450,000 knee replacements are performed in the United States each year (CDC, 2008). Several prosthetic devices involving removal of varying amounts of bone are available for knee joint replacement. The femoral side of the joint is replaced with a metallic surface, and the tibial side is replaced with polyethylene. More than 80% of patients obtain significant or total relief of pain with a total knee replacement. They must, however, engage in a vigorous program of rehabilitation to achieve the best results. Joint failure is more common with knee replacement than with a total hip replacement. Loosened joint components, often on the tibial side, are the most common cause of failure. The possible complications following a total knee replacement are the same as those for a total hip replacement.
- Total shoulder replacement is indicated for unremitting pain and marked limitation of range of motion because of arthritic involvement of both the humeral and glenoid joint surfaces of the shoulder. The joint is immobilized in a sling or an abduction splint for two to three weeks following arthroplasty. Dislocation, loosening of the prosthesis, and infection are potential problems associated with total shoulder replacement.
- Total elbow replacement involves replacement of the humeral and ulnar surfaces of the elbow joint with a metal and polyethylene prosthesis. Pain and disabling stiffness of the joint are indications for an elbow arthroplasty. Complications, including dislocation, fracture, tricep weakness, loosening, and infection, occur frequently.

Infection is the major complication associated with total joint replacement. Besides interfering with healing and prolonging recovery, infection also may necessitate removal of the prosthesis and lead to loss of joint function. Other potential complications include circulatory impairment to the affected limb, thromboembolism, nerve damage, and dislocation of the joint.

Refer to Chapter 4 for further discussion of care for the patient undergoing surgery. The Moving Evidence into Action box on page 67 provides evidence nurses can use in planning and providing individualized care for patients undergoing joint replacement surgery.

2. Osteoporosis is both preventable and treatable; therefore, nursing care focuses primarily on planning and implementing interventions to prevent the disease, its manifestations, and the resulting injuries. An important aspect of preventing osteoporosis is educating patients under age 35.

Osteoarthritis (OA) is a chronic process for which there is no cure. The focus of nursing care for the patient with OA is providing comfort, helping maintain mobility and activities of daily living (ADL), teaching, and assisting with adaptations to maintain life roles.

Conservative measures, including regular exercise and weight loss as indicated, are primary components of the treatment plan for OA.

The goals of OA treatment are to relieve pain and maintain as much normal joint function as possible. Conservative treatment may include any or all of the following:
- ROM exercises, muscle strengthening exercises, aerobic exercises, walking, quadriceps strengthening exercises, yoga, tai chi, and water-based exercises are recommended (Blackham, Garry, Cummings, & Russell, 2008).
- Heat and ice
- A balance between exercise and rest
- Use of a cane, crutches, or a walker as needed
- Weight loss if indicated

Care of the patient with Paget's disease focuses on relieving pain, suppressing active disease, and preventing or minimizing the effects of complications. Many patients with Paget's disease are asymptomatic and do not require treatment. For more severely affected patients, pharmacologic agents are usually effective. Rarely, surgery may be required.

Once the diagnosis of rheumatoid arthritis (RA) has been established, the goals of therapy are to relieve pain, reduce inflammation, slow or stop joint damage, and improve well-being and ability to function. No cure currently exists for RA; the goal of treatment is to relieve its manifestations. An interdisciplinary approach is used with a balance of rest, exercise, physical therapy, and suppression of the inflammatory processes.

Because a cure is not available and traditional therapies may not be fully effective, the patient with RA is vulnerable to quackery. Many nontraditional treatments, including diets, topical preparations, vaccines, hormones, plant extracts, and copper bracelets, have been put forth. These treatments are often costly and none has been shown to be effective.

The following complementary therapies are those that people with OA may use to relieve pain and stiffness. These same therapies are also used by people with rheumatoid arthritis.
- Biomagnetic therapy
- Acupuncture. Studies have demonstrated a beneficial effect of acupuncture for OA of the shoulder and the knee (Lathia, Jung, & Chen, 2009; McPhee et al., 2008).
- Elimination of nightshade foods such as potatoes, tomatoes, peppers, eggplant, and tobacco
- Nutritional supplements such as glucosamine, chondroitin, boron, zinc, copper, selenium, manganese, flavonoids, and/or SAM-e. The evidence supporting use of glucosamine and chondroitin is mixed. Analysis of multiple studies shows that these agents may be helpful in reducing pain for some people with mild to

moderate OA of the knee (Seed, Dunican, & Lynch, 2009).

- Herbal therapy
- Massage therapy
- Osteopathic manipulation
- Vitamin therapy
- Yoga

3. Osteoporosis: Bisphosphonates inhibit bone resorption, increasing the mineral density of bones and reducing the incidence of fractures. They are used both in the prevention and treatment of osteoporosis.

Health education for the patient and family—bisphosphonates:

- Take the medication as directed with clear water only. Consuming other beverages or food within 30 minutes of taking the drug may interfere with its absorption and effectiveness.
- Do not lie down until after you have eaten, as the drug can irritate the esophagus.
- Report symptoms to your primary care provider (for example, new or worsening heartburn, difficult or painful swallowing, or jaw pain).
- Keep in mind that fever with or without chills and flulike symptoms may occur while receiving intravenous bisphosphonates; this will subside when treatment ends.
- Report any abnormal symptoms, such as tingling around the mouth or numbness and tingling of the fingers or toes, which may indicate an imbalance of electrolytes in the blood.
- Take calcium and vitamin D supplements as instructed by your primary care provider.
- Keep in mind that response to these medications is gradual and continues for months after the drug is stopped.

In postmenopausal osteoporosis, calcitonin prevents further bone loss and increases bone mass when the patient consumes adequate amounts of calcium and vitamin D. Calcitonin may be used in postmenopausal women who cannot or will not take estrogen.

Health education for the patient and family—calcitonin:

- Take the medication in the evening to minimize side effects.
- Warm nasal spray to room temperature before using.
- Keep in mind that rhinitis (runny nose) is the most common side effect with calcitonin nasal spray. Other possible side effects include sores, itching, or other nasal symptoms. Report nosebleeds to your primary care provider.
- Keep in mind that nausea and vomiting may occur during initial stages of therapy; they disappear as treatment continues.
- While taking the medication, consume adequate amounts of calcium and vitamin D.

Paget's disease: When used for Paget's disease, bisphosphonates slow the accelerated bone turnover associated with this disease.

Health education for the patient and family—bisphosphonates:

- Take the medication as directed with clear water only. Consuming other beverages or food within 30 minutes of taking the drug may interfere with its absorption and effectiveness.
- Do not lie down until after you have eaten, as the drug can irritate the esophagus.
- Report symptoms such as new or worsening heartburn, difficult or painful swallowing, or jaw pain to your primary care provider.
- Keep in mind that fever with or without chills and flulike symptoms may occur while receiving intravenous bisphosphonates; this will subside when treatment ends.
- Report any abnormal symptoms, such as tingling around the mouth or numbness and tingling of the fingers or toes, which may indicate an imbalance of electrolytes in the blood.
- Take calcium and vitamin D supplements as instructed by your primary care provider.
- Keep in mind that response to these medications is gradual and continues for months after the drug is stopped.

Gout: Allopurinol acts on purine metabolism, reducing the production of uric acid and decreasing serum and urinary concentrations of uric acid. It is used for patients with manifestations of primary or secondary gout, including acute attacks, tophi, joint destruction, urinary stones, and nephropathy. It is not indicated for use in the treatment of asymptomatic hyperuricemia.

Health education for the patient and family—allopurinol:

- Stop taking the drug and report any skin rash, painful urination, blood in the urine, eye irritation, or swelling of the lips or mouth to the physician immediately.
- Take the medication after meals to minimize gastric distress.
- Drink 3–4 quarts of fluid daily to maintain a urinary output greater than 2 L/day.
- Keep in mind that acute gouty attacks may occur during the initial stages of allopurinol therapy; continue therapy prescribed for attacks (such as colchicine) to minimize acute episodes.
- Do not take a double dose of medication if you miss a dose.

Colchicine is used to prevent recurrent episodes of the disease. Colchicine does not alter serum uric acid levels, but appears to interrupt the cycle of urate crystal deposition and inflammatory response. It is given once or twice daily by mouth. Colchicine is also available as a fixed-dose combination with a uricosuric agent: probenecid (Benemid®). Plain colchicine may, on rare occasion, be used to treat an acute attack of gout; combination therapy is employed to prevent further attacks.

Health education for the patient and family—colchicine:

- Drink 3–4 quarts of liquid per day.

- Report adverse responses, including gastrointestinal problems, fatigue, bleeding, easy bruising, or recurrent infections, to the physician.
- Do not drink alcohol.

Probenecid is a uricosuric drug that inhibits the tubular reabsorption of urate, promoting the excretion of uric acid and decreasing serum uric acid levels. Sulfinpyrazone is a uricosuric drug that potentiates the renal excretion of uric acid, reducing serum uric acid levels. It is used to prevent recurrent attacks of acute gouty arthritis and to treat chronic gout. Health education for the patient and family— uricosuric:

- Do not take aspirin or products containing aspirin while taking probenecid. Use acetaminophen for relief of mild pain.
- Drink at least 3 quarts of fluids per day to minimize the risk of kidney stone formation.
- Take sulfinpyrazone with meals to minimize gastric distress and report epigastric pain, nausea, or black stools to the physician promptly.

Osteomalacia: Therapeutic management of osteomalacia usually involves administration of calcium and vitamin D (800 IU daily) supplements. Patients in whom metabolic activation of vitamin D is impaired may require a metabolite of the vitamin that does not require activation (Fauci et al., 2008). Phosphate supplements may be indicated. Radiologic evidence of healing often is apparent within weeks of initiating therapy.

Osteoarthritis: The pain of OA often can be managed through the use of mild analgesics such as acetaminophen. Acetaminophen (Tylenol®) is generally preferred for long-term use because it has fewer toxic side effects. NSAIDs such as ibuprofen (Motrin®), naproxen (Aleve®), and ketoprofen (Orudis® KT™) are prescribed to relieve the pain and stiffness associated with OA of the hip or knee. However, Osteoarthritis Research Society International (OARSI) guidelines specify that NSAIDs are to be given at the lowest effective dose and are not to be considered long-term treatment (Gutierrez, 2008). A selective COX-2 inhibitor [celecoxib (Celebrex®)] may be ordered for patients who have a history of gastrointestinal bleeding or who do not tolerate other NSAIDs. See Chapter 40 and the section on rheumatoid arthritis beginning on page 1363 for more information about these drugs.

Strong evidence also supports the use of topical NSAIDs [for example, diclofenac topical gel (Pennsaid®)] and capsaicin (Capzasin™, Zostrix®) for relief of OA pain. These drugs have the advantage of minimizing systemic adverse effects. The patient should be taught to keep the medications away from the eyes, the nose, the mouth, or any open skin and not to bandage or apply heat to the treated area. The products should be used no more than three or four times a day and discontinued immediately if severe irritation occurs.

Potent anti-inflammatory medications such as systemic corticosteroids are seldom prescribed for patients with OA, although intra-articular corticosteroid injections may be used. With intra-articular injections, a long-acting corticosteroid medication, often mixed with a local anesthetic such as lidocaine, is injected directly into the joint space of the affected joints. Although this procedure may provide marked pain relief, it can hasten the rate of cartilage breakdown if performed more frequently than every four to six months. Intra-articular hyaluronic acid (HA) is an option for patients with OA of the knee joint. HA is a component of synovial fluid; it also appears to have anti-inflammatory effects.

Prescription analgesics such as tramadol or an opioid analgesic may be necessary for patients with advanced OA and moderate to severe pain. See Chapter 9 for more information about these drugs.

Rheumatoid arthritis (RA): Three general approaches are used in the pharmacologic management of patients with RA:

- NSAIDs and mild analgesics are used to reduce the inflammatory process and manage manifestations of the disease. Although these drugs may relieve symptoms of RA, they appear to have little effect on disease progression.
- The second approach uses low-dose oral corticosteroids to reduce pain and inflammation. Recent studies suggest that low-dose oral corticosteroids also may slow the development and progression of bone erosions associated with RA. Intra-articular corticosteroids may be used to provide temporary relief in patients for whom other therapies have failed to control inflammation.
- A diverse group of drugs classified as disease-modifying antirheumatic drugs (DMARDs) are employed in the third approach to treating RA. These drugs, which include synthetic (or nonbiologic) DMARDs such methotrexate, sulfasalazine, and antimalarial agents, and biologic DMARDs such as anti-tumor necrosis factor-α, abatacept, and rituximab, appear to alter the course of the disease, reducing its destruction of joints. Current guidelines from the American College of Rheumatology (2008) advocate early use of DMARDs, particularly for patients with high disease activity, functional limitation, or extra-articular disease.

Gastrointestinal side effects and interference with platelet function are the greatest hazards of aspirin therapy. Patients are instructed to take aspirin with meals, milk, or antacids to minimize gastrointestinal distress and reduce the risk of GI bleeding. Enteric-coated forms of aspirin and nonacetylated salicylate compounds produce less gastric distress than plain or buffered aspirin do and reduce the risk of gastric ulceration, but they are more expensive. Salsalate (Disalcid®, Mono-Gesic®, Salflex®) and choline magnesium trisalicylate (Trilisate®, Tricosal) are examples of nonacetylated salicylate products. All salicylate products are contraindicated for patients with a history of aspirin allergy.

NONSTEROIDAL ANTI-INFLAMMATORY DRUGS A number of NSAIDs are available for use in the management of RA. All NSAIDs act by inhibiting prostaglandin synthesis. Although the efficacy of all NSAIDs, including aspirin, is equivalent, patient responses are individual. Several trials of different NSAIDs may be necessary to find the most effective drug.

Aspirin is an inexpensive and effective anti-inflammatory and analgesic agent. It is, however, associated with a significant risk for gastrointestinal bleeding, due in part to its antiplatelet effects. Some NSAIDs are considerably more expensive than aspirin but may cause less gastrointestinal distress and require fewer doses per day. Gastric irritation, ulceration, and bleeding remain the most common toxic effects of NSAIDs. They can also affect the lower intestinal tract, leading to perforation or aggravation of inflammatory bowel disorders. All NSAIDs can be toxic to the kidneys. With the exception of the COX-2 inhibitor celecoxib, most NSAIDs also inhibit platelet function, increasing the risk for bleeding.

NSAIDs commonly prescribed for patients with RA are listed in Table 40–5. The FDA has asked drug manufacturers to increase label warnings about the potential serious adverse cardiovascular and gastrointestinal effects of nonselective NSAIDs and COX-2 inhibitors. Nursing implications for the administration of NSAIDs are described in Chapter 12.

CORTICOSTEROIDS Systemic corticosteroids can dramatically relieve the symptoms of RA and appear to slow the progression of joint destruction. The long-term use of corticosteroids is associated with multiple side effects, such as poor wound healing, increased risk of infection, osteoporosis, and gastrointestinal bleeding. Severe rebound manifestations can occur when these medications are discontinued. For these reasons, the use of systemic corticosteroids is limited to low dosages daily. The nursing implications for corticosteroid therapy are discussed in Chapter 13.

DISEASE-MODIFYING ANTIRHEUMATIC DRUGS Disease-modifying antirheumatic drugs are a diverse group of medications, including drugs that modify immune and inflammatory responses (Table 40–6). They share characteristics that make them useful in the treatment of RA. The DMARDs may be used individually (monotherapy) or in combination. Although beneficial effects are not apparent for several weeks or months following the initiation of therapy, they can produce not only clinical improvement, but also evidence of decreased disease activity. Because their anti-inflammatory effect is minimal, NSAIDs are continued during therapy. As many as two-thirds of

patients taking disease-modifying drugs show improvement, although these drugs have not been shown to slow bone erosion or facilitate healing. All of these drugs are fairly toxic, and close monitoring is necessary during the course of therapy. Most are contraindicated for patients who have an active bacterial or herpes zoster infection, active or latent tuberculosis, or hepatitis B or C (Bergman, 2008). Nonbiologic DMARDS. Commonly used nonbiologic DMARDs include methotrexate, sulfasalazine, leflunomide (Arava®), hydroxychloroquine, and minocycline.

Methotrexate often is the first DMARD used to treat patients with aggressive RA. A weekly dose can produce a beneficial effect in as few as two to four weeks. Gastric irritation and stomatitis are the most frequent side effects associated with methotrexate, but side effects may be better controlled if folic acid is taken at the same time. Alcoholism, diabetes, obesity, advanced age, and renal disease increase the risk of toxic effects (hepatotoxicity, bone marrow suppression, interstitial pneumonitis).

Sulfasalazine, a drug regularly prescribed for chronic inflammatory bowel disease, may also be prescribed for RA. Adverse effects such as neutropenia and thrombocytopenia are relatively common with sulfasalazine, necessitating frequent CBCs to monitor its effects. See Chapter 24 for further discussion of this drug and its nursing implications. Leflunomide reversibly inhibits an enzyme involved in the autoimmune process. Because this drug is teratogenic, it is contraindicated for premenopausal women and for men who want to have children.

Hydroxychloroquine (Plaquenil®) is an antimalarial agent sometimes employed in the treatment of RA. Three to six months of therapy is required to achieve the desired response, and many patients do not experience significant benefit. Although hydroxychloroquine has a relatively low toxicity, it can cause pigmentary retinitis and vision loss. Patients receiving this drug require a thorough vision examination every six months. Minocycline, related to tetracycline, has a modest anti-inflammatory effect and inhibits destructive enzymes such as collagenase. Because its effect is less dramatic than that of other DMARDs, it generally is used early in the treatment plan (during the first year) (McPhee et al., 2008).

For patients not responding to the preceding preparations, penicillamine or gold salts may be prescribed. Although these agents may be effective in the management of RA, toxic reactions are common and can be severe, including bone marrow suppression, proteinuria, and nephrosis.

Biologic DMARDs. Biologic DMARDs generally are used for patients who (1) have moderate or high disease activity, (2) have had active RA for a longer period of time, or (3) have failed to respond adequately to methotrexate and/or other nonbiologic DMARDs (Bergman, 2008). Biologic DMARDs act by inhibiting components of the immune or inflammatory response, such as TNF or interleukin-1. They control the manifestations of RA in most patients, slow the progression of joint damage, and reduce disability (Fauci et al., 2008). Biologic DMARDs increase the risk for infection and have been associated with an increased risk for reactivation tuberculosis. Patients are screened for tuberculosis prior to treatment.

Three biologic DMARDs act by inhibiting tumor necrosis factor, thus interrupting the inflammatory cascade of RA. Etanercept (Enbrel®) inhibits the binding of tumor necrosis factor to receptor sites. Infliximab (Remicade®) is a biologic response modifier and TNF α receptor antagonist. Given by intravenous infusion, the drug is administered to reduce infiltration of inflammatory cells and TNF α production. Adalimumab (Humira®), given by subcutaneous injection, binds with TNF receptor sites. Abatacept (Orencia®) and rituximab (Rituxan®) generally are reserved for patients with high levels of disease activity. Abatacept acts by interfering with the formation of T cells, whereas rituximab is a monoclonal antibody that depletes B cells. Like other biologic DMARDs, these drugs are given parenterally, by intravenous infusion.

Systemic lupus erythematosus: Certain cytotoxic or antineoplastic drugs are effective as immunosuppressive agents. They act by decreasing the proliferation of cells in the immune system and are widely used to prevent rejection following a tissue or organ transplant. They are usually administered concurrently with corticosteroid therapy, allowing lower doses of both preparations and resulting in fewer side effects.

Health education for the patient and family—cytotoxics:

• Avoid large crowds and situations where you might be exposed to infections.

• Report signs of infection such as chills, fever, sore throat, fatigue, or malaise to the physician.

• Use contraceptive measures to prevent pregnancy while you are taking these drugs because they cause birth defects.

• Avoid the use of aspirin and ibuprofen while taking these drugs. Report any signs of bleeding to the physician.

• Do not be concerned if you stop menstruating while taking cyclophosphamide. The menses will resume after the drug is discontinued.

• If you are taking cyclophosphamide, report difficulty in breathing or cough to the physician.

Osteomyelitis: Antibiotic therapy is mandatory to prevent acute osteomyelitis from progressing to the chronic phase. Parenteral antibiotic therapy begins as soon as cultures (blood and/or wound) are obtained. A penicillinase-resistant semisynthetic penicillin (for example, nafcillin or oxacillin) may be given until the culture and sensitivity results are known. These antibiotics are used initially because many cases of osteomyelitis are caused by *Staphylococcus aureus.* When the detailed sensitivity report is obtained from the cultures, more definitive antibiotics are prescribed.

For the patient with acute or chronic osteomyelitis, antibiotics are continued for four to six weeks. Intravenous antibiotic administration or oral therapy is common. Oral therapy with twice-daily ciprofloxacin has been shown to be as effective as parenteral therapy for treating adult patients with chronic osteomyelitis caused by susceptible organisms (McPhee et al., 2008).

Bone tumors: Chemotherapeutic agents are administered to shrink the malignant tumor before surgery, to control recurrence of tumor growth after surgery, and to treat metastasis of the tumor.

Scleroderma: Medications to treat systemic sclerosis are chosen based on the patient's symptoms. Immunosuppressive agents and corticosteroids are of limited benefit but may be used to slow or prevent pulmonary fibrosis and to treat life-threatening disease. Penicillamine may be used to treat scleroderma and pulmonary fibrosis. Calcium channel blockers such as nifedipine (Procardia®) or alpha-adrenergic blockers such as prazosin (Minipress®) may be prescribed for patients with Raynaud's phenomenon. When manifestations of esophagitis accompany systemic sclerosis, H_2-receptor blockers such as cimetidine (Tagamet®) or ranitidine (Zantac®), antacids, or omeprazole (Prilosec®), which blocks all gastric secretion, may be ordered. Tetracycline or another broad-spectrum antibiotic may be prescribed to suppress intestinal flora and relieve symptoms of malabsorption. Patients with kidney disease are usually treated with angiotensin-converting enzyme (ACE) inhibitors such as captopril (Capoten®) to control hypertension and preserve renal function. End-stage kidney disease is managed with dialysis and transplantation.

Low back pain: The medications of choice for low back pain include NSAIDs and analgesics. NSAIDs block prostaglandin production and reduce inflammation, thus relieving the pain. Muscle relaxants such as cyclobenzaprine (Flexeril®), methocarbamol (Robaxin®), and carisoprodol (Soma®) may be used, but little evidence supports their efficacy.

Epidural steroid injections may be used to help reduce intense, intractable pain. A steroid solution is injected into the epidural space, which helps decrease the swelling and inflammation of the spinal nerves.

4. Because there is no cure or specific treatment for MD, care focuses on preserving and promoting mobility. An interdisciplinary approach involving many members of the healthcare team is necessary to meet the physical and psychologic needs of these patients and their families. Diagnosis and classification of the muscular dystrophies are most often based on the manifestations and the pattern of muscle involvement. Biochemical examination, muscle biopsy, and electromyography confirm the diagnosis. Diagnostic tests are described in Chapter 38.

Tests include measuring creatine kinase (CK-MM, the isoenzyme found in skeletal muscle), which is elevated in the patient with suspected MD; performing a muscle biopsy to identify fibrous connective tissue and fatty deposits that displace functional muscle fibers; and conducting an electromyogram (EMG), which shows a decrease in amplitude in MD.

Nursing care for a patient with MD focuses on promoting independence and mobility and providing psychologic support for both the patient and family. A holistic approach is essential in planning and implementing care.

Case Study

1. *"What are the unmodifiable risk factors for osteoporosis?"*
   - Being older
   - Having a family history of osteoporosis
   - Having a history of fracture in a first-degree relative
   - Being female, especially Caucasian or Asian
   - Being thin and/or having a small frame
2. *"What are the modifiable risk factors for osteoporosis?"*
   - Low estrogen levels in women (amenorrhea, menopause)
   - Low testosterone levels in men
   - Dietary: low lifetime calcium intake, vitamin D deficiency
   - Medication use: corticosteroids, some anticonvulsants
   - Lifestyle: inactivity, cigarette smoking, excessive alcohol use
3. *"What are the most common signs and symptoms of osteoporosis?"* The most common manifestations of osteoporosis are loss of height; progressive curvature of the spine; low back pain; and fractures of the forearm, spine, or hip. Osteoporosis is often called the silent disease because bone loss occurs without symptoms.
4. *"Are there complications of osteoporosis? Explain."* Fractures are the most common complication of osteoporosis, with the disease being responsible for an estimated 2 million fractures each year. Some fractures are spontaneous; others may result from everyday activities. Persistent pain results in many patients and may restrict the patient's activities or interfere with activities of daily living (ADL). Hip fractures are associated with in increased risk for mortality.

Care Plan Critical-Thinking Activity

1. The onset of RA occurs most frequently between the ages of 30 and 50.
2. The cause of RA is unknown. Genetic factors are believed to play a role in its development, likely in combination with environmental factors. It is speculated that an infectious agent such as mycoplasma, Epstein-Barr virus, or another virus may

play a role in initiating the abnormal immune responses present in RA. Several studies have found that heavy smokers are at increased risk for developing RA.
3. Helpful resources:
   - National Institute of Arthritis and Musculoskeletal and Skin Diseases
   - American College of Rheumatology
   - Arthritis Foundation
   - The Arthritis Society
   - American Physical Therapy Foundation
   - American Chronic Pain Association.

Short Answers

Fill in the table differentiating between the features of osteoporosis and osteomalacia.

Differentiating Features	Osteoporosis	Osteomalacia
Pathophysiology	Bone resorption that outpaces bone formation	Inadequate mineralization of bone matrix
Calcium level (serum)	Normal	Low or normal
Phosphate level (serum)	Normal	Low or normal
Parathyroid hormone level (serum)	Normal	High or normal
Alkaline phosphatase level (serum)	Normal	Elevated
Hydroxyproline (urine)	Not applicable	Not applicable
Radiographic findings	Osteopenia, fractures	Decreased bone density, radiolucent bands known as Looser's zones, or pseudofractures

NCLEX-RN® Review Questions

1. Answer: 2
   Rationale: The most common manifestations of osteoporosis are loss of height; progressive curvature of the spine; low back pain; and fractures of the forearm, spine, or hip. Calcitonin (Miacalcin®) is a hormone that increases bone formation and decreases bone resorption. Fractures are the most common complication of osteoporosis. Care of the patient with osteoporosis focuses on identifying the risk early, stopping or slowing the process, alleviating symptoms, and preventing complications. Proper nutrition and exercise are important components of treatment.
   Nursing Process: Planning
   Patient Need: Health Promotion and Maintenance

2. Answer: 2

Rationale: Paget's disease is a progressive metabolic skeletal disorder of the osteoclast that results from localized excessive metabolic activity in bone, with excessive bone resorption followed by excessive bone formation. The most common manifestation is localized pain of the long bones, spine, pelvis, and cranium. This chronic remodeling results in the affected bones being larger and softer, causing bone pain, arthritis, obvious skeletal deformities, and fractures. Paget's disease is also called osteitis deformans.

Nursing Process: Assessment

Patient Need: Physiological Integrity

3. Answer: 4

Rationale: The serum uric acid level is normally maintained between 3.5 and 7.0 mg/dL in men and 2.8 and 6.8 mg/dL in women. At levels greater than 7.0 mg/dL, the serum is saturated with urate, the ionized form of uric acid. Over time, urate deposits in subcutaneous tissues cause the formation of small white nodules called tophi). Gout typically has an abrupt onset, usually at night, and often involves the first metatarsophalangeal joint. Kidney disease may occur in patients with untreated gout, particularly when hypertension is present.

Nursing Process: Assessment

Patient Need: Physiological Integrity

4. Answer: 1

Rationale: Hypophosphatemia can result from insufficient dietary intake, excessive losses through the urine or stool, or a shift into the cells. The manifestations of osteomalacia include bone pain and tenderness. The two main causes of osteomalacia are (1) insufficient calcium absorption in the intestine due to a lack of calcium intake or vitamin D deficiency and (2) increased losses of phosphorus through the urine. Osteomalacia is a metabolic bone disorder characterized by inadequate or delayed mineralization of bone matrix in mature compact and spongy bone, resulting in softening of bones.

Nursing Process: Assessment

Patient Need: Health Promotion and Maintenance

5. Answer: 4

Rationale: At an earlier age, men are affected more frequently than women are, but the rate of OA in women exceeds men by the middle adult years. The onset of OA is usually gradual and insidious, and the course is slowly progressive. Osteoarthritis is the most common form of arthritis and is a leading cause of pain and disability in older adults (CDC, 2008). Increasing age is the primary risk factor for OA.

Nursing Process: Assessment

Patient Need: Physiological Integrity

6. Answer: 2

Rationale: Manifestations of SLE are as follows:

• Painful or swollen joints and muscle pain
• Unexplained fever
• Red rash, especially on the face
• Alopecia
• Pale, cyanotic fingers or toes
• Sensitivity to the sun
• Edema in legs and around eyes
• Ulcers in the mouth
• Enlarged glands
• Extreme fatigue

Nursing Process: Assessment

Patient Need: Physiological Integrity

7. Answer: 2

Rationale: Hallux valgus is commonly referred to as hammertoe.

Nursing Process: Assessment

Patient Need: Physiological Integrity

8. Answer: 1

Rationale: Scoliosis is a lateral curvature of the spine. Kyphosis is an exaggerated posterior curvature of the thoracic spine. In kyphosis, an increased curvature of the thoracic spine as viewed from the side is referred to as hunchback. Along with loss of height, characteristic dorsal kyphosis and cervical lordosis develop, accounting for the dowager's hump often associated with aging. The abdomen tends to protrude and knees and hips flex as the body attempts to maintain its center of gravity.

Nursing Process: Assessment

Patient Need: Physiological Integrity

Chapter 41

Terms Matching

1. F
2. K
3. C
4. L
5. G
6. M
7. A
8. P
9. I
10. D
11. N
12. H
13. O
14. B
15. E
16. J

Focused Study

1.
   1. Assess level of consciousness (response to auditory and/or tactile stimulus).
   2. Obtain vital signs (BP, P, R).
   3. Check pupillary response to light.
   4. Assess strength of hand grip and movement of extremities bilaterally.
   5. Determine ability to sense touch/pain in extremities.
2. If the patient has problems with neurologic structure or function, analyze its onset, characteristics, course, severity, precipitating and relieving factors, and any

associated symptoms, noting the time and circumstances. For example, ask the patient the following questions:
- Describe the location and intensity of the pain you have experienced in your left leg. Is it made worse by coughing, sneezing, or walking?
- When did you first notice numbness in your fingers?
- Describe the difficulty you have when you try to walk.

3. The nervous system is divided into two regions: the central nervous system (CNS), which consists of the brain and spinal cord, and the peripheral nervous system (PNS), which consists of the cranial nerves, the spinal nerves, and the autonomic nervous system.

The CNS consists of the brain and spinal cord, highly evolved clusters of neurons that act to accept, interconnect, interpret, and generate a response to nerve impulses originating throughout the body.

The PNS links the CNS with the rest of the body. It is responsible for receiving and transmitting information from and about the external environment. The PNS consists of nerves, ganglia (groups of nerve cells), and sensory receptors located outside—or peripheral to—the brain and spinal cord. The PNS is divided into a sensory (afferent) division and a motor (efferent) division.

4.

Age-Related Change	Significance
• ↓ number of brain cells, cerebral blood flow, and metabolism • Slower nerve conduction velocity • Slower retrieval of information from long-term memory • Slower response to changes in balance • Possibility of exhibiting less readiness to learn and depending on prior experiences to solve problems • More easily distracted and a decreased ability to maintain attention	Delayed response to multiple stimuli and slower reflexes; may need additional time to process and respond to verbal stimuli Some age-related forgetfulness, which can be improved by using memory aids such as making lists May contribute to increased risk for falls Improvement in learning new skills or knowledge when they are related to previously learned information and when limits are set on times for learning (for example, no more than 30 minutes at one time)

Case Study

1. *"What are the four major regions of the brain?"* The cerebrum, the diencephalon, the brainstem, and the cerebellum
2. *"What does the brainstem consist of?"* It consists of the thalamus, hypothalamus, and epithalamus.
3. *"What protects and surrounds the spinal cord?"* Cerebrospinal fluid
4. *"How many pairs of spinal nerves are there? Where are they located?"* There are 31 pairs of spinal nerves. The spinal nerves are named by their location: cervical, 8 pairs; thoracic, 12 pairs; lumbar, 5 pairs; sacral, 5 pairs; and coccygeal, 1 pair.

Short Answers

Fill in the table regarding the functions of the cranial nerves.

Name	Function
I Olfactory	Sense of smell
II Optic	Vision
III Oculomotor	Eyeball movement
	Raising of upper eyelid
	Constriction of pupil
	Proprioception
IV Trochlear	Eyeball movement
V Trigeminal	Sensation of the upper scalp, upper eyelid, nose, nasal cavity, cornea, and lacrimal gland
	Sensation of the palate, upper teeth, cheek, top lip, lower eyelid, and scalp; sensation of the tongue, lower teeth, chin, and temporal scalp
	Chewing
VI Abducens	Lateral movement of the eyeball
VII Facial	Movement of facial muscles
	Secretions of lacrimal, nasal, submandibular, and sublingual glands
	Sensation of taste
VIII Acoustic	Sense of equilibrium
	Sense of hearing
IX Glossopharyngeal	Swallowing
	Gag reflex
	Secretions of parotid salivary gland
	Sense of taste
	Touch, pressure, and pain from pharynx and posterior tongue
	Pressure from carotid arteries
	Receptors to regulate blood pressure
X Vagus	Swallowing
	Regulation of cardiac rate
	Regulation of respirations
	Digestion
	Sensation from thoracic and abdominal organs
	Proprioception
	Sense of taste
XI Accessory	Movement of head and neck
	Proprioception
XII Hypoglossal	Movement of tongue for speech and swallowing

NCLEX-RN® Review Questions

1. Answer: 4

   Rationale: Each neuron consists of a dendrite, a cell body, and an axon.

   Nursing Process: Assessment

   Patient Need: Physiological Integrity

2. Answer: 3

   Rationale: Cell bodies, most of which are located in the CNS, are clustered in ganglia or nuclei. The dendrite is a short projection from the cell body that conducts impulses toward the cell body. Many axons are covered with a myelin sheath, a white lipid substance. The myelin sheath serves to increase the speed of nerve impulse conduction in axons and is essential for the survival of larger nerve processes.

   Nursing Process: Assessment

   Patient Need: Physiological Integrity

3. Answer: 2

   Rationale: The excitatory neurotransmitter is usually acetylcholine (ACh). The neurotransmitter may be either inhibitory or excitatory. Norepinephrine (NE), which may be either excitatory or inhibitory, is another major neurotransmitter. Neurotransmitters are the chemical messengers of the nervous system.

   Nursing Process: Assessment

   Patient Need: Physiological Integrity

4. Answer: 2

   Rationale: The left hemisphere has greater control over nonverbal perceptual functions. The brain is the control center of the nervous system, generating thoughts, emotions, and speech. The brain has four major regions: the cerebrum, the diencephalon, the brainstem, and the cerebellum. The brain contains four ventricles, which are chambers filled with cerebrospinal fluid (CSF).

   Nursing Process: Evaluation

   Patient Need: Health Promotion and Maintenance

5. Answer: 4

   Rationale: The brain contains four ventricles, which are chambers filled with cerebrospinal fluid (CSF). The brain has four major regions: the cerebrum, the diencephalon, the brainstem, and the cerebellum. The brainstem consists of the midbrain, pons, and medulla oblongata.

   Nursing Process: Assessment

   Patient Need: Physiological Integrity

6. Answer: 3

   Rationale: The brain contains four ventricles, which are chambers filled with cerebrospinal fluid (CSF).

   Nursing Process: Assessment

   Patient Need: Physiological Integrity

7. Answer: 3

   Rationale: The usual amount of CSF ranges from 80–200 mL and is replaced several times each day. CSF is a clear and colorless liquid. It forms a cushion for the brain tissue, protects the brain and spinal cord from trauma, helps provide nourishment for the brain, and removes waste products of cerebrospinal cellular metabolism. CSF is normally produced and absorbed in equal amounts.

   Nursing Process: Assessment

   Patient Need: Physiological Integrity

8. Answer: 4

   Rationale: At least three metabolic factors affect cerebral blood flow: carbon dioxide, hydrogen ion, and oxygen concentrations.

   Nursing Process: Assessment

   Patient Need: Physiological Integrity

9. Answer: 3

   Rationale: The spinal cord is surrounded by 33 vertebrae: 7 cervical; 12 thoracic; 5 lumbar; 5 sacral; and 4 fused vertebrae, which form the coccyx.

   Nursing Process: Assessment

   Patient Need: Physiological Integrity

10. Answer: 4

    Rationale: VII = Able to smile, frown, wrinkle forehead, show teeth, puff out cheek, purse lips, raise eyebrows, and close eyes against resistance.

    Nursing Process: Assessment

    Patient Need: Physiological Integrity

Chapter 42

Terms Matching

1. G
2. Y
3. L
4. P
5. I
6. C
7. B
8. H
9. N
10. J
11. V
12. O
13. T
14. S
15. A
16. K
17. E
18. X
19. M
20. W
21. R
22. Q
23. U
24. D
25. F

Focused Study

1. Goals of medication therapy include protecting the patient from harm and reducing or preventing seizure activity without causing impairment of cognitive function. AEDs are used to reduce or control seize activity. These medications usually work by raising

the seizure threshold or by limiting the spread of abnormal activity in the brain.

Because the FDA issued a warning that AEDs have been associated with suicidal thoughts and behaviors, nurses should assess patients on AEDs for these thoughts and behaviors. Furthermore, nurses should educate family members to alert the healthcare provider should any unusual changes in the patient's mood or behavior occur.

2. Generally recognized criteria include unresponsive coma with absent motor reflex movements, no spontaneous respirations, pupils fixed and dilated, absent ocular responses to head turning and caloric stimulation, flat EEG, no cerebral blood flow, and persistence of these manifestations for 30 minutes to 1 hour and for 6 hours after the onset of coma and apnea.

3. Sudden weakness or numbness of the face, arm, or leg, especially on one side of the body; sudden confusion, trouble speaking or understanding speech; sudden trouble walking, dizziness, loss of balance or coordination; sudden trouble with vision in one or both eyes; sudden severe headache without a cause.

4. The purpose of ICP monitoring is to preserve brain function and prevent secondary damage due to an ICP. The criteria associated with the use of ICP monitoring can vary depending on the patient's condition. Generally, ICP monitoring is utilized for patients who are comatose and have a Glasgow Coma Scale of 8 or less.

Case Study

1. *Discuss the clinical manifestations of a migraine.* In a migraine headache, the pain is unilateral and throbbing but can become bilateral as the headache continues. Doing physical activity or even moving the head can intensify pain. Chills; nausea and vomiting; fatigue; and sensitivity to light, sound, or odor are often present. Other manifestations may include blurred vision, anorexia, hunger, diarrhea, abdominal cramping, facial pallor, sweating, and stiffness or tenderness of the neck. The headache lasts 4–72 hours and then gradually subsides. The patient may be acutely ill and is often extremely irritable. The sensory organs often become hypersensitive, and the patient withdraws from sound and light. The scalp is tender. After the headache, the headache area is sensitive to touch and a deep aching is present. The patient is exhausted.

2. *What factors are believed to trigger an onset of a migraine?* Rapid changes in blood glucose levels, stress, emotional excitement, fatigue, alcohol intake, stimuli such as bright lights, and food high in tyramine or other vasoactive substances (for example, aged cheese, nuts, chocolate, and alcoholic beverages) have been associated with migraine attacks. Caffeinated foods have also been implicated. Hypertension and fever may make the disorder worse. The menstrual cycle is a trigger for many women.

3. *List suggestions to decrease the incidence of migraines.* Wake up at the same time every morning. Eat meals and exercise on a regular schedule. Do not smoke or consume caffeine after 3 PM. Do not consume artificial sweeteners or MSG. Reduce or eliminate red wine, cheese, alcohol, caffeine, and chocolate. Practice relaxation techniques such as yoga, meditation, and biofeedback.

Short Answers
Fill in the table regarding the manifestations of brain tumors by location.

Lobe	Manifestations
Frontal Lobe Tumors	• Inappropriate behavior • Recent memory loss • Personality changes • Headache • Inability to concentrate • Expressive aphasia • Impaired judgment • Motor dysfunctions
Parietal Lobe Tumors	• Sensory deficits: paresthesia, loss of two-point discrimination, visual field deficits
Temporal Lobe Tumors	• Psychomotor seizures
Occipital Lobe Tumors	• Visual disturbances
Cerebellum Tumors	• Disturbances in coordination and equilibrium
Pituitary Tumors	• Endocrine dysfunction • Visual deficits • Headache

NCLEX-RN® Review Questions

1. Answer: 4
   Rationale: It is suggested to avoid caffeine after 3 PM. It is also suggetsed to wake up at the same time each morning and to eat meals and exercise on a regular schedule. Furthermore, it is suggested to avoid artificial sweeteners and MSG.
   Nursing Process: Planning
   Patient Need: Health Promotion and Maintenance

2. Answer: 1
   Rationale: Doll's eye movements are reflexive movements of the eyes in the opposite direction of head rotation; they are an indicator of brainstem function.
   Nursing Process: Assessment
   Patient Need: Physiological Integrity

3. Answer: 1
   Rationale: Brain death is the cessation and irreversibility of all brain functions, including the brainstem. Although the exact criteria for establishing brain death may vary somewhat from

state to state, it is generally agreed that brain death has occurred when there is no evidence of cerebral or brainstem function for an extended period (usually 6–24 hours) in a patient who has a normal body temperature and is not affected by a depressant drug or alcohol poisoning.

Generally recognized criteria are as follows:
- Unresponsive coma with absent motor and reflex movements
- No spontaneous respiration (apnea)
- Pupils fixed (unresponsive to light) and dilated
- Absent ocular responses to head turning and caloric stimulation (Caloric stimulation is performed by irrigating the ear with ice-cold water to test the oculovestibular reflex, a reflex controlled by the brainstem. Normally, the cold causes the eyes to first move toward the irrigated side, followed by a return to midline.)
- Flat electroencephalogram (EEG) and no cerebral blood circulation present on angiography (if performed)
- Persistence of these manifestations for 30 minutes to 1 hour and for 6 hours after onset of coma and apnea

Nursing Process: Assessment
Patient Need: Physiological Integrity

4. Answer: 1
Rationale: Cerebral edema is an increase in the volume of brain tissue due to abnormal accumulation of fluid. Cerebral edema is associated with increased intracranial pressure; it may occur as a local process in the area of a tumor or an injury, or it may affect the entire brain. Cerebral blood flow may decrease as cerebral edema increases, which in turn increases the ICP.
Nursing Process: Assessment
Patient Need: Physiological Integrity

5. Answer: 2
Rationale: The two most common types of migraine headaches are migraine without an aura (occurring in about 85% of cases) and classic migraine with aura (Porth & Matfin, 2009).
Nursing Process: Planning
Patient Need: Health Promotion and Maintenance

6. Answer: 3
Rationale: It is contraindicated to hold the patient down or to force anything into the patient's mouth. It is appropriate to cushion the head, loosen anything tight around the neck, and turn the patient on his or her side.
Nursing Process: Implementation
Patient Need: Safe, Effective Care Environment

7. Answer: 1
Rationale: Teach family members to call for medical assistance if the seizures lasts for more than five minutes, recovery is slow, a second seizure occurs, the individual has difficulty breathing after recovery, or there are signs of injury (such as bleeding from the mouth).
Nursing Process: Planning
Patient Need: Health Promotion and Maintenance

8. Answer: 2
Rationale: Acute subdural hematomas are usually located at the top of the head and develop within 48 hours of the initial head injury.
Nursing Process: Assessment
Patient Need: Physiological Integrity

Chapter 43

Terms Matching
1. E
2. I
3. G
4. P
5. H
6. J
7. B
8. C
9. O
10. N
11. L
12. Q
13. F
14. K
15. D
16. A
17. M

Focused Study
1. This condition is characterized by flaccid paralysis, loss of skin reflexes and deep tendon reflexes, and loss of all sensations below the level of injury. There is loss of urinary bladder tone, intestinal peristalsis, perspiration, and vasomotor tone. In addition, the autonomic dysfunction results in hypotension, bradycardia (50–70 beats/minute), warm skin, and body temperature that responds to the immediate environment (Hickey, 2009).
2. A ruptured intervertebral disk is usually managed conservatively unless the patient is experiencing severe neurologic deficits. The goals of treatment are pain relief and healing of the involved disk by fibrosis. Conservative treatment is usually prescribed for two to six weeks. If the patient continues to have pain after that time, surgery may be considered. The treatment regimen depends on the severity of the manifestations. Decreasing activity level with bedrest is no longer recommended; in many cases, the patient is advised to continue with normal activities while taking prescribed medications for pain, inflammation, and muscle spasms.

Medications used to treat back pain include nonnarcotic analgesics, anti-inflammatory drugs such as the NSAIDs, muscle relaxants, and sedative/tranquilizers.
3. Time, location, and type of event-causing injury; location, duration, quality, and intensity of pain; dyspnea; sensation; and paresthesia

4. Elevate the head of the patient's bed and remove compression stockings or boots. These measures increase pooling of blood in the lower extremities and decrease venous return, thus decreasing blood pressure. Assess blood pressure every two to three minutes while at the same time assessing for stimuli that initiated the response (such as a full bladder, impacted stool, or skin pressure). The most serious danger in dysreflexia is elevated blood pressure, which could precipitate a stroke, a myocardial infarction, dysrhythmias, or seizures. If the patient has a Foley catheter, ensure that there are no kinks in the tubing. If the patient does not have a Foley catheter, drain the bladder with a straight catheter. If manifestations persist, assess for a fecal impaction. If an impaction is present, insert Nupercaine cream into the anus, wait 10 minutes, and manually remove the impaction.

Case Study

1. *In an effort to differentiate the cause of the back injury, what diagnostic tests are anticipated?* Diagnostic tests are ordered to differentiate the cause of back pain; for example, back and leg pain may be caused by spinal tumors, degenerative processes, or abdominal diseases. Assessing pain is an important part of diagnosis. The tests include x-rays and CT scans of the lumbosacral or cervical area to identify skeletal deformities and narrowing of the disk spaces (see Chapter 41). Electromyography (EMG), which measures electrical activity of skeletal muscles at rest and during voluntary contraction, may be conducted to identify specific muscles affected by the pressure of the herniation on the nerve roots. A myelogram with contrast medium is done to rule out tumors and to illustrate areas of herniation, although it does not provide the detail found with CT or MRI.

    Muscle strength and reflexes are tested, with the straight leg-test being an important diagnostic test. It is conducted by placing the patient in the supine position and passively raising the leg or by having the patient sit on a table and slowly extending the knee with both hip and knee flexed at a 90° angle. This movement places traction on the nerve root, which increases the pain if the nerve root is inflamed.

2. *What medications are used in the management of pain and muscle spasms?* Medications used to treat back pain include nonnarcotic analgesics, anti-inflammatory drugs such as the NSAIDs, muscle relaxants, and sedative/tranquilizers. Muscle spasms are treated with muscle relaxants.

3. *What are the goals of conservative treatment?* The goals of treatment are pain relief and healing of the involved disk by fibrosis.

4. *What data is collected in the health history and physical assessment?* Health history: Type of employment, risk factors, pain (location, duration, intensity). Physical assessment: Muscle strength and coordination, sensation, reflexes.

Crossword Puzzle

question	term answer
Administered to prevent vomiting	ANTIEMETICS
A forcible bending forward	HYPERFLEXION
External force applied in rear-end collision	ACCELERATION
A medication used to treat spasticity	LIORESAL
Used to treat bradycardia	ATROPINE
A medication used to treat hypoten-sion in shock	DOPAMINE
External force applied in head-on collision	DECELERATION
An example of a proton pump inhibitor	PROTONIX
What corticosteroids may be used to decrease	INFLAMMATION

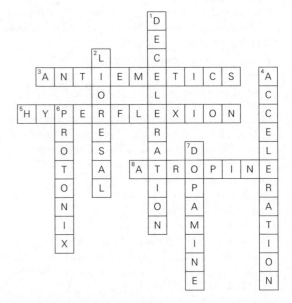

NCLEX-RN® Review Questions

1. Answer: 4

    Rationale: Although all of the listed nursing diagnoses may apply, the diagnosis of pain should be considered a priority. The pain of the ruptured disk is often discouraging and debilitating and may well affect the patient's ability to work. Pain will also affect the patient's tolerance of activity, mobility, and ability to perform self-care. Therefore, pain should be addressed as a priority.

    Nursing Process: Diagnosis

    Patient Need: Physiological Integrity

2. Answer: 2

    Rationale: All of the choices listed promote bowel elimination with the exception of maintaining a high-fluid, low-fiber diet. When considering dietary needs of a patient on a bowel retraining program, it is imperative to include a high-fluid, high-fiber diet. A high-fiber diet promotes bowel elimination and regularity.

Nursing Process: Planning

Patient Need: Safe, Effective Care Environment

3. Answer: 1

Rationale: Hypertension, bradycardia, and cool skin below the level of injury are clinical manifestations of autonomic dysreflexia. In autonomic dysreflexia, there is an exaggerated nervous system response. As baroreceptor function and parasympathetic control of heart rate travel via the cranial nerves, these responses remain intact (Porth & Matfin, 2009). Continued hypertension produces a baroreflex-mediated vagal slowing of the heart and bradycardia. There is also a baroreceptor-mediated vasodilation, with warm, flushed skin and profuse sweating above the level of injury and pale, cold, and dry skin below it (Porth & Matfin, 2009).

Nursing Process: Assessment

Patient Need: Physiological Integrity

4. Answer: 3

Rationale: A positive Babinski reflex is often present in patients with CJD. This reflex assessment is utilized to indicate CNS damage or dysfunction. Another clinical manifestation often characteristic of CJD is hyperreflexia. Battle signs and an increased white blood cell count are not factors in the clinical manifestations specific to CJD.

Nursing Process: Assessment

Patient Need: Physiological Integrity

5. Answer: 2

Rationale: Amphotericin B (Amphotec®) is an antifungal agent that may be used in the treatment of fungal meningitis. Phenytoin (Dilantin®) is an anticonvulsant. Rifampin (Rifadin®) is one of the preferred antibiotics in the treatment of bacterial meningitis. Dexamethasone (Decadron®) is a steroid that is often given with the antibiotics to suppress inflammation.

Nursing Process: Implementation

Patient Need: Safe, Effective Care Environment

6. Answer: 1

Rationale: All are manifestations that could be found in a patient with tetanus. Early manifestations of tetanus include pain at the infection site, stiffness of the jaw and neck, dysphagia, profuse perspiration, drooling, and increased salivation. Later manifestations as the infection progresses include hyperreflexia; facial or jaw muscle spasms; and rigidity or spasms of the neck, abdominal, and back muscles.

Nursing Process: Assessment

Patient Need: Physiological Integrity

7. Answer: 3

Rationale: When a patient at risk is assessed for fluid volume deficit, a 1 lb weight loss is equal to approximately 500 mL of fluid loss. A fluid loss of 1500 mL would be estimated as a 3 lb weight loss. A fluid loss of 1000 mL would be estimated as a 2 lb weight loss. A fluid loss of 100 mL would be estimated as a 0.2 lb weight loss.

Nursing Process: Assessment

Patient Need: Physiological Integrity

Chapter 44

Terms Matching

1. E
2. H
3. L
4. J
5. C
6. F
7. G
8. A
9. K
10. D
11. B
12. I

Focused Study

1. Assess the corneal reflex by lightly touching the cornea with a wisp of cotton. If the reflex is intact, the patient will blink. Severing the ophthalmic division of the trigeminal nerve destroys the corneal reflex and leaves the cornea at risk for dryness and injury.

   Assess the facial nerve by asking the patient to blow out the cheeks, wrinkle the forehead, frown, wink, and close both eyes tightly. Test taste by placing bitter, salty, and sweet substances on the anterior portion of the tongue. Facial weakness is evidenced by changes in movement in the involved side of the face. The facial nerve also innervates the anterior two-thirds of the tongue.

   Assess the function of the oculomotor muscles by asking the patient to follow your finger through the cardinal positions of vision. The eyes should move together; alterations in movement indicate an abnormal response.

   Assess the motor portion of the trigeminal nerve by asking the patient to clench the teeth while you palpate the tightness of the contracted masseter and temporal muscles. Loss of motor function is indicated by loss of bulk and tightness of these muscles.

2. The diagnosis must include decline in memory and at least one of the following cognitive abilities:
   1. Ability to generate coherent speech or understand spoken or written language
   2. Ability to recognize or identify objects, assuming intact sensory function
   3. Ability to execute motor activities, assuming intact motor abilities, sensory function, and comprehension of the required task
   4. Ability to think abstractly, make sound judgments, and carry out complex tasks

The decline in cognitive abilities must be severe enough to interfere with daily life.

Many different diseases and conditions may cause dementia, including Alzheimer's disease, vascular dementia, Parkinson's disease, normal pressure hydrocephalus, Creutzfeldt-Jakob disease, metabolic disorders, medications, poisoning, and anoxia. Even though the actual cause of dementias may not be known, factors that increase the risk of developing one or more kinds of dementia have been identified. These risk factors include aging, a family history of a disease that causes dementia, smoking and alcohol use, atherosclerosis, high cholesterol and plasma homocysteine levels, diabetes mellitus, and Down syndrome.

3. The acute stage is characterized by severe and rapid weakness, especially in the lower extremities; loss of muscle strength progressing to quadriplegia and respiratory failure; decreasing deep tendon reflexes; decreasing vital capacity; paresthesias, numbness; pain, especially nocturnal; and facial muscle involvement (inability to wrinkle forehead or change expressions). There is also involvement of the autonomic nervous system manifested by bradycardia, sweating, and fluctuating blood pressure (notably hypotension), which may last two weeks. The stabilizing/plateau stage occurs two to three weeks after initial onset. This stage marks the end of changes in condition, characterized by a "leveling off" of symptoms. Generally, the labile autonomic functions stabilize.

The recovery stage may take from several months to two years. This stage is marked by improvement in symptoms. Generally, muscle strength and function return in descending order.

4. Thymectomy is often recommended for patients younger than 60. The two surgical approaches used are the transcervical approach, which is considered less invasive, and the transsternal approach. The latter approach allows a more extensive removal of the gland; however, it also poses more potential complications because it involves splitting the sternum. Preoperatively, patients may be tapered from steroid therapy. Usually, pyridostigmine is administered to prevent muscular manifestations during the perioperative period. Postoperative nursing care focuses on preventing complications and controlling pain. Nursing implications for the patient undergoing thymectomy are presented in the box on page 1541. Remission may take several years to achieve. A tracheostomy may be required when the diaphragm or intercostal muscles are involved.

A rhizotomy is the surgical severing of a nerve root. Closed surgical interventions by percutaneous rhizotomy involve inserting a needle through the cheek into the foramen ovale at the base of the brain and partially destroying the trigeminal nerve with glycerol (an alcohol), radiofrequency-induced heat, or balloon compression of the trigeminal ganglion. These procedures carry less risk and result in shorter hospital stays than do open procedures, but recurrence of pain is a possibility. Following surgery, the patient may have some facial numbness, but there usually is no residual paralysis. The involved side of the face is insensitive to pain. The patient will have some loss of facial sensation (for example, to temperature and/or touch) and is at risk for loss of the corneal reflex.

Plasma exchange in myasthenia gravis may be used in conjunction with other therapies; for example, it may be performed prior to surgical intervention or after administration of high-dose intravenous immune globulin (Myasthenia gravis fact sheet, 2009). The goal of therapy is to remove the antiacetylcholine receptor antibodies, thus improving severe muscle weakness, fatigue, and other manifestations. The procedure is frequently performed when respiratory muscle involvement is evident.

Case Study

1. *"What are the risk factors of Alzheimer's disease?"* Alzheimer's disease (AD) develops from the interaction of multiple factors. Age is the major risk factor, but other risk factors include head trauma, inflammatory factors, and oxidative stress. In addition, other risk factors being considered include low educational level, lack of mental stimulation, migraines, and heavy smoking and alcohol consumption. People who develop AD under age 65 are said to have early-onset AD; those who develop AD after age 65 have late-onset AD. A small percentage of AD is caused by a genetic variation and is characterized by an early onset—sometimes to people as young as 30. Research into the genetics of early-onset AD has identified mutations of at least three genes: APP gene on chromosome 21, PSI gene on chromosome 14, and PS2 on chromosome 1. The ApoE gene on chromosome 19 increases the risk for development of late-onset AD and lowers the age of onset, but it is not yet known how this occurs.

2. *"What are the warning signs of Alzheimer's disease?"* The 10 warning signs of AD are memory loss, difficulty performing familiar tasks, problems with language, disorientation to time and place, poor or decreased judgment, problems with abstract thinking, habit of misplacing things, changes in mood or behavior, changes in personality, and loss of initiative (Alzheimer's Association, 2009).

Memory loss is usually the first sign of Alzheimer's disease. Memory deficits are initially subtle, and family members and friends may not suspect a problem until the disease progresses and manifestations become more noticeable. Family members and patients with AD may also deny the manifestations and hide deficits until the person exhibits unsafe or extremely unusual behavior. Progression of the disease varies, but the course is one of deteriorating cognition and judgment with eventual physical decline and total inability to perform activities of daily living (ADL). With the loss of the ability to perform even the most basic ADLs, the burden of meeting the patient's needs shifts to the caregiver.

3. *"What are the stages of Alzheimer's disease?"*

   Stage 1: No cognitive impairment. Memory problems are neither experienced nor evident to others.

   Stage 2: Very mild decline. People find themselves having memory lapses, forgetting familiar names, or losing everyday objects such as keys and glasses. These memory problems are not evident to others, nor are they detectable during a medical examination.

   Stage 3: Mild cognitive decline. Early-stage AD may be diagnosed in some, but not all, people with AD in this stage. Family and friends begin to notice problems, and the deficits may be measured or detected during a medical examination. Common problems include trouble finding words or names, decreased ability to remember names when introduced to new people, tendency to retain little information when reading a passage, decreased ability to plan or organize, habit of losing or misplacing valuable objects, and performance issues in social and work setting that are noticeable to others.

   Stage 4: Moderate cognitive decline. A careful medical interview will identify deficiencies is knowledge of recent events, impaired ability to perform challenging mental arithmetic (such as counting backward from 100 by 7s), decreased capacity to perform complex tasks (such as buying groceries or paying bills), and a reduced memory for personal history. The person often appears subdued and withdrawn, especially in social or mentally challenging situations.

   State 5: Moderately severe cognitive decline. Major deficits in memory and a decline in cognitive function emerge. Some assistance with ADL becomes essential, but the person can usually eat and use the toilet. People do usually retain knowledge about themselves and know their name and the name of family members. Problems include inability to recall current address or telephone number; confusion about where they are as well as the date, day, or the week or season; and trouble with less challenging mental arithmetic (such as counting backward by 4s from 40).

   Stage 6: Severe cognitive decline. This stage is characterized by worsening memory, emergence of personality changes, and the need for extensive help for ADL. There is loss of most awareness of recent experiences and events as well as of the surroundings. The person generally knows his or her name, but has problems recalling most personal history. People do sometimes forget the names of family members, but they can usually distinguish familiar from unfamiliar faces. Without supervision they may, for example, put pajamas over daytime clothing or shoes on the wrong feet. They need help with details of toileting (flushing, wiping, disposing of tissue) and are increasingly incontinent of urine or feces. There is

disruption of their normal sleep/waking cycle. They tend to wander and get lost. Significant personality and behavior changes occur, such as suspiciousness and delusions, hallucinations, and compulsive/repetitive behavior (such as hand-wringing and tissue shredding).

   Stage 7: Very severe cognitive decline. This is the final stage. These individuals lose the ability to respond to their environment, the ability to speak, and the ability to control movement. Some words or phrases may be spoken, but they are not recognizable. Total care is needed for eating and toileting. (There is general incontinence.) The ability to walk without assistance is lost first, followed by the ability to sit without support, the ability to smile, and the ability to hold up the head. Reflexes become abnormal, muscles grow rigid, and swallowing is impaired. There are many possible causes of death as the person with AD reaches the final stage. The affected person is at increased risk for aspiration pneumonia from impaired swallowing. Loss of neurons impairs sensations such as hunger and thirst, leading to complications of malnutrition and dehydration. Infections can result in sepsis.

Word Search

word	definition
Baclofen	muscle relaxant
Imuran	immunosuppressant
Levodopa	dopamine precursor
Symmetrel	glutamate antagonist
Parlodel	dopamine agonist
Cogentin	anticholinergic
Dilantin	anticonvulsant
Rilutek	antiglutamate
Leustatin	anticancer drug
Prednisone	glucocorticoid

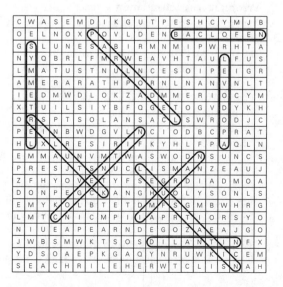

NCLEX-RN® Review Questions

1. Answer: 3

   Rationale: The 10 warning signs of Alzheimer's disease are memory loss, difficulty performing familiar tasks, problems with language, disorientation to time and place, poor or decreased judgment, problems with abstract thinking, habit of misplacing things, changes in mood or behavior, changes in personality, withdrawal from work or social activities, and loss of initiative (Alzheimer's Association, 2009).

   Nursing Process: Assessment

   Patient Need: Physiological Integrity

2. Answer: 2, 3, 4

   Rationale: The manifestations of MS vary according to the areas destroyed by demyelination and the affected body system. Multiple sclerosis (MS) is a chronic demyelinating disease of the CNS (brain, optic nerves, and spinal cord). The initial onset may be followed by a total remission, making diagnosis difficult. The onset of MS is usually between 20 and 40 years of age, but the disease has been diagnosed in individuals as young as 2 years and as old as 75 years.

   Nursing Process: Assessment

   Patient Need: Physiological Integrity

3. Answer: 3, 4

   Rationale: Men and women are affected equally. Parkinson's disease begins with subtle manifestations. PD is one of the most common neurologic disorders, affecting more than 1 million people in North America and more that 4 million people worldwide. The disorder usually develops after age 50 (called late-onset PD), but it does occur in younger adults. (PD before age 50 is called early-onset PD.) Drug induced Parkinsonism is usually reversible.

   Nursing Process: Planning

   Patient Need: Health Promotion and Maintenance

4. Answer: 2

   Rationale: Diagnosis is based primarily on a thorough history and physical examination and is made based on having two of the three cardinal manifestations: tremor at rest, bradykinesia, and rigidity.

   Nursing Process: Assessment

   Patient Need: Physiological Integrity

5. Answer: 4

   Rationale: Malnutrition is related to dysphagia. The following complications are associated with Parkinson's disease:

   • Oculogyric crisis, in which the eyes become fixed with a lateral and upward gaze

   • Paranoia and hallucinations, which may accompany dementia

   • Impaired communication due to changes in speech, handwriting, and expressiveness

   • Falls from balance, posture, and motor changes

   • Infections such as pneumonia related to immobility

   • Malnutrition related to dysphagia and inability to prepare meals

   • Altered sleep patterns due to loss of dopamine, L-dopa side effects (nightmares, dreams), side effects of anticholinergics (hyperreflexia, muscle twitching), and depression

   • Skin breakdown and pressure ulcers associated with urinary incontinence, malnutrition, and sweat reflex changes

   • Depression and social isolation

   Nursing Process: Assessment

   Patient Need: Physiological Integrity

6. Answer: 3

   Rationale: Huntington's disease (HD) is a familial disease. Each child of an HD parent has a 50% chance of inheriting the HD gene; if a child does inherit the gene, he or she will eventually develop the disease (NINDS, 2009c). HD is a progressive, degenerative, inherited neurologic disease characterized by increasing dementia and chorea (jerky, rapid, involuntary movements). Early signs of personality change include severe depression, memory loss with decreased ability to concentrate, emotional lability, and impulsiveness. HD causes destruction of cells in the caudate nucleus and putamen areas of the basal ganglia.

   Nursing Process: Evaluation

   Patient Need: Safe, Effective Care Environment

7. Answer: 3

   Rationale: There is no cure for amyotrophic lateral sclerosis (ALS). It is a rapidly progressive and fatal degenerative neurologic disease characterized by weakness and wasting of muscles under voluntary control without any accompanying sensory changes. ALS is also known as Lou Gehrig's disease (named for a famous baseball player who died of the disease), ALS affects motor neurons in three locations: the anterior horn cells, which are the lower motor neurons (LMNs) of the spinal cord; the motor nuclei of the brainstem; and the upper motor neurons (UMNs) of the cerebral cortex.

   Nursing Process: Planning

   Patient Need: Health Promotion and Maintenance

8. Answer: 1

   Rationale: Myasthenia gravis (MG) is a chronic autoimmune neuromuscular disorder characterized by fatigue and severe weakness of skeletal muscles. The manifestations of MG correspond to the muscles involved. Initially, the eye muscles are affected and the patient experiences either diplopia (unilateral or bilateral double vision) or ptosis (drooping of the eyelid). In MG, antibodies destroy or block neuromuscular junction receptor sites, resulting in a decreased number of acetylcholine receptors. In most patients with MG, the thymus gland, which is usually inactive after puberty, continues to produce antibodies because of hyperplasia of the gland or because of tumors. It is believed that the thymus is a source of an autoantigen that triggers an autoimmune response in MG. The exact mechanism and reason for the thymus gland's antibody production are unknown. MG is sometimes associated with thyrotoxicosis (hyperthyroidism), rheumatoid arthritis, and lupus erythematosus.

Nursing Process: Evaluation

Patient Need: Safe, Effective Care Environment

9. Answer: 1, 3

Rationale: Trigeminal neuralgia (TN) is more common in women than in men, occuring most often in middle or late adult life. There are no specific diagnostic tests for TN. The disorder is diagnosed by the characteristic location and type of pain. The disorder is treated by pharmacologic or surgical interventions. TN, also called *tic douloureux*, is a chronic disease of the trigeminal cranial nerve (V) that causes unilateral excruciating facial pain. Trigeminal neuralgia is characterized by brief (lasting a few seconds to a few minutes), repetitive episodes of sudden severe facial pain. The pain may occur as often as hundreds of times a day to as infrequently as a few times a year. The pain is experienced over the surface of the skin. It most often begins near one side of the mouth and rises toward the ear, eye, or nostril on the same side of the face. The disease goes into spontaneous remission for periods lasting from days to years.

Nursing Process: Assessment

Patient Need: Physiological Integrity

Chapter 45

Terms Matching

1. E
2. I
3. G
4. B
5. A
6. C
7. K
8. H
9. J
10. D
11. F

Focused Study

1. Throughout the interview, the nurse should be alert to nonverbal behaviors such as squinting and abnormal eye movements. These behaviors may suggest that the patient is experiencing problems with eye function. The nurse should also explore problems such as watery, irritated eyes and changes in vision.

2. Age-related changes of the eye:

Lens:
- ↓ elasticity, decreasing focus and accommodation for near vision (presbyopia)
- ↑ density and size, making the lens more stiff and opaque
- Yellowing of the lens and changes in the retina, which affect color perception

Cornea:
- Possibility of fat deposits around the periphery and throughout the cornea
- ↓ corneal sensitivity

Pupil:
- ↓ size and responsiveness to light; hardening of the sphincter

Retina and visual pathways:
- Narrowing of visual fields
- Lost photoreceptor cells
- Less effective rods
- Risk of macular degeneration
- Distorted depth perception
- Increased adaptation to dark and light

Lacrimal apparatus:
- ↓ reabsorption of intraocular fluid
- ↓ production of tears

Posterior cavity:
- Visible debris and condensation
- Possibility of vitreous body pulling away from the retina

Age-related changes of the ear:

Inner ear:
- Loss of hair cells, ↓ blood supply, less flexible basilar membrane, degeneration of spiral ganglion cells, and ↓ production of endolymph that result in progressive hearing loss with age (presbycusis)
- Loss of high-frequency sounds; possible loss of or decrease in middle and low-frequency sounds
- Degeneration of vestibular structures, organ of Corti, and cochlea

Middle ear:
- Weakened and stiffened muscles and ligaments, decreasing the acoustic reflex

External ear:
- Higher keratin content of the cerumen, contributing to increased cerumen in the ear canal

3. Eyes:
- Glaucoma is a term used for a group of diseases that damage the optic nerve and cause blindness. The diseases are primarily the result of increased intraocular pressure on the optic nerve.
- Gyrate atrophy of the choroid and retina is a genetic disorder resulting in a progressive vision loss, with total blindness occurring between ages 40 and 60.
- Best's disease is a familial disorder found most often in Caucasians who originated in Europe. The disease causes gradual loss of vision beginning during the teenage years.

Ears:
- Deafness is a common disorder with genetic implications that is seen from newborns to the elderly.
- Penred syndrome is an inherited disorder that accounts for as much as 10% of hereditary deafness. The deafness is usually accompanied by a thyroid goiter.
- Neurofibromatosis, a rare inherited disorder, is characterized by the development of acoustic neuromas and malignant central nervous system tumors.

4. Diagnostic Tests of Eye Disorders

Computed Tomography (CT) Scan of the Eye
Radiologic examination used to identify foreign objects or tumors in the eyeball or orbit. The head is positioned in a cradle, and a wide strap is applied around the head to keep it immobilized during the test. Tell the patient to remove all hairpins, clips, and earrings before the test. If a contrast dye is used, dentures must also be removed. Assess for allergies to iodine and, if present, notify the physician; medications such as diphenhydramine (Benadryl®) and rantidine (Zantac®) may be given one hour before the procedure. Assess medications: Oral hypoglycemic agents are contraindicated for use with iodinated contrast. Inform patient that the test takes from 5 to 10 minutes. Instruct the patient to increase oral fluid intake after the examination.

Refraction, Retinoscopy, Refractometry
These tests are used to measure refractive error. Either a handheld retinoscope or an instrument with multiple lenses is used; with the latter method, patient chooses lenses that provide the best vision.
No special preparation is needed; tell the patient that his or her pupils will be dilated with medication and may be enlarged for several hours.

Tonometry
This test is used to diagnose increased intraocular pressure in glaucoma. A computerized device is used to evaluate refraction. The cornea is anesthetized prior to being touched with the device. Normal value is 10–22 mmHg.
No special preparation is needed. Instruct the patient not to rub his or her eyes.

Diagnostic Tests of Ear Disorders

Audiometry
Audiometry is used to evaluate and diagnose conductive and sensorineural hearing loss. The patient sits in soundproof room and responds by raising his or her hand when sounds are heard.
No special preparation is needed.

Auditory Evoked Potential (AEP)
This test is used to identify electrical activity of the auditory nerve. Electrodes are placed on various areas of the ear and on the forehead, and a graphic recording is made.
No special preparation is needed.

Auditory Brainstem Response (ABR)
An ABR measures the electrical activity of the auditory pathway from the inner ear to the brain to diagnose brainstem pathology, stroke, and acoustic neuroma.
No special preparation is needed.

Caloric Test
A caloric test is used to assess vestibular system function. Cold or warm water is used to irrigate the ear canals one at a time, and the patient is observed for nystagmus. Normally, the nystagmus occurs opposite the ear being irrigated. If no nystagmus occurs, the patient needs further testing for brain lesions.

Assess patient for use of alcohol, central nervous system depressants, and barbiturates. These chemicals may alter the test results.

Case Study

1. *What is the colored part of the eye? What is its function?* The colored part of the eye is the iris. It is a disc of muscle tissue that surrounds the pupil and lies between the cornea and the lens. The iris gives the eye its color and regulates light entry by controlling the size of the pupil. The pupil is the dark center of the eye through which light enters. The pupil constricts when bright light enters the eye and when it is used for near vision; it dilates when light conditions are dim and when the eye is used for far vision. In response to intense light, the pupil constricts rapidly in the pupillary light reflex.

2. *Where is the lens located? What is its function?* The lens is a biconvex, avascular, transparent structure located directly behind the pupil. It can change shape to focus and refract light onto the retina. The posterior cavity lies behind the lens.

3. *What is the best way to assess the central visual field?* The central visual field may be assessed with an Amsler grid. The most basic form has black lines on a white grid, forming squares that measure 5 mm. A black dot is in the center of the grid. The Amsler grid is useful for identifying early changes in vision from macular degeneration and diabetes mellitus. To use the Amlser grid, ask the patient to hold the grid at normal reading distance (about 12–14 inches), cover one eye, and stare at the center dot. Ask the patient if any of the lines look crooked or bent; if any of the boxes are different in size or shape; and if any of the lines are wavy, missing, blurry, or discolored. Repeat with the other eye. The test should be conducted before the pupils are dilated, and the patient should be wearing their best correction.

4. *How are sound waves transmitted through the ear so that the patient can perceive and interpret the sounds?* Sound waves enter the external auditory canal and cause the tympanic membrane to vibrate at the same frequency. The ossicles not only transmit the motion of the tympanic membrane to the oval window, but also amplify the energy of the sound wave. As the stapes moves against the oval window, the perilymph in the vestibule is set in motion. The increased pressure of the perilymph is transmitted to fibers of the basilar membrane and then to the organ of Corti. The up-and-down movements of the fibers of the basilar membrane pull the hair cells in the organ of Corti, which in turn generates action potentials that are transmitted to cranial nerve VIII and then to the brain for interpretation.

Several brainstem auditory nuclei transmit impulses to the cerebral cortex. Fibers from each ear cross, with each auditory cortex receiving impulses from both ears. Auditory processing is so finely tuned that a wide variety of sounds of different pitch and loudness can be heard at any one time. In addition, the source of the sound can be localized.

5. *Explain equilibrium.* The inner ear provides information about the position of the head. This information is used to coordinate body movements so that equilibrium and balance are maintained. The types of equilibrium are static balance and dynamic balance. Receptors called maculae in the utricle and the saccule of the vestibule detect changes in the position of the head. Maculae are groups of hair cells; these cells have protrusions that are covered with a gelatinous substance. Embedded in this gelatinous substance are tiny particles of calcium carbonate called otoliths, which make the gelatin heavier than the endolymph that fills the membranous labyrinth. As a result, when the head is in the upright position, gravity causes the gelatinous substance to bear down on the hair cells. When the position of the head changes, the force on the hair cells also changes, bending them and altering the pattern of stimulation of the neurons. Thus, a different pattern of nerve impulses is transmitted to the brain, where stimulation of the motor centers initiates actions that coordinate various body movements according to the position of the head. The receptor for dynamic equilibrium is in the crista, a crest in the membrane that lines the ampulla of each semicircular canal. The cristae are stimulated by rotatory head movement as a result of changes in the flow of endolymph and of movement of hair cells in the maculae. The direction of endolymph and hair cell movement is always opposite the motion of the body.

6. *What is a tympanogram? What does an abnormal tympanogram indicate?* A tympanogram is used to measure the pressure of the middle ear and to observe the tympanic membrane's response to waves of pressure. Insert the device into the ear canal. Ask the patient not to speak, move, swallow, or jump when hearing a sound. Tell the patient that he or she will hear a loud tone as the measurements are taken. Repeat for the other ear. The normal pressure inside the middle ear is a 100 daPa. Abnormal findings may include fluid in the middle ear, a perforated eardrum, impacted earwax, or a tumor of the middle ear.

Short Answers
Label the following figures.

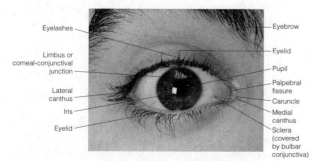

Figure 45–1 ■ Eyebrows, eyelids, eyelashes, conjunctiva, lacrimal apparatus, extrinsic eye muscles.

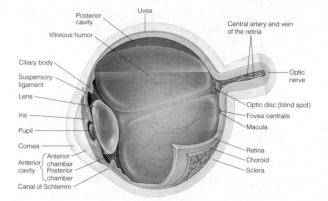

Figure 45–3 ■ Sclera, cornea, iris, pupil, anterior cavity.

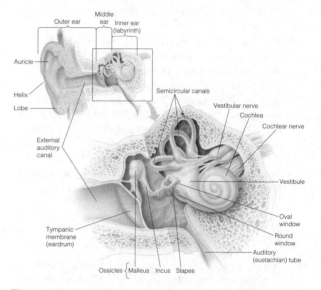

Figure 45–10 ■ External ear, middle ear, inner ear.

NCLEX-RN® Review Questions

1. Answer: 1

   Rationale: The iris gives the eye its color and regulates light entry by controlling the size of the pupil. The pupil is the dark center of the eye through which light enters. The pupil constricts when bright light enters the eye and when the eye is used for near vision. It dilates when in dim light and when the eye is used for far vision. In response to intense light, the pupil constricts rapidly in the pupillary light reflex. The white sclera lines the outside of the eyeball and protects and gives shape to the eyeball. The sclera gives way to the cornea over the iris and pupil. The cornea is transparent, avascular, and sensitive to touch. The cornea forms a window that allows light to enter the eye and is a part of its light-bending apparatus.

   Nursing Process: Assessment

   Patient Need: Physiological Integrity

2. Answer: 4

   Rationale: The anterior cavity is filled with aqueous humor. Aqueous humor is a clear fluid. It provides nutrients and oxygen to the cornea and the lens. It is constantly formed and drained to maintain a relatively constant pressure of 15–20 mmHg in the eye.

Nursing Process: Assessment

Patient Need: Physiological Integrity

3. Answer: 1

Rationale: When the eye focuses on an image, it is called accommodation. Refraction is the bending of light rays as they pass from one medium to another medium of different optical density. Convergence (which is the medial rotation of the eyeballs so that each is directed toward the viewed object) allows the eye to focus on an image in the retinal fovea of each eye. In the pupillary light reflex, the pupil constricts rapidly in response to intense light.

Nursing Process: Assessment

Patient Need: Physiological Integrity

4. Answer: 1

Rationale: To measure visual fields, sit directly opposite the patient at a distance of 18–24 inches. Ask the patient to cover one eye with the opaque cover while you cover your own eye opposite the patient. (For example, if the patient covers the right eye, you cover your left eye.) Ask the patient to look directly at you. Move the penlight from the periphery toward the center from right to left, above and below, and from the middle of each of these directions. If you have normal peripheral vision, both you and the patient should see the penlight enter the field of vision at the same time.

Nursing Process: Implementation

Patient Need: Physiological Integrity

5. Answer: 4

Rationale: The tympanic membrane is a part of the external ear. The middle ear contains three auditory ossicles: the malleus, the incus, and the stapes. The external ear consists of the auricle (or pinna), the external auditory canal, and the tympanic membrane.

Nursing Process: Assessment

Patient Need: Physiological Integrity

6. Answer: 4

Rationale: The human ear is most sensitive to sound waves with frequencies between 1000 and 4000 cycles per second, but it can detect sound waves with frequencies between 20 and 20,000 cycles per second. Hearing is the perception and interpretation of sound. Sound is produced when the molecules of a medium are compressed, which results in a pressure disturbance evidenced as a sound wave. Sound waves enter the external auditory canal and cause the tympanic membrane to vibrate at the same frequency.

Nursing Process: Assessment

Patient Need: Physiological Integrity

7. Answer: 4

Rationale: The tympanic membrane should be pearly gray, shiny, and translucent without bulging or retraction.

Nursing Process: Assessment

Patient Need: Physiological Integrity

Chapter 46

Terms Matching

1. E
2. N
3. V
4. CC
5. I
6. C
7. AA
8. L
9. R
10. DD
11. T
12. A
13. P
14. Z
15. B
16. D
17. F
18. Y
19. S
20. Q
21. X
22. O
23. U
24. W
25. BB
26. M
27. K
28. H
29. G
30. J

Focused Study

1. Infectious conjunctivitis may be bacterial, viral, or fungal in origin. Bacterial conjunctivitis is often caused by *Staphylococcus* and *Haemophilus*. Adenovirus infection is the leading cause of conjunctivitis in adults. Systemic infections that may affect the eyes include herpes simplex and other viral infections. Contact with genital secretions infected with *Gonococcus* can cause gonococcal conjunctivitis, a medical emergency that can lead to corneal perforation.

2. Keratitis is described as either nonulcerative or ulcerative. In nonulcerative keratitis, all layers of corneal epithelium are affected but remain intact. Viral infections, tuberculosis, and autoimmune disorders such as lupus erythematosus may cause nonulcerative keratitis. Ulcerative keratitis, in contrast, affects the epithelium and stroma of the cornea, leading to tissue destruction and ulceration. Bacterial conjunctivitis (for example, *Staphylococcus*, *S. pneumoniae*, and *Chlamydia*) may lead to ulcerative keratitis.

3. The following diagnostic studies may be ordered:
   • Caloric testing (electronystagmography) evaluates the vestibulo-ocular reflex by identifying eye

movements (nystagmus) in response to caloric testing. In patients with impaired vestibular function, the normal nystagmus response is blunted or absent. This portion of the test is contraindicated in patients who have a perforated tympanic membrane.

- Rinne and Weber tests of hearing show decreased air and bone conduction on the affected side when a sensorineural hearing loss is present. In Ménière's disease, audiology shows sensorineural hearing loss involving the low tones.
- X-rays and CT scans of the petrous bones are used to evaluate the internal auditory canal. In patients with Ménière's disease, the vestibular aqueducts may be shorter and straighter than normal.
- The glycerol test is conducted by giving the patient oral glycerol to decrease fluid pressure in the inner ear. An acute temporary hearing improvement is considered diagnostic for Ménière's disease.

4. Reconstructive surgeries of the middle ear, such as a stapedectomy and tympanoplasty, may help restore a conductive hearing loss. Stapedectomy is the removal and replacement of the stapes. This procedure is used to treat hearing loss related to otosclerosis.

In a tympanoplasty, the structures of the middle ear are reconstructed to improve conductive hearing deficits. Chronic otitis media with necrosis and scarring of the middle ear is a common indication for this type of surgery.

For the patient with a sensorineural hearing loss, a cochlear implant may be the only hope for restoring sound perception. The cochlear implant consists of a microphone, a speech processor, a transmitter and receiver/stimulator, and electrodes. Compared to a hearing aid, its function is more similar to the way the ear normally receives and processes sounds. The microphone picks up sounds, sending them to the speech processor, which selects and processes useful sounds. The transmitter and receiver/stimulator receive signals from the speech processor, convert them to electrical impulses, and send these impulses to the electrodes for transmission to the brain.

Case Study

1. *"Is conjunctivitis the same as pink eye?"* Yes, bacterial conjunctivitis is also known as pink eye.
2. *"Is pink eye contagious?"* Bacterial conjunctivitis, also known as pink eye, is highly contagious and often is caused by *Staphylococcus* and *Haemophilus*.
3. *"What do most people with pink eye experience?"* Redness and itching of the affected eye are common manifestations of acute conjunctivitis. The patient may also complain of a scratchy, burning, or gritty sensation. Photophobia may occur. Tearing and discharge accompany the inflammatory process. The discharge may be watery, purulent, or mucoid depending on the cause of conjunctivitis. The patient may have associated manifestations such as

pharyngitis, fever, malaise, and swollen preauricular lymph nodes.
4. *"How is it normally treated?"* Bacterial conjunctivitis is treated with antibiotics and anti-inflammatory drugs as appropriate. Topical anti-infectives applied as eyedrops or ointment may include erythromycin, gentamicin, penicillin, and bacitracin. For severe infections or cellulitis, anti-infectives may be administered by subconjunctival injection or systemic intravenous infusion. Antihistamines are used to minimize symptoms of conjunctivitis when an allergic response underlies the inflammatory process. Frequent eye irrigations may be ordered to remove the copious purulent discharge associated with conjunctivitis. Soaking the lids with warm saline compresses prior to cleansing promotes comfort and facilitates the removal of crusts and exudate in conjunctivitis.
5. *"What are some things I need to know so that I don't give this to my girlfriend?"* Teach Mr. Smith to wash his hands thoroughly before instilling eye medications. Hand hygiene is the single most important measure to prevent transmission of infection to the eye. He should avoid touching or rubbing his eyes. Touching or rubbing the eyes increases the risk of infection and corneal trauma. Advise him to use a new, clean cotton-tipped swab or cotton ball for cleaning each eye. Using a new swab or cotton ball prevents cross-contamination between eyes. Teach him to instill prescribed eyedrops as ordered. The prescribed medications will reduce inflammation and eliminate infection. Discuss with him the importance of avoiding contact lens use until the infectious process has cleared and of completing the prescribed treatment. Use of contact lenses in the inflamed eyes can lead to further damage and impair healing.
6. *My eyes are really sensitive to the sunlight right now. Should I just wear sunglasses until this gets better?* Instruct him to use dark sunglasses with appropriate UV protection when out of doors, even on cloudy days. Photophobia is a common manifestation of conjunctivitis and causes eye pain with increased light intensity.

Care Plan Critical-Thinking Activity

1. All of these activities may increase Mrs. Rainey's intraocular pressure and increase her risk for damaging the optic nerve. This may further impair her ability to see clearly.
2. Mrs. Rainey should avoid caffeinated drinks and foods. She should avoid stimulants. She should drink plenty of water and eat fresh fruits and vegetables to prevent constipation. She should eat a diet rich in vitamins and minerals.

Short Answers
Fill in the table regarding the differences between open-angle and angle-closure glaucoma.

	Open-Angle Glaucoma	**Angle-Closure Glaucoma**
Incidence	Accounts for 90% of all cases of glaucoma	Uncommon
Risk Factors	Over age 35 Genetic link African American ancestry	Narrow anterior chamber angle Aging Asian ancestry
Pathophysiology	Impaired aqueous outflow through the canal of Schlemm Unknown cause Usually unilateral	Pupil dilation or lens accommodation that causes already narrowed angle to close, blocking aqueous outflow Rapid rise in intraocular pressure Usually bilateral
Manifestations	No initial manifestations Frequent lens changes in glasses Impaired dark adaptation Halos around lights Gradual reduction of visual fields with preservation of central vision until late in the disease Mild to severe increased intraocular pressure	Abrupt onset of eye pain, headache Decreased visual acuity Nausea and vomiting Reddened conjunctiva Cloudy cornea Fixed pupil Rapid, significant increase in intraocular pressure
Management	Topical medications such as beta blockers, adrenergics, prostaglandin analogs Carbonic anhydrase inhibitors Laser trabeculoplasty, trabeculectomy	Topical miotics or beta blockers Systemic osmotic agents, carbonic anhydrase inhibitors Laser iridotomy or peripheral iridectomy

NCLEX-RN® Review Questions

1. Answer: 3
   Rationale: In myopia (nearsightedness), the objects at close range are seen clearly, and those at a distance are blurred. Nystagmus is rapid involuntary eye movements. A cataract is an opacification (clouding) of the lens of the eye. The eyeball is too short in hyperopia (farsightedness), which causes the image to focus behind the retina. People with this condition see objects clearer at a distance than they see objects close to them.
   Nursing Process: Assessment
   Patient Need: Physiological Integrity

2. Answer: 2
   Rationale: A chalazion is a granulomatous cyst or nodule of the lid. Infection of one or more of the sebaceous glands of the eyelid may cause a hordeolum (sty). Hyphema, which is bleeding into the anterior chamber of the eye, is a potential result of blunt eye trauma. A cataract is an opacification (clouding) of the eye lens.
   Nursing Process: Assessment
   Patient Need: Physiological Integrity

3. Answer: 4
   Rationale: Critical proliferative retinopathy is not a stage of diabetic retinopathy. Diabetic retinopathy progresses through four stages: (1) mild nonproliferative or background retinopathy, (2) moderate nonproliferative retinopathy, (3) severe nonproliferative retinopathy, and (4) proliferative retinopathy.
   Nursing Process: Assessment
   Patient Need: Physiological Integrity

4. Answer: 2
   Rationale: Otitis externa is commonly known as swimmer's ear (not diver's ear). It is inflammation of the ear canal and is most prevalent in people who spend significant time in the water. Competitive athletes, including swimmers, divers, and surfers, are particularly prone to otitis externa. Wearing a hearing aid or ear plugs, which hold moisture in the ear canal, is an additional risk factor.
   Nursing Process: Evaluation
   Patient Need: Physiological Integrity

5. Answer: 3
   Rationale: Otosclerosis is a hereditary disorder with an autosomal dominant pattern of inheritance. Otosclerosis occurs most commonly in females, not males. Otosclerosis is a common cause of conductive hearing loss. The progressive hearing loss typically begins in adolescence or early adulthood and seems to be accelerated by pregnancy.
   Nursing Process: Assessment
   Patient Need: Physiological Integrity

6. Answer: 3
   Rationale: Ménière's disease, also known as endolymphatic hydrops, is a chronic disorder characterized by recurrent attacks of vertigo with tinnitus and a progressive unilateral hearing loss. An acoustic neuroma, or schwannoma, is a benign tumor of cranial nerve VIII. Labyrinthitis, also called otitis interna, is inflammation of the inner ear. Otitis externa is inflammation of the ear canal.
   Nursing Process: Assessment
   Patient Need: Physiological Integrity

7. Answer: 2

Rationale: Higher-pitched (not lower-pitched) tones and conversational speech are lost initially. Because the hearing loss of presbycusis is gradual, the patient and family may not realize the extent of the deficit. Hearing acuity begins to decrease in early adulthood and progresses as long as the individual lives. Hearing aids and other amplification devices are useful for most patients with presbycusis.

Nursing Process: Planning

Patient Need: Physiological Integrity

Chapter 47

Terms Matching

1. B
2. J
3. K
4. M
5. A
6. E
7. H
8. D
9. G
10. I
11. L
12. F
13. C

Focused Study

1. Female patient:
   - Presence of vaginal bleeding, itching, or discharge
   - Obstetrical history
   - Menstrual history
   - Use of contraceptives
   - Sexual history
   - Medication use
   - History of cancer
   - History of tobacco use

   Male patient:
   - Presence of penile discharge
   - Presence of rashes or lesions
   - Voiding difficulties
   - Concerns with sexual performance
   - Medical history
   - Medication use
   - History of cancer

2. Female reproductive system:
   - External genitalia
     - Mons pubis
     - Labia
     - Clitoris
     - Vaginal and urethral openings
     - Glands
   - Internal organs
     - Vagina
     - Cervix
     - Uterus
     - Fallopian tubes

Male reproductive system:
- External genitalia
  - Penis
  - Scrotum
  - Internal organs
  - Testes
  - Ducts
  - Seminiferous tubules
  - Epididymis
  - Vas deferens
  - Ampulla
  - Seminal fluid and semen
- Prostate gland
  - Prostatic urethra
  - Urethra

3. The male sex hormones are called androgens. Most androgens are produced in the testes, although the adrenal cortex also produces a small amount.
   - Testosterone, the primary androgen produced by the testes, is essential for the development and maintenance of sexual organs and secondary sex characteristics and for spermatogenesis. It also promotes metabolism, growth of muscles and bone, and libido (sexual desire).
   - The ovaries produce estrogens, progesterone, and androgens in a cyclic pattern. Estrogens are steroid hormones that occur naturally in three forms: estrone (E_1), estradiol (E_2), and estriol (E_3). Estradiol, the most potent, is the form secreted in greatest amount by the ovaries. Estrogens are essential for the development and maintenance of secondary sex characteristics; in conjunction with other hormones, they stimulate the female reproductive organs to prepare for growth of a fetus. Estrogens are responsible for the normal structure of skin and blood vessels. They decrease the rate of bone resorption, promote increased high-density lipoproteins, reduce cholesterol levels, and enhance the clotting of blood. Estrogens also promote the retention of sodium and water.
   - Progesterone primarily affects the development of breast glandular tissue and the endometrium. During pregnancy, progesterone relaxes smooth muscle to decrease uterine contractions. It also increases body temperature. Androgens are responsible for normal hair growth patterns at puberty and may have metabolic effects.

   The ovaries produce estrogens, progesterone, and androgens in a cyclic pattern.
   - Estrogens are steroid hormones that occur naturally in three forms: estrone (E_1), estradiol (E_2), and estriol (E_3). Estradiol, the most potent, is the form secreted in greatest amount by the ovaries. Estrogens are essential for the development and maintenance of secondary sex characteristics; in conjunction with other hormones, they stimulate the female reproductive organs to prepare for growth of a fetus. Estrogens are responsible for the normal structure of skin and blood vessels. They decrease the rate of bone resorption, promote increased high-density

lipoproteins, reduce cholesterol levels, and enhance the clotting of blood. Estrogens also promote the retention of sodium and water.

- Progesterone primarily affects the development of breast glandular tissue and the endometrium. During pregnancy, progesterone relaxes smooth muscle to decrease uterine contractions. It also increases body temperature. Androgens are responsible for normal hair growth patterns at puberty and may have metabolic effects.

Case Study

1. *"What is the ovarian cycle?"* The ovarian cycle has three consecutive phases that occur cyclically each 28 days (although the cycle may be longer or shorter), as follows:
   - The follicular phase lasts from the 1st to the 10th day of the cycle.
   - The ovulatory phase lasts from the 11th to the 14th day of the cycle and ends with ovulation.
   - The luteal phase lasts from the 14th to the 28th day.
2. *"Why do I need estrogen?"* Estrogens are essential for the development and maintenance of secondary sex characteristics; in conjunction with other hormones, they stimulate the female reproductive organs to prepare for growth of a fetus. Estrogens are responsible for the normal structure of skin and blood vessels. They decrease the rate of bone resorption, promote increased high-density lipoproteins, reduce cholesterol levels, and enhance the clotting of blood. Estrogens also promote the retention of sodium and water.
3. *"What is the difference between the vagina and the cervix?"* The vagina is a fibromuscular tube about 3–4 inches (8–10 cm) in length that is located posterior to the bladder and urethra and anterior to the rectum. The upper end contains the uterine cervix in an area called the fornix. The walls of the vagina are membranes that form folds, called rugae. These membranes are composed of mucus-secreting stratified squamous epithelial cells. The vagina serves as a route for the excretion of secretions, including menstrual fluid, and is an organ of sexual response. The walls of the vagina are usually moist and maintain a pH that ranges from 3.8–4.2. This pH is bacteriostatic and is maintained by the action of estrogen and normal vaginal flora. Estrogen stimulates the growth of vaginal mucosal cells so that they thicken and have increased glycogen content. The glycogen is fermented to lactic acid by Döderlein's bacilli (lactobacilli that normally inhabit the vagina), which slightly acidifies the vaginal fluid. The cervix projects into the vagina and forms a pathway between the uterus and the vagina. The uterine opening of the cervix is called the internal os; the vaginal opening is called the external os. The space between these openings, which is the endocervical canal, serves as a route for the discharge of menstrual fluid and the entrance for sperm. The cervix is a firm structure protected by mucus that changes consistency and quantity during the menstrual cycle and during pregnancy.

NCLEX-RN® Review Questions

1. Answer: 1
   Rationale: Each testis surrounded by two coverings: an outer tunica vaginalis and an inner tunica albuginea. Each testis is divided into 250–300 lobules, and each lobule contains one to four seminiferous tubules. The testes produce sperm and testosterone. The testes develop in the abdominal cavity of the fetus and then descend through the inguinal canal into the scrotum. They are homologous to the female's ovaries. Each of these paired organs is about 1.5 inches (4 cm) long and 1 inch (2.5 cm) in diameter. They are suspended in the scrotum by the spermatic cord.
   Nursing Process: Evaluation
   Patient Need: Physiological Integrity
2. Answer: 4
   Rationale: Secretions from the prostate gland make up about one-third the volume of semen and enter the urethra through several ducts during ejaculation. The prostate gland is about the size of a walnut (not a pea). It encircles the urethra just below the urinary bladder (see Figure 47–1). It is made up of 20–30 tubuloalveolar glands surrounded by smooth muscle.
   Nursing Process: Evaluation
   Patient Need: Physiological Integrity
3. Answer: 3
   Rationale: The optimum temperature for sperm production is about 2–3 degrees below body temperature. The scrotum is a sac or pouch made of two layers. When the testicular temperature is too low, the scrotum contracts to bring the testes up against the body. The scrotum hangs at the base of the penis, anterior to the anus, and regulates the temperature of the testes.
   Nursing Process: Evaluation
   Patient Need: Physiological Integrity
4. Answer: 2
   Rationale: The clitoris is an erectile organ that is analogous to the penis in the male. Collectively, the external genitalia are called the vulva. The external genitalia include the mons pubis, the labia, the clitoris, the vaginal and urethral openings, and glands. The labia majora, which are folds of skin and adipose tissue covered with hair, are outermost; they begin at the base of the mons pubis and end at the anus. The labia minora, which are located between the clitoris and the base of the vagina, are enclosed by the labia majora. After puberty, the mons is covered with hair in a diamond-shaped distribution.
   Nursing Process: Assessment
   Patient Need: Physiological Integrity
5. Answer: 3
   Rationale: Men taking a variety of medications may be at an increased risk for the development of erectile

dysfunction. Classifications of medications that may be associated with erectile dysfunction include antispasmodics, antihypertensive agents, antidepressants, beta blockers, tranquilizers, and sedatives.

Nursing Process: Assessment

Patient Need: Physiological Integrity

6. Answer: 1

Rationale: Prostate specific antigen (PSA) is a blood test used to diagnose prostate cancer and to monitor treatment of prostate cancer. Venereal disease research laboratory (VDRL), rapid plasma reagin (RPR), and fluorescent treponemal antibody absorption (FTA-ABS) are blood tests that screen for syphilis.

Nursing Process: Assessment

Patient Need: Physiological Integrity

7. Answer: 2

Rationale: The ovaries in the adult woman are flat, almond-shaped structures located on either side of the uterus below the ends of the fallopian tubes. They are homologous to the male's testes. The other answer selections are not homologous to the male's testes.

Nursing Process: Assessment

Patient Need: Physiological Integrity

8. Answer: 2

Rationale: The corpus luteum is the site from which the mature ovum is expelled. The role of the corpus luteum is the production and secretion of hormones until the placenta becomes effective.

Nursing Process: Assessment

Patient Need: Physiological Integrity

Chapter 48

Terms Matching

1. D
2. J
3. A
4. M
5. O
6. B
7. C
8. P
9. G
10. N
11. F
12. I
13. H
14. L
15. K
16. E

Focused Study

1. Penile Cancer
   - Risk factors
     - Phimosis
     - Poor genital hygiene
     - Human papillomavirus (HPV)
   - HIV infections
   - Ultraviolet radiation exposure (such as that used to treat psoriasis) also may play a role

   Testicular Cancer
   - Age
   - Cryptorchidism (undescended testicle)
   - Family history of testicular cancer
   - Cancer of the other testicle
   - Potential risk factors under investigation include occupational risks, the presence of multiple atypical nevi, HIV infection, cancer *in situ*, and age

   Prostate Cancer
   - Age
   - Race
   - Family history
   - Vasectomy surgery
   - Dietary factors, including a diet high in animal fat and excessive supplemental vitamin A

2. Radical prostatectomy: The removal of the prostate, the prostate capsule, the seminal vesicles, and a portion of the bladder neck. In a laparoscopic radical prostatectomy (LRP), small incisions are made in the abdomen and a laparoscope is inserted and used to remove the prostate. The most common radical prostatectomy techniques are as follows:
   - Retropubic prostatectomy
   - Perineal prostatectomy
   - Suprapubic prostatectomy

   Radical orchiectomy: The surgical removal of the affected testicle and spermatic used as treatment in all forms and stages of testicular cancer

   Partial or total amputation of the penis: Surgery used to manage invasive penile cancer

   Circumcision: Surgical removal of the penile foreskin

3. When treating erectile dysfunction, the cause must be determined first. A variety of diagnostic tests may be employed, as follows:
   - Laboratory studies
     - Complete blood count
     - Lipid profile
     - Urinalysis
     - Testosterone level
     - Prolactin level
     - Thyroxin levels
     - Prostate specific antigen (PSA) levels
   - Penile monitoring
     - Noctornal penile tumescence and rigidity (NPTR) monitoring
   - Penile blood flow
     - Cavernosometry and cavernosography

   The management of erectile dysfunction may include medications, mechanical devices, or alterations in lifestyle.

   Medications
   - Oral medications
     - Sildenafil citrate (Viagra®)
     - Vardenafil hydrochloride (Levitra®)
     - Tadalafil (Cialis®)

- Injectable medications
  - Testosterone injections IM Q 3 weeks
  - Papaverine
  - Prostaglandin E
- Topical patches
  - Testosterone
- Uretheral suppository
  - Alprostadil (Caverject®)

Mechanical Devices
- Vacuum constriction device (VCD)
  - Used to draw blood into the penis
- O-ring
  - Used at the base of the penis to trap blood in the shaft and maintain the erection

Surgery
- Revascularization procedures
- Implantation of penile prosthetic devices

Lifestyle Changes
- Smoking cessation
- Diet
- Exercise
- Stress reduction
- Reduced alcohol intake

Case Study

1. *"What is the cause of testicular cancer?"* The cause of testicular cancer is unknown, but both congenital and acquired factors have been associated with tumor development. About 5% of testicular cancers develop in a man with a history of undescended testicle (cryptorchidism). Testicular cancer is more common on the right side, which parallels the incidence of cryptorchidism (Tierney et al., 2004).
2. *"What are the risk factors for testicular cancer?"*
   - Age
   - Cryptorchidism
   - Genetic predisposition, especially in identical twins and brothers
   - Cancer of the other testicle

   Other risk factors under investigation include occupational risks, presence of multiple atypical nevi, HIV infection, cancer *in situ*, body size, and maternal hormone use (ACS, 2004).
3. *"What are the manifestations of testicular cancer?"* The first sign of testicular cancer may be a slight enlargement of one testicle with some discomfort. The man may also have an abdominal ache and a feeling of heaviness in the scrotum. Local spread of cancer to the epididymis or spermatic cord is inhibited by the outer covering of the testicles, the tunica albuginea. Therefore, spread by lymphatic and vascular channels to other organs often causes distant disease before large masses develop in the scrotum. Lymphatic dissemination usually leads to disease in retroperitoneal lymph nodes, whereas vascular dissemination can lead to metastasis in the lungs, bone, or liver. Bilateral presentation of testicular cancer is unusual. Manifestations of metastasis include lower extremity edema, back pain, cough, hemoptysis, or dizziness. Tumors that produce HCG may cause breast enlargement (gynecomastia).

Short Answers

Complete the chart by indicating the appropriate cause of erectile dysfunction for each category.

Medications	Procedures
1. Antihypertensives	1. Coronary bypass
2. Psychotropic agents	2. Radiation therapy
3. Antihistamines	3. Prostatectomy
4. Immunosuppressive agents	4. Transplant surgeries
5. Anticholinergic agents	

Inflammatory Causes	Neurogenic Causes	Arterial Causes
1. Prostatitis	1. Spinal cord injury	1. Atherosclerosis
2. Cystitis	2. Stroke	2. Hypertension
	3. Parkinson's disease	3. Sickle cell anemia
	4. Multiple sclerosis	
	5. Diabetes mellitus	

NCLEX-RN® Review Questions

1. Answer: 4
   Rationale: Erectile dysfunction (ED) can be treated with oral medications or medications injected directly into the penis or into the urethra at the tip of the penis. ED is the inability of the male to attain and maintain an erection sufficient to permit satisfactory sexual intercourse. *Impotence*, a term often used synonymously with *erectile dysfunction*, may involve a total inability to achieve erection, an inconsistent ability to achieve erection, or the ability to sustain only brief erections. It has many possible causes.
   Nursing Process: Evaluation
   Patient Need: Physiological Integrity
2. Answer: 2
   Rationale: Phimosis is constriction of the foreskin so that it cannot be retracted over the glans penis. In paraphimosis, the foreskin is tight and constricted and does not cover the glans penis. Priapism is an involuntary, sustained, painful erection that is not associated with sexual arousal. A hydrocele, which is the most common cause of scrotal swelling, is a collection of fluid in the tunica vaginalis.
   Nursing Process: Assessment
   Patient Need: Physiological Integrity
3. Answer: 3
   Rationale: A hydrocele, which is the most common cause of scrotal swelling, is a collection of fluid in the tunica vaginalis. Testicular torsion, which is twisting of the spermatic cord with scrotal swelling and pain, is a potential medical emergency. A spermatocele is a mobile, usually painless mass that forms when efferent ducts in the epididymis dilate

and form a cyst. A varicocele is an abnormal dilation of a vein in the spermatic cord.

Nursing Process: Assessment

Patient Need: Physiological Integrity

4. Answer: 2

Rationale: Orchitis most commonly occurs as a complication of a systemic illness or as an extension of epididymitis. Orchitis is an acute inflammation or infection of the testes. The most common infectious cause of orchitis in postpubertal men is mumps (not measles). The manifestations have a sudden onset, usually within three to four days after the swelling of the parotid glands.

Nursing Process: Assessment

Patient Need: Physiological Integrity

5. Answer: 1

Rationale: Testicular cancer is more common on the right side, which parallels the incidence of cryptorchidism. Testicular cancer accounts for only 1% of all cancers in men; however, it is the most common cancer in men between the ages of 15 and 40. The first sign of testicular cancer may be a slight enlargement of one testicle with some discomfort.

Nursing Process: Assessment

Patient Need: Physiological Integrity

6. Answer: 2

Rationale: Testicular torsion, which is twisting of the spermatic cord with scrotal swelling and pain, is a potential medical emergency. The two necessary preconditions for BPH are age of 50 and older and the presence of testes. The exact cause of BPH is unknown. Risk factors of BPH include age, family history, race (highest in African Americans and lowest in native Japanese), and a diet high in meat and fats.

Nursing Process: Assessment

Patient Need: Physiological Integrity

7. Answer: 1

Rationale: A spermatocele is a mobile, usually painless mass that forms when efferent ducts in the epididymis dilate and form a cyst. Testicular torsion, which is the twisting of the spermatic cord with scrotal swelling and pain, is a potential medical emergency. A hydrocele, which is the most common cause of scrotal swelling, is a collection of fluid in the tunica vaginalis. A varicocele is an abnormal dilation of a vein in the spermatic cord.

Nursing Process: Assessment

Patient Need: Physiological Integrity

8. Answer: 1

Rationale: Epididymitis is an infection or inflammation of the epididymis, which is the structure that lies along the posterior border of the testis. When the diagnosis is confirmed, a urethral swab culture may be obtained.

Nursing Process: Assessment

Patient Need: Physiological Integrity

Chapter 49

Terms Matching

1. G
2. A
3. J
4. L
5. E
6. M
7. H
8. C
9. F
10. D
11. K
12. B
13. I

Focused Study

1. Alternative and complementary therapies include the following:
   • Acupuncture
   • Biofeedback
   • Massage
   • Herbs: *Cimicifuga racemosa* (black cohosh), *Vitex agnus castii* (chaste tree), *Rehmannia*, ginseng, kava, dong quai, golden seal, flaxseed, valerian, and evening primrose
   • Meditation and yoga

2. *Therapeutic D and C:* A procedure in which the cervical canal is dilated and the uterine wall is scraped. The procedure is used to diagnose and treat dysfunctional uterine bleeding and other disorders of the female reproductive system. It may be performed to correct excessive or prolonged bleeding.

   Endometrial ablation: A procedure that destroys the endometrial layer of the uterus using a laser, a thermal balloon, or electrocautery. It is performed in women who do not respond to pharmacological management or to a D and C.

   Hysterectomy: The surgical removal of the uterus. It is a treatment option for bleeding disorders and the presence of cancer.

   Anterior colporrhaphy: A procedure used to repair cystoceles. The procedure shortens the pelvic muscles, providing tighter support for the bladder.

   Marshall-Marchetti-Krantz: A surgical procedure used to resuspend the urinary bladder in correct anatomic position.

   Posterior colporrhaphy: A surgical procedure used to repair a rectocele by shortening the pelvic muscles, providing a tighter support for the rectum.

3. The menopausal period marks the natural biologic end of reproductive ability. Menopause may be the result of aging, surgical intervention, or chemicals. Surgical menopause occurs when the ovaries are removed in premenopausal women, dramatically reducing the production of estrogen and progestins. Chemical menopauseoften occurs during cancer chemotherapy, when cytotoxic drugs arrest ovarian function.

As ovarian function decreases, the production of estradiol decreases and is replaced with estrone as the body's major ovarian estrogen. Estrone is produced in small amounts and has only about one-tenth the biologic activity of estradiol. With decreased ovarian function, the second ovarian hormone, progesterone, which is produced during the luteal phase of the menstrual cycle, also is markedly reduced.

4. Risk Factors:
   • Infection of the external genitalia and anus with HPV
   • First intercourse before 16 years of age
   • Multiple sex partners or male partners with multiple sex partners
   • History of sexually transmitted infections
   • HIV infection
   • Smoking
   • Poor nutritional status
   • Obesity
   • Multiple pregnancies
   • Long-term use of birth control pills
   • Family history of cervical cancer
   • Exposure to diethylstilbestrol (DES) in utero

   Manifestations:
   • Preinvasive cancer limited to the cervix and rarely causing manifestations
   • Invasive cancer that causes vaginal bleeding after intercourse or between menstrual periods and a bloody or brown vaginal discharge that increases as the cancer progresses
   • Manifestations of advanced disease that include referred pain in the back or thighs, hematuria, bloody stools, anemia, and weight loss

   Diagnostic Tests:
   • Pap smear
   • Colposcopy
   • Cervical biopsy
   • A loop diathermy technique [loop electrosurgical excision procedure (LEEP)]

   Treatment:
   • Colposcopy
   • Laser surgery, a viable treatment method when the cancer is limited to the cervical epithelium
   • Also used for noninvasive lesions, cryosurgery, which involves the use of a probe to freeze tissue, causing necrosis and sloughing
   • Conization to treat microinvasive carcinoma when colposcopy cannot define the limits of the invasion
   • Hysterectomy or radical hysterectomy (removal of the uterus, fallopian tubes, lymph nodes, and ovaries) performed for invasive lesions

Case Study

1. *How often does the American Cancer Society recommend that women have Pap tests?* The American Cancer Society (2005) recommends that women should begin annual screenings for cervical cancer with the Pap test about three years after they begin having vaginal intercourse, but no later than 21 years of age. Screening should be done every year with regular Pap tests or every two years using liquid-based tests. At or after the age of 30, after three consecutive normal Pap tests, screening can be performed every two to three years at the discretion of the healthcare provider. As an alternative, cervical cancer screening with HPV DNA tests and Pap tests may be performed every three years. Women 70 years of age and older who have had three or more normal Pap smears in the last 10 years may choose to stop cervical cancer screening. Screening for women who have had a total hysterectomy (including the cervix) is not recommended unless the surgery was done as a treatment for cancer. Women who have had a hysterectomy without removal of the cervix should continue to follow ACS guidelines (ACS, 2006a).

2. *Is Elizabeth a good candidate to receive Gardasil®? Why or why not?* Elizabeth Baldwin is older than the normally recommended age to receive the vaccine. The vaccine is normally given to girls who are not yet sexually active. There are ongoing studies to review the benefit of administering the vaccine to women in her age group.

3. *What are the instructions for performing a breast self-examination?*
   • Lie down on your back and place your right arm behind your head. (BSE should be done while lying down because this position spreads breast tissue evenly over the chest wall, which makes it easier to feel all of the breast tissue.)
   • Use the finger pads of the middle fingers on your left hand to feel for lumps in the right breast. Use overlapping dime-sized circular motions of the finger pads to feel the breast tissue.
   • Use three different levels of pressure to feel all of the breast tissue. Light pressure is needed to feel the tissue closest to the skin; medium pressure, to feel a little deeper; and firm pressure, to feel the tissue closest to the chest and ribs. A firm ridge in the lower curve of each breast is normal. Use each pressure level to feel the breast tissue before moving on to the next spot.
   • Move around the breast in an up-and-down pattern starting at an imaginary line drawn straight down your side from the underarm, moving across the breast to the middle of the chest bone (sternum, breastbone). Check the entire breast area before going down until you feel only ribs then feel up to the neck or collar bone.
   • Repeat the exam on your left breast using the finger pads of your right hand.
   • Stand in front of the mirror with your hands pressing firmly down on your hips. Look at your breasts for any changes in size, shape, contour, or dimpling.
   • Examine your underarm while sitting or standing, with your arm only slightly raised.
   • If you find any changes, see your healthcare provider as soon as possible.

Crossword Puzzle

question	term answer
Fluid-filled sac	CYST
Removable devise used to support the uterus	PESSARY
Exercises used to strengthen pelvic muscles	KEGAL
Abnormal opening between two organs	FISTULA
Vascular solid tumor attached by a pedicle	POLYP
Tumor removal leaving the uterus intact	MYOMECTOMY
Vaccine administered to prevent cervical cancer as a result of HPV	GARDISAL
Progesterone-like medications	PROGESTINS

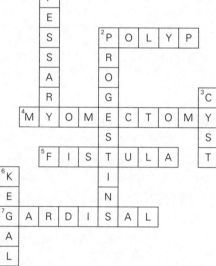

NCLEX-RN® Review Questions

1. Answer: 2
   Rationale: Menopause is the permanent cessation of menses. Menopause is neither a disease nor a disorder, but a normal physiological process. Earlier menopause is associated with genetics, smoking, higher altitude, and obesity. The average woman will live one-third of her life after menopause.
   Nursing Process: Planning
   Patient Need: Health Promotion and Maintenance

2. Answer: 2
   Rationale: Metrorrhagia is bleeding between menstrual periods. Menorrhagia is excessive or prolonged menstruation. Oligomenorrhea is scant menses. Amenorrhea is the absence of menstruation.
   Nursing Process: Assessment
   Patient Need: Physiological Integrity

3. Answer: 3
   Rationale: Anteversion is an exaggerated forward tilting of the uterus. Retroversion of the uterus is a backward tilting of the uterus toward the rectum. Retroflexion involves a flexing or bending of the uterine corpus in a backward manner toward the rectum. Anteflexion is a flexing or folding of the uterine corpus upon itself.
   Nursing Process: Assessment
   Patient Need: Physiological Integrity

4. Answer: 3
   Rationale: Use overlapping dime-sized (not quarter-sized) circular motions of the finger pads to feel the breast tissue. Lie down on your back and place your right arm behind your head. Use three different levels of pressure to feel all of the breast tissue. Look at your breasts for any changes in size, shape, contour, or dimpling.
   Nursing Process: Evaluation
   Patient Need: Health Promotion and Maintenance

5. Answer: 3
   Rationale: There are several types of ovarian cancers: epithelial tumors, germ cell tumors, and gonadal stromal tumors. Ovarian cancer is the fourth most common gynecologic cancer in women in the United States. An enlarged abdomen with ascites signals *later*-stage disease. In early stages, ovarian cancer generally causes no warning signs or manifestations.
   Nursing Process: Planning
   Patient Need: Physiological Integrity

6. Answer: 2
   Rationale: FCC is most common in women 30–50 years of age and is rare in postmenopausal women who are not taking hormone replacement. Fibrocystic changes (FCC), or fibrocystic breast disease, is the physiological nodularity and breast tenderness that increases and decreases with the menstrual cycle. FCC includes many different lesions and breast changes. Women with fibrocystic changes experience bilateral or unilateral pain or tenderness in the upper, outer quadrants of their breasts and report that their breasts feel particularly thick and lumpy the week prior to menses.
   Nursing Process: Assessment
   Patient Need: Physiological Integrity

7. Answer: 4
   Rationale: Alternative and complementary therapies that a woman with premenstrual syndrome (PMS) may find helpful focus on diet, exercise, relaxation, and stress management. PMS can be a factor in absenteeism at school or work, decreased productivity, difficulties in interpersonal relationships, and disruption in lifestyle. Manifestations of PMS occur during the *luteal* phase of the menstrual cycle (7–10 days prior to the onset of the menstrual flow) and abate when the menstrual flow begins. The treatment of PMS integrates a self-monitored record of manifestations, regular exercise, caffeine, and a diet low in simple sugars and high in lean proteins.
   Nursing Process: Assessment
   Patient Need: Physiological Integrity

8. Answer: 4

Rationale: A third-degree prolapse, or procidentia, is complete prolapse of the uterus outside the body, with inversion of the vaginal canal. First-degree, or mild, prolapse involves a descent of less than half the uterine corpus into the vagina. Second-degree, or marked, prolapse involves the descent of the entire uterus into the vaginal canal so that the cervix is at the introitus to the vagina.

Nursing Process: Assessment

Patient Need: Physiological Integrity

Chapter 50

Terms Matching

1. E
2. J
3. A
4. K
5. L
6. D
7. C
8. G
9. F
10. B
11. H
12. I

Focused Study

1. The nursing implications of medications and treatments used to treat STIs involves the following:
   - Education
     - The nurse must provide the patient with information needed to successfully complete the course of prescribed therapy.
   - The nurse must provide information concerning actions to take to prevent spread of infection.
2. Risk Factors:
   - Hormonal-based contraceptives
   - Obesity
   - Diabetes
   - Unprotected sexual activity
   - Multiple sexual partners
   Complications:
   - PID
   - Ectopic pregnancy
   - Infertility
   - Chronic pelvic pain
   - Neonatal death and illness
   - Genital cancer
3. The care of the patient with a sexually transmitted infection focuses on the following:
   - Treatment, prevention of complications, and prevention of further transmission to others
   - Pharmacologic therapies used in the management of each condition
     - Education on the correct manner to administer the treatments
     - Adverse signs and symptoms to report

4. The prevention of sexually transmitted infection begins with protection from pathogens. This can be accomplished by the use of condoms and reduced number of sexual contacts. Sexually active individuals should be aware of symptoms to report and should have regular physical examinations.

Case Study

1. *"What cause genital herpes?"* Genital herpes is a viral infection caused by the herpes simplex virus (HSV).
2. *"How will this be cured?"* Genital herpes is a viral infection. There is no cure for this disease. Management is focused on the prevention of spread and development of complications and symptom management.
3. *"What happens with the virus between outbreaks?"* The period between outbreaks is known as latency. During latency, the virus retreats into the nerve fibers that lead from the infected site to the lower spine. The virus remains latent until it is reactivated.
4. *"Am I required to provide the names of my sexual contacts to anyone?"* The names of the sexual contacts of a patient with genital herpes do not have to be reported.
5. *"How long will it take for the related symptoms to go away?"* The manifestations of the initial outbreak are the most severe and may take 12 days to resolve. Future outbreaks are milder and may resolve in four to five days.

Short Answers

Fill in the table regarding sexually transmitted diseases.

Infection	Characteristics of Discharge
Candidiasis	Thick, cheesy white discharge
Bacterial vaginosis	Thin, white, or grayish
Trichomoniasis	Frothy, yellow or white
Gonorrhea	Serous, milky or purulent penile discharge

NCLEX-RN® Review Questions

1. Answer: 1

Rationale: Many sexually transmitted infections (STIs) are more easily transmitted from a man to a woman than from a woman to a man. The incidence of STIs is highest in young adults aged 15–24. STIs are caused by bacteria, *Chlamydia*, viruses, fungi, protozoa, and parasites. Infections that are transmitted by vaginal, oral, and anal intimate contact and intercourse are referred to as STIs.

Nursing Process: Assessment

Patient Need: Physiological Integrity

2. Answer: 3

Rationale: HSV-1 is associated with cold sores but may be transmitted to the genital area by oral intercourse or by self-inoculation through poor handwashing practices. HSV-2 is transmitted by sexual activity or during childbirth and is the virus that causes genital herpes. Genital warts, caused by human papillomavirus (HPV), are transmitted by vaginal, anal, or oral–genital contact. Gonorrhea, also known as GC or "the clap," is caused by *Neisseria gonorrhoeae*, a gram-negative diplococcus.

Nursing Process: Assessment

Patient Need: Physiological Integrity

3. Answer: 1

Rationale: Genital warts are not a reportable disease. Gonorrhea, syphilis, and AIDS are reportable diseases in every state. Note that chlamydial infections are reportable in most states.

Nursing Process: Assessment

Patient Need: Physiological Integrity

4. Answer: 2

Rationale: Chlamydia may be present for months or years without producing noticeable symptoms in women. Because chlamydia is asymptomatic in most women until the uterus and fallopian tubes have been invaded, treatment may be delayed, which results in devastating, long-term complications. The infections caused by chlamydia include acute urethral syndrome, nongonococcal urethritis, mucopurulent cervicitis, and pelvic inflammatory disease (PID). Complications of chlamydial infections in men include epididymitis, prostatitis, sterility, and Reiter's syndrome.

Nursing Process: Assessment

Patient Need: Physiological Integrity

5. Answer: 3

Rationale: The primary stage of syphilis is characterized by the appearance of a chancre and by regional enlargement of lymph nodes with little or no pain accompanying these warning signs. Manifestations of secondary syphilis may appear any time from two weeks to six months after the initial chancre disappears. These symptoms can include a skin rash, especially on the palms of the hands or soles of the feet; mucous patches in the oral cavity; sore throat; generalized lymphadenopathy; condyloma lata (flat, broad-based papules, unlike the pedunculated structure of genital warts) on the labia, anus, or corner of the mouth; flulike symptoms; and alopecia. The latent stage of syphilis begins 2 or more years after the initial infection and can last up to 50 years. During this stage, no symptoms of syphilis are apparent and the disease is not transmissible by sexual contact. It can be transmitted by infected blood, however; thus, all prospective blood donors must be screened for syphilis. There are two types of tertiary, or final, stage of syphilis. Benign late syphilis is characterized by rapid onset, localized development of infiltrating tumors. A more insidious, diffuse inflammatory response involves the central nervous system and the cardiovascular system. Though still treatable at this stage, much of the cardiovascular and central nervous system damage is irreversible.

Nursing Process: Assessment

Patient Need: Physiological Integrity

6. Answer: 1

Rationale: Pelvic inflammatory disease (PID) is not a reportable disease in the United States. PID is usually polymicrobial (caused by more than one microbe) in origin; gonorrhea and chlamydia are common causative organisms. Manifestations of PID include fever, purulent vaginal discharge, severe lower abdominal pain, and a painful cervical movement. Complications include pelvic abscess, infertility, ectopic pregnancy, chronic pelvic pain, pelvic adhesions, dyspareunia, and chronic pelvic pain. Abscess formation is common.

Nursing Process: Assessment

Patient Need: Physiological Integrity

7. Answer: 3

Rationale: Flat warts are slightly raised lesions that are often invisible to the naked eye and develop on keratinized skin. Keratotic warts are thick, hard lesions that develop on keratinized skin such as the labia major, penis, and scrotum. Papular warts are smooth lesions that also develop on keratinized skin. Condyloma acuminata are cauliflower-shaped lesions that appear on moist skin surfaces such as the vagina and anus.

Nursing Process: Assessment

Patient Need: Physiological Integrity

8. Answer: 1

Rationale: Trichomoniasis is caused by *Trichomonas vaginalis*, a protozoan parasite. It is the most common curable STI in young, sexually active women. Symptoms usually appear within 5–28 days of exposure. Women have a frothy, green-yellow vaginal discharge with a strong fishy odor that is often accompanied by itching and irritation of the genitalia.

Nursing Process: Assessment

Patient Need: Physiological Integrity